KU-105-161

THE PRACTICAL HANDBOOK OF HOMOEOPATHY

*The Who, What, Where, Why and How
of Homoeopathy*

COLIN GRIFFITH

WATKINS PUBLISHING

LONDON

This edition published in the UK 2006 by
Watkins Publishing, Sixth Floor, Castle House,
75–76 Wells Street, London W1T 3QH

Text Copyright © Colin Griffith 2006

Colin Griffith has asserted his right under the Copyright, Designs
and Patents Act 1988 to be identified as the author of this work.

All rights reserved.
No part of this book may be reproduced or utilized in any form
or by any means, electronic or mechanical,
without prior permission in writing from the Publishers.

1 3 5 7 9 10 8 6 4 2

Designed and typeset by Jerry Goldie

Printed and bound in Great Britain

British Library Cataloguing-in-Publication data available

ISBN-10: 1-84293-191-1
ISBN-13: 9-781842-931912

www.watkinspublishing.com

This book is not to be used as a substitute for professional medical care and
treatment. The ultimate decision concerning care should be between you
and your doctor. The information in this book is offered with no guarantees
on the part of the author and Publisher.

CONTENTS

Acknowledgements

This book would never have been written if it were not for the encouragement and support of my agent, Fiona Spencer-Thomas, and my publisher, Michael Mann. Fiona, a homoeopath herself, has been unstinting with her time and expertise and I cannot thank her enough for believing in my literary efforts. Michael, a champion of practical alternative thinking, has given me invaluable help all through the publishing process. I was too late to acknowledge Annie Wilson for her tact and skill in editing *The Companion to Homoeopathy*; only she knows how demanding that job was. I should like to make amends by thanking her wholeheartedly for her work on this volume. I am grateful, too, for the help and encouragement Penny Stopa has given me through countless emails and phone calls. I particularly owe special thanks to my fellow homeopath, Linda Rogerson-Heath, for her careful reading and painstaking correction of the text. Her many years of hospital nursing experience give her an authority I am glad to draw on.

Acknowledgement is due too to all my patients who have found homoeopathy so helpful – and in the process taught me so much. Even after all these years in practice I still find it remarkable and encouraging that so many want to follow a way of well-being that is demanding and that requires strength of mind in the face of some pretty tough opposition.

Foreword

When first asked to produce a first-aid book on homoeopathy, I was daunted by the sheer number of excellent examples already on the shelves. I often recommend patients to get several of them so that if one book might be short on something another would fill the gap. Those by D. M. Gibson, Phyllis Speight, Dorothy Shepherd and Miranda Castro are all highly recommendable and there are many others that serve us well. As the ground rules of homoeopathy are not subject to any appreciable evolutionary change, it would seem superfluous to add yet another title to the list. It has taken me a while to see what might be useful to people who have an interest in using homoeopathy in the home that has not been covered already.

Two things have helped me to get past this little block. Firstly, having taken eight years to write *The Companion To Homoeopathy,* a hefty tome on the philosophy on which homoeopathy depends and how it works in practice, a complementary book on the practical application of homoeopathy in the home was suggested. Secondly, I remembered the pleas of many of my patients (chiefly mothers) over the years as to when I would write a book to answer the queries they kept ringing me about. People want to know about home practice; they want to participate in their own healing; they want to understand what and why and when to take responsibility.

The home practice of homoeopathic first aid – what exactly could this cover? There are so many people who have come to use and trust homoeopathic medicines for first aid that the demand for more information has spawned an industry that would surprise many by its size – and profitability! Nowadays you can walk into any health food store and buy homoeopathic remedies to treat all manner of complaints from colds and hay fever to gastric 'flu and muscle strain. You can go to any of the homoeopathic pharmacies and ask for any one of literally hundreds of different remedies that might be used for the treatment of any conceivable complaint. A glance through the book at the chapter headings will show you just how wide home practice can be. Home practice should be more though: it is also the recognition of when to call the homoeopath, of when another complementary therapy would speed progress, of when expert help is needed for problems outside the normal range of medicines and even of when to leave well alone.

For acute problems many people just plunge in and try out the remedies on a 'hope for the best' basis. There's nothing wrong with that – it's a good place to start. It is virtually impossible to do any harm with homoeopathic medicines; even if you do choose an inappropriate remedy no one will suffer more for it, unless delay causes a serious condition to be left untreated. However, the 'suck it and see' school of first aid is not really satisfactory after a while. Once a home prescriber has tasted the sweet satisfaction of success in dealing with a cold or a headache or a menstrual cramp, she will want to do more. Homoeopathy is moreish. Once you've got the bug, it doesn't let go. This is when first-aid books come in handy. Much thumbed booklets are ready on the kitchen shelf to indicate what remedies to use for a deep cut or a bad fall, an irritating cough or an incipient cold. Bolder prescribers want to be able to tackle a high fever or a bout of food poisoning. But what do you do if little Mark's fever has not lifted despite giving **Belladonna**; if Mary's rash was responding to **Pulsatilla** very nicely but is now coming back again; if Nick's indigestion hasn't cleared up on the usual dose of **Nux Vomica** and so on. Professional support in dealing with conditions that might shake your confidence is important.

'I've looked it up in the books but I just don't know what I should do now. Should I go to the doctor? Or is there something else I can try?'

Although this book covers the familiar territory of common and not so common acute ailments; all the first-aid remedies that I believe every household in the land should have, as well as how to maintain and administer them, and suggested potencies of the medicines, it also goes into explanations of why and when the remedies might not work as expected and what one can do about that – including recognising the times when you do need professional help. There are also explanatory sections on problems frequently encountered in the home which seem to have little to do with medicine but which impinge on the health of the patient and possibly of the family as a whole: behavioural problems, eating disorders, learning difficulties and so on. Finding out where to go and who to talk to can ease frustration and the loneliness of doubt. This book seeks to help you to do several things:

- to take some of the frustration and anxiety out of home prescribing by showing you how to think 'homoeopathically'
- to recognise when to seek the help of your chosen practitioner
- to know what sort of information would help the practitioner when you do need to go for a consultation
- to recognise signs and symptoms of more serious pathology that should not be ignored
- to see when it might be a good idea to consider other alternative therapies that complement homoeopathy
- to know when to risk making a fuss because your instinct is that there is an emergency
- to learn about conditions that you may suspect are developing but which make you feel helpless such as eating disorders and obsessive compulsive behaviour.

In short, it is intended as a book of 'homoeopathic household management'. It is not intended to make the homoeopath redundant. It is not about what is called 'constitutional treatment' – the progressive, ongoing, regular visits one makes to the practitioner as part of one's healing journey and personal self-development; that is a whole (holistic) body experience which one cannot and should not try to do for oneself (or for loved ones). First aid is about specific therapeutic treatment of acute or sub-acute conditions (flare-ups in chronic illness) that might arise at any time. There are some homoeopaths who would rather their patients did not do too much home practice, as they feel that the long term benefits of the constitutional remedies they have prescribed might be compromised. There is truth in this. Some people become addicted to prescribing for anything and everything indiscriminately. Homoeopathy is about practising discrimination – with discretion and patient observation. It is always best to talk about this issue with your homoeopath if you are in doubt. I shall mention certain caveats that will help you avoid messing up someone else's prescribing. If you make working with a book like this a team effort with your practitioner then you will soon be able to take responsibility for the health of the family without feeling inadequate and suspecting that homoeopathy is too difficult or just a 'curate's egg'.

Remember that it takes time to think homoeopathically but the best way to learn how is to practise.

Part I

THE WHO, WHAT, WHERE, WHY AND HOW OF HOMOEOPATHY

Who is this book for?

Everyone who cares about natural healing and wants to use natural medicines; who knows that within each one of us there is the means to self-heal; who has the imagination to see that any illness is never solely of the *part* but of the *whole* body; who believes that chemical drugs only suppress symptoms and change the course of illnesses so that chronic poor health is the eventual result. In short, for anyone who wants to be responsible for the household management of their day-to-day well-being. (I hope that it is also useful as a handy aide-memoire to those just setting out in practice.)

What does the book contain?

There is detailed information about first aid for emergencies, acute conditions and acute flare-ups in chronic problems; diagnostic signs of longer-term problems which are not suitable for home prescribing but which are included here to demonstrate the potential of homoeopathy. There are clear indications of conditions which should be treated in hospital, with safe suggestions on using remedies in such emergencies. There is information about everyday illnesses that affect the different systems of the body and about the remedies associated with the conditions and supplementary practical tips. In addition, there is a list of 50 of the most useful homoeopathic remedies with a thumbnail sketch of each, details of how to obtain and maintain a first-aid kit and of how to administer the remedies with confidence.

What medical knowledge do I need to use this book?

Virtually none. Prescribing remedies is about observing symptoms and matching them with remedy 'pictures', not about labelling parts of the body or having a working knowledge of organ functions.

What is a remedy picture?

Remedies have personalities and characteristics; each one has its own individual sphere of influence and is associated with symptoms that manifest in ways peculiar to the remedy. **Rhus-tox.**, for example, has rheumatic pains that are better for massage, heat and keeping moving to prevent stiffness while **Bryonia** has rheumatic pains that are better for keeping still; **Arsen-alb.** covers diarrhoea and vomiting with anxiety, restlessness and thirst for sips of cold water, while **Veratrum Album** has the same problem with cold sweats, insatiable thirst and utter exhaustion. It is the unique symptom picture of remedies that we match with the individual symptom picture of the patient.

What do I need to use this book?

A first-aid kit, observation skills, discrimination, trust in your intuition, patience, tact and plenty of common sense. It is also strongly advised that you work with this book in tandem with a professional homoeopath to give you additional support.

How reliable are the remedies?

Very – as long as you keep them out of harm's way and the patient's energy is not compromised by one of the substances that can antidote remedies (see part III).

How safe is homoeopathy?

It is one of the safest systems of treatment available. Remedies cannot do anyone harm even if they are inappropriate to the condition being treated. Curative reactions to remedies may sometimes be unexpected (a profuse sweat, a bout of diarrhoea, a streaming nose) but such events (called aggra-vations) are eliminative and therefore beneficial to a system that is always ready to throw out what is toxic or harmful.

How do homoeopathic remedies differ from orthodox medicine?

Homoeopathy belongs to physics while allopathy (conventional medicine) belongs to chemistry. Homoeopathy is the application of so-called 'energy medicine' while allopathy depends on chemicals. Though remedies appear to be little white pills or a bottle of colourless drops this belies the fact that the medicine that effects the curative changes is invisible; just as radio waves are. The pills and drops are only *vehicles* for dynamic energy, not medicine in themselves. This answers the question as to why the pills all look the same. Chemical drugs are synthesised in a laboratory and effect changes on the body by overriding the body's own chemical reactions, the very ones that are creating the symptoms.

How does homoeopathy differ from allopathy?

Allopathy is based on the philosophy of suppression. Symptoms are observed and treated as if *they* were the disease; as such, a set of symptoms is given an identifying label and the patient is prescribed a drug known for its ability to remove the symptoms. There are always two reactions to chemicals: the primary effect (of suppressing symptoms) and the secondary reaction which, unless the dosage is very mild, is a measure of the body's recognition of and intolerance to alien toxicity; the reaction can be anything from a rash or constipation to dizziness, headache or worse.

Homoeopathy is based on the philosophy of elimination; of ridding the body of whatever 'toxicity' (including negative mental and emotional feelings) may be creating an imbalance in the Whole. A remedy chosen for the individual in the particular state of the moment only ever creates healing if the body recognises it and is stimulated by it to hasten the elimination of negative energy in the form of discharges, either physical (sweat, mucus etc.) or emotional (words, tears).

How is homoeopathy complementary to allopathy if it is alternative?

Sometimes patients who have been taking drugs for a chronic condition for some time (such as with asthma or high blood pressure) want to avoid putting any further chemicals in their overloaded system so they seek help from a homoeopath for acute ailments. An asthma patient may ask for help to deal with a cold that would otherwise lead to an increased dose of steroids; a patient with high blood pressure might need help for stress headaches. The homoeopathy does not interfere with the necessary effects of the drugs and the proprietary drugs do not necessarily prevent the remedies from working.

What are the remedies made from?

Animal, vegetable and mineral: homoeopathy finds its remedies wherever there is a source of dynamic energy that can be rendered into medicine by homoeopathic pharmacology. **Apis** is made from the common bee; **Belladonna** is a plant poison (deadly nightshade); **Lycopodium** is made from a type of moss; calcium carbonate is a form of lime. A remedy is made because someone has recognised inherent and latent dynamic energy that is peculiarly characteristic of the raw material substance and intuitively has felt that it would be beneficial when given to a patient suffering in a way that has similar characteristics. Given this there is no surprise that **Apis** covers stinging pains in parts that are hot and swollen. The bark of the cinchona tree is the origin of quinine and is curative of certain types of malaria; **China Officinalis**, the remedy made from the bark, is curative of malarial type fevers. Rather more controversially, **Amethyst** has been known since ancient times as a healing stone that limits the damaging effects of alcohol; as a remedy it is indicated for alcoholic depression.

Where are the remedies made?

In pharmacies dedicated to making homoeopathic medicines. The pharmacists who run them have studied pharmacology as well as homoeopathic philosophy. (See page 354 for a list of pharmacies.)

What is the principle on which a remedy is chosen?

Like cures like. All remedies have been tested on people. A test (called a proving) is carried out according to a rigorous protocol (even if it is unconventional in orthodox terms). People, called provers, take the remedy daily until they produce symptoms. These are recorded as being symptoms of the remedy, not of the patient. When all the provers have finished taking the remedy (because the allotted time is up or because the symptoms are too uncomfortable to continue) the information on the symptoms is collated and written up. Once the provers stop taking the remedy, the symptoms subside fairly quickly or an antidote is found to relieve them of any discomfort. From the trial there will be found some universal symptoms that everyone suffered and these form the core of the remedy picture and contribute most to our understanding of it; other people will have experienced different and more abstruse symptoms which are also included. The remedy can now be used when a person *with closely similar symptoms* comes for treatment. If the symptoms of a disease or condition generally match those of a remedy then that remedy will act curatively.

How do the remedies work on the body if they are not material doses?

While allopathic drugs work by being processed by the liver (the body's post office), homoeopathic remedies work via the central nervous system. This all-pervading network of message pathways is alive to every event in the body. It organises the body's functions in response to essential hormones which are relayed from deep in the brain. The body, when stuck in its problem and unable to find a solution to its own distress, recognises via the CNS the similar energy pattern of the chosen remedy which galvanises the self-healing process into reaction. **Belladonna** produces a high fever, red face, pulsating arteries and cold hands and feet. By giving the patient this remedy, the effect of which is *stronger than the disease* in a person with the same symptoms, they are able to respond to it and in the process the natural symptoms are over-come. An aggravation of symptoms may initially be set up as a primary reaction to the remedy stimulus but it is eliminative and thus curative. If a remedy seems to initiate a beneficial result but this then fails, the remedy was only a 'partial cure' and reassessment of the symptoms is necessary.

Which remedies should I start my first-aid kit with?

Start small and build a collection. Though they are comparatively inexpensive, getting more than 10 or 12 to start with can be daunting. Look at the list in part III and choose from those with an asterisk the ones which seem most appropriate to your family's needs. The list is bound to include **Aconite, Arnica, Arsen-alb., Rhus-tox., Ruta** and **Hypercal Ø** (mother tincture). If you have children then **Belladonna, Pulsatilla** and **Chamomilla** will also be indispensable.

What is meant by 'potency'?

Remedies are produced at different levels of energy and these levels are numbered according to the centesimal or 'c' scale: 6, 30, 200, 1M, 10M (M is the Latin sign for 1000). There are others, including 'x' or decimal potencies (6x being the most common), but the 'c' scale is the usual one in Britain. Despite the numbers it is best to think of them as describing depth and speed of action rather than strength; 'strength' can lead you to fear using high potencies. Traditionally, in first aid, '6' is regarded as the potency used for minor complaints that are essentially physical. The 30 is viewed as middle-of-the-road and most useful for acute complaints as it is deep acting enough to reach into the psyche as well as to deal with physical symptoms. The 200 is seen as fast acting and is often used by practitioners when an acute has 'fast' symptoms such as a high fever or a dramatic gastric bug. Both the 200 and 1M feature regularly in constitutional prescribing but sometimes the latter is useful when even a 200 is insufficient to hold any improvement in an acute. The 10M is an eyebrow raiser only if seen as a 'big gun'. Actually 10M is fast and very thorough and is sometimes necessary for situations that would otherwise become emergencies. (**Ignatia** 10M is invaluable in situations heavy with acute grief, for example.) Some homoeopaths use the 100 as it goes some way to bridge the gap between the 30 and 200. In this book you will find suggestions for the use of some remedies in higher potencies because they are so frequently called for in acute illness, especially among children. To have them in the first-aid kit ensures there is no disappointment when the indications demand a deep response.

How do I know which potency to order?

If you are a patient then you can talk to your practitioner about the potencies that suit you and your family best. If you are not, then you could ask the pharmacy for help. Generally the 30 is the best place to start except in particular cases. Throughout the book I make potency suggestions. You will see that certain remedies are regularly needed in other potencies: **Aconite**, **Arnica** and **Belladonna** are all useful in 200 as well as in 30 while **Pulsatilla** (particularly frequently indicated by children) is useful in 30, 200 and 1M.

What do I need to know and do to choose a remedy?

You need to know that there are several types of symptoms:
- general (those which affect the whole body such as excessive thirst, chilliness, fever): these symptoms (diarrhoea, say, or teething) often tell us no more than where to look for more particular and individualising symptoms.
- mental and emotional (those which affect the psyche such as grief, mood swings, fury): these are of the utmost importance and, when they are present, are always indicative of the chosen remedy.
- particular (those which are specific to a part of the body such as a yellow

tongue, sciatica in the left leg, chilblains on the right foot): these are useful as they usually indicate the patient's focus of distress. (Good observation will sometimes reveal how this focus can change during the course of treatment.)

• 'strange, rare and peculiar' symptoms: these have considerable significance because of their oddity. For example, a red triangle on the tip of the tongue; excessive thirst for cold water though the patient is salivating profusely; burning pains that are better for hot applications.

• 'modalities': those things that qualify symptom pictures such as 'cough worse entering a warm room', 'wheezing worse in damp weather', 'feeling better for massaging the part and having a hot bath'; 'fever that begins at 3 p.m.'. Modalities are of great use and if they are not initially obvious should be elicited by careful questioning.

Certain symptomatic attributes make remedy selection easier: location, pain, intensity, discharges, colour, distribution, time factors and temperament.

• Location helps you find what system of the body to look up for information but also needs to be assessed in conditions that might cause you to worry in case you need professional help. Symptoms that only appear on the right or left side or that cross from one side to the other are worth noticing.

• Pain can vary: aching, bearing down, burning, smarting, searing, stabbing, stinging, digging, cutting, twisting, throbbing, exploding, darting, wandering (from one part to another).

• Intensity is important as it can assist in choosing a potency to match.

• Discharges are vital as they show us how the body is expressing its distress or how it is reacting to a remedy curatively. Diarrhoea can be black, green, bloody, watery or can fit a wide range of other descriptions. Mucus, pus, urine, wax and vomit can be similarly varied.

• The colour of the affected part is always important if it is abnormal. Certain remedies are associated with particular colours and sometimes colour will lead you to select one of just a few remedies (**Belladonna** = red; **Carbo-veg**. = blueness; **Lachesis** = purple or dark blue-red).

• Distribution can be useful especially when considering skin problems as certain remedies are identified with particular parts of the body. It is also useful to note how certain pains are distributed (for example,

Berberis Vulgaris has kidney pains that radiate down to the groin and thigh while urinating).
- Symptoms of certain remedy states have characteristic time factors: **Aconite's** croup will come on at midnight; **Lycopodium's** worst time of day is between 4 and 8 p.m.; **Apis** and **Belladonna** fevers usually come on or intensify at around 3 p.m.; **Pulsatilla**'s mucus-laden cough is worse on waking and in the evening.
- The way that an illness is expressed in mood is all important in many cases. If a patient who is normally cheerful becomes irritable then the remedy indicated will have this negative mood characteristic in its picture. If a contented child becomes tearful and clingy then this fact should be central to the selection. If a worried businessman becomes intolerant and morose then these characteristics are of the disease he is producing.

Objective symptoms are those that you can observe without asking questions. They include things such as the degree of thirst and temperature, body odours and expression, even language. Notice whether the patient is restless or not, sweating or not, sensitive to anything extraneous or not (such as noise or being fussed) and observe their body language (such as the posture any pain might oblige the patient to adopt).

Subjective symptoms are those you will need to ask about. They include the location, quality and intensity of pain and how the patient feels. What you cannot see, ask about:
- What does it feel like?
- What is the pain like? How does it feel? (You are looking for burning, stinging, throbbing etc.)
- Where is the pain exactly?
- Does the pain go anywhere else? (Left and right or alternation of them are very important.)
- When is the pain at its worst? (The time of day or night; after or before eating etc.)
- What makes it better? What makes it worse? (Hot or cold; rubbing or holding still; a warm drink; a brisk walk in fresh air etc.)

Try not to ask direct questions such as 'Do you have a metallic taste in your mouth?' or 'Do you have a burning pain?'

Sometimes you will be able to recognise a remedy from its general picture; **Pulsatilla** is easy to identify because of its weepy and dependent mood, whatever the pathology. Others are more difficult to spot. When you have chosen one of the remedies listed under the condition you are assessing, cross reference that with its more general description in part III. Remember, you are looking for a *similar* description not an exact match. Some symptoms described under a remedy may not be expressed by the patient; this does not necessarily mean that it is not indicated for the problem.

What are those symbols homoeopaths use when describing symptoms?

- < means 'worse for' or ' aggravated by'
- > means 'better for' or 'ameliorated by'
- + means 'desires'
- = means 'leads to' or 'causes'

For example:
- **Bryonia**: < from the slightest movement; > keeping still; + cold water.
- **Rhus-tox.**: < for initial movement; > massaging the part; > and + hot bath.
- **Ipecac.**: coughing = watery eyes.

What do I need to do after prescribing?

Watch and wait. The patient might fall asleep, be sick, have diarrhoea, feel hungry, become very cross or calm right down. Elimination is good if sometimes messy. Here are a few rules of thumb:
- Do not repeat a remedy if reactions happen straight away; wait till a reaction has finished.
- If one dose seems to clear the problem leave well alone.
- The faster and more violent the symptoms, the more frequent the dosage (and the higher the potency).
- If the patient improves but then slips back repeat the remedy. If there is no reaction within 4 hours (sooner in worrying conditions) then reassess. If you are sure of your choice, repeat. If not, check the other listed remedies.

- If a second remedy does nothing, get in touch with your homoeopath for advice.
- If the patient is on the mend do not give a lower potency of the same remedy thinking that the patient still needs something but less of it; you risk undoing the effects of the original potency. Stay with what works.

Why are remedies sometimes mentioned in the book when the instruction tells me to see the homoeopath?

Some remedy pictures are given to describe difficult situations which are best dealt with by the homoeopath but this will give you an idea of what you are dealing with and, in some cases, show you that there are remedies for circumstances that you might otherwise think were beyond the scope of homoeopathy. This will encourage you to seek homoeopathic help where previously you might have felt there was none and so save the patient from suppressive treatment. There are other circumstances in which you are advised to see the homoeopath but you are given remedy suggestions in case there is a delay in getting an appointment or a callback.

Is there anything I should not do?

- Don't give **Bryonia** before or after **Calc-carb.**
- Don't give **Nat-mur.** before or after **Nit-ac.**
- Don't go down in potency from, say, a 200 to a 30.
- Don't keep bothering the patient with questions after prescribing; let the patient come and tell you how they are unless the condition requires constant monitoring.
- Don't become a slave to the book; if your instinct tells you something then follow it and if you get it wrong don't be afraid to ask for help.

Why does homoeopathy sometimes fail?

Sometimes there are situations where remedies, even if well indicated, do not effect any change. There might be various reasons:

- Antidoting substances: the patient has negated the effects with peppermint, say, or eucalyptus.
- Dud remedies: the remedy may have been rendered ineffectual by a mobile phone, say, or direct sunlight.
- Making the wrong selection: sometimes symptom pictures are indistinct

or at other times you may have gone strictly with the book and suppressed your 'gut feeling'.

• There is an emotional impediment; some unresolved emotional state underlies the symptom picture.

• There is a structural impediment to the remedy: sometimes a body that has earlier sustained a traumatic injury is unable to respond fully because the injury has forced the body to find a compensatory posture to deal with pain.

• There is a hereditary impediment: the genetic make-up of each individual carries the influence of unresolved disease patterns. These, the so-called miasms, are a core part of a professional homoeopath's study.

What are the miasms and why are they so important?

The miasms are inherited influences that dictate how each individual symptomatically responds negatively to the environment, to physical trauma, to emotional turmoil, to pollution and defective nutrition, to inappropriate medical intervention, to upbringing in general and to any unresolved family issues from a previous generation. For a fuller appraisal of the miasms see my book, *The Companion to Homoeopathy* (Watkins, 2005). Though the miasms are given names that relate them to specific diseases, you should understand that they are essentially states of energy from which any similar diseases may arise. They are:

Psora: (from which we get the word 'psoriasis') which is related to dryness, itching, allergic reactions, skin conditions, slowness of recovery, slow but pathological changes to the structure of the body. (Typically, it underlies conditions such as eczema, for example.)

Syphilis: in which the body is subject to diseases of festering tissue destruction, haemorrhaging, violent or self-destructive behaviour. (Typically it underlies conditions that are always worse at night, for example, ulcerating or related to behavioural disorders.)

Sycosis: which influences the body to produce diseases characterised by mucus and pus production, inflammations and deformity of tissue, addictive behaviour and delusional states (mild or profound). (Typical of 'wet' asthma or childhood warts, for example.)

Tuberculosis: which is often influenced in its turn by the previous 3 miasms but in its own right causes glandular, lung, throat and digestive disorders and multiple allergies along with restlessness and dissatisfaction about one's lot. (Typical of such conditions as frequent nosebleeds or winter sore throats with swollen glands.)

Leprosy: which shares many of the features of syphilis, psora and TB and is much the hardest to recognise. It is responsible for slowness of recovery from conditions of the five senses, skin, tendons, bones and glands; it is the origin of feelings of resignation in the face of ill-starred inevitability. (Typical of ganglia or fungal infections.)

Cancer: which holds aspects of all the others. It is where the body has lost its sense of direction and integrity to such a degree that it compromises the general purposefulness and creative drive of the person; it can be implicated in any kind of pathology whatever. (Typical of, say, frequent high fevers in childhood or recurrent infestation by intestinal worms.)

None of these should in any way be alarming. They are just as much a force for good as they might seem to be otherwise. Without the knowledge of their significance we should be unable to understand the important purpose that disease has for us. By recognising a characteristic symptom picture of disease we are able to find the remedial strategy for its elimination, the result being the promotion of our creative well-being. Because of the years of study devoted to understanding these miasms, it is part of the homoeopath's work to treat these underlying states with constitutional prescribing and this is a fundamental reason for undergoing regular treatment. Sometimes, when a patient comes to an impasse with their treatment (usually in chronic states but occasionally in acute conditions), a homoeopath will resort to prescribing a nosode, a remedy made from the disease material associated with one of the miasms. As there is no material in the medicine, only the energy, there is no risk to the patient whatever. Do not be surprised if your practitioner needs to use Psorinum, Syphilinum, Medorrhinum (sycosis), Tuberculinum, Leprosinum or Carcinosin at some point. Mention is made of the miasms and nosodes in Part II where you will need to consult the homoeopath to help you over a block to cure.

What is constitutional treatment?

Constitutional treatment is the taking of remedies that match the condition of the body, mind and spirit (i.e. creative purposefulness) at any given time. No one's constitution naturally remains unchanging. No one is ever in stasis for long without chronic patterns of pathology beginning to emerge (even if they are no more than minor tendencies). For those who wish to maintain the flow of well-being in order to be creative, productive and purposeful, regular reviews of general progress are vital. Homoeopathy is a system of wellness; it uses the description of illness to find the way back to health.

Where can I find a homoeopath to suit me?

In the appendix of the book there is a list of various organisations which can help. Ask for a recommendation from one of the registers of qualified homoeopaths. You could look in Yellow Pages. Best of all is to go by personal recommendation. Not all homoeopaths work in the same way; some have soft furnishings, coffee tables and casual clothing, others wear suits; some use computers to work everything out, others behave more like counsellors and just listen. Homoeopathy is an art form as well as a science and individual style may be important to you. Go by instinct; only you know what makes you feel comfortable. When you have found a practitioner who suits you ask if there are any other households locally who use homoeopathy; it can be very helpful to know others in your area who think about health in the way you do and sometimes in an emergency it is good to be able to call on neighbours who might have a remedy that is missing from your kit.

Part II

PRESCRIBING THE REMEDIES

1   ACCIDENT AND EMERGENCY

Traumatic Injuries

Blows and trauma to any part of the body often need your knowledge of only a small number of remedies: **Arnica, Aconite, Rhus-tox., Ruta, Hypericum, Ledum, Bryonia, Symphytum, Bellis Perennis** and **Oak**. As injuries to the various parts of the body do require distinct remedies it is useful to differentiate between them. Some remedies have a stronger affinity for soft tissue (muscle, abdomen, breast) while others are associated with hard tissue (bones, tendons and ligaments).

When treating any injury assess first how the patient feels 'in himself' and then check where the main impact occurred. The first remedy given for any trauma might need to be for shock and the choice can make the difference between a short recovery and a long one. There are two principal remedies to consider: **Aconite** and **Arnica**. They are not interchangeable; they have distinct pictures. The difference between them can be a source of confusion, so to know which one treats what kind of shock is important.

Aconite is indicated when the shock of the trauma has created an intensity even to the point of fear and panic or dread in the patient – and possibly in everyone else who was a witness. If you can see this state in the patient then **Aconite** comes first; if it doesn't, remedies chosen for bruising, cuts or broken bones will not work or will be compromised. Remember that fear can override pain and injury in any of us. Shock with fear can be so severe that it can be held in the body's tissues for life and influence future health. A traumatised person in **Aconite** is one with a fearful expression and, if it's a child, they might be screaming and crying. This is not like **Arnica**.

Arnica is indicated for a different type of shock pattern: the patient is stunned as if from a blow to the head. Rather than having a facial expression of fear, **Arnica** looks drained and drawn, stunned as if they are unable to find the words to express how they feel. When asked how they feel, **Arnica** will reply: 'No, I'm fine; really I'm OK. Leave me to it and I'll sort myself out.'

Yet you can see that they are not fine and may even become irritable with your efforts to help. Oversensitivity makes touch or approach unbearable.

If you have trouble remembering this difference then visualise these two images: **Aconite** is like a pickaxe – sharp, sudden and scary. **Arnica** is like a sledgehammer – blunt, stunning and debilitating. **Aconite** patients can produce enough adrenalin in the system to express their fears but **Arnica** patients have far less energy; indeed, an indication for **Arnica** is that after the injury the patient becomes quite drowsy and might fall asleep or even become unconscious.

One or other of these two remedies is needed as the first prescription in a high percentage of common injuries. What determines the potency used is the seriousness of the accident. Gauge the reactions of the patient; on an arbitrary scale of 1 to 10 give 30 for anything up to 5 out of 10, and 200 for anything from 6 out of 10 to 9 out of 10. If an injury is really so serious that the patient needs hospital treatment then it is perfectly justifiable to give 1M or 10M. One does not always have the luxury of choice in serious accidents; do what you can with what you have to hand. However, though the **Aconite** state can quite quickly get swallowed up by procedure (i.e. in hospital) and thus lost to view, **Arnica** does not go away so readily. It is still a good idea to use the potency of choice later even though other (orthodox) treatment may have been started.

It is usually unnecessary to give any more than one dose of **Aconite**; it is only going to work on the system to remove the fear element. You do not have to wait long to prescribe whatever other remedy is indicated for the actual injury to the flesh or bones. Anything from 2 to 10 minutes later it is reasonable to go in with the next remedy – and often, after **Aconite**, **Arnica** is indicated for the bruising and body-shock. (Remember that **Aconite** antidotes or modifies **Arnica**. If you have missed **Aconite** and given **Arnica** instead and then realise that there is fear, then give a dose of **Aconite** and follow it with **Arnica** when the fear is gone. Do not alternate **Aconite** and **Arnica**; they cancel each other out.)

Another point about **Arnica** that is important: there are many injuries where you would expect there to be bruising and **Arnica** is the main remedy to bring bruising out to the surface – where it should be. When bruising does not come out it can be the source of aching and soreness in muscles for many years and can even be the trigger for accident-proneness. Always report accident-proneness to the homoeopath as it is, in its own right, a very important symptom! It may indicate the need for deep constitutional treatment.

Rhus-tox. is useful in injuries to muscle tissue. **Ruta** is indicated in damage to the periosteum (the protective covering of bone), joints and their flexor tendons. **Ledum** works on joints and tendons and is especially indicated when rheumatic pains result from the injury. **Bryonia**, too, is a remedy for injured bones and is most characterised by the patient's extreme reluctance to move the part, as pains are worse on movement. **Hypericum** is needed in injury to parts rich in nerves: fingertips, lips, the teeth, the spine. **Symphytum** is called for in injury to periosteum and bone especially when there are fractures or breaks; it is particularly useful in damage to bone which is thinly covered in flesh such as the bone around the eye or the shins. **Bellis Perennis** is needed in injuries to the soft tissues and organs of the abdominal cavity and specifically the breasts. **Oak** is a remedy for injuries to the spine especially the coccyx (the tail bone – see page 21). In relatively minor injuries use the 30c potency. In more serious injuries use the 200 and let the homoeopath know about the circumstances.

There is another remedy to be aware of in the aftermath of injuries – either sooner or later – that may *seem* not to be indicated. This is **Pulsatilla**. If the typical emotional picture of this ubiquitous remedy is present then without it the rest of your prescribing might be compromised. If the patient becomes very tearful, dependent, needy and clingy and feels overheated and in need of fresh air then nothing else but **Pulsatilla** will do. It is a different kind of emotional shock remedy and is quite often needed.

Injuries to different parts of the body will often produce symptoms indicating different remedies. To help you select the remedy for particular injuries here is a list that differentiates them.

Blows to the Head

For injuries to the head always contact your homoeopath as soon as possible even if you have the necessary remedies or have to take the patient to

hospital! An injury to a baby's head is often the result of dropping the child. If it was onto a sharp corner or a stone-hard surface, **Aconite** often comes first and then **Arnica** in quick succession. The still soft cranium can withstand a blow sometimes better than an adult's but the fear of insecurity brings on **Aconite**. **Arnica** can often bring out the bruising very quickly; this is a good sign. Look out for drowsiness, falling asleep and especially vomiting, all of which can be signs that something is wrong. If in doubt, take the child to hospital and do not concern yourself with worrying about whether or not you are wasting anyone's time; you are being responsible and making sure. Head injuries is one of those categories where you must make certain.

In other injuries, vertigo, headaches and visual disturbances are all to be looked into. If the blow to the head has been severe enough telephone your homoeopath and make an emergency appointment to see a cranial osteopath. This hands-on treatment will complement the remedies that you may have given already and the second opinion can add to your confidence.

If there are visual disturbances after head injuries, it is useful to know that **Cicuta Virosa** is the most indicated remedy for this. The patient may roll the eyes a lot as if to clear the vision and also find it hard to focus on words; there might be double vision. Sometimes this is accompanied by jerking movements of the head. If you have to wait to see the homoeopath get **Cicuta** 200 and give one dose in the meantime.

Another remedy state resulting from a head injury which you need to consult the homoeopath about is one in which the patient becomes torpid, sluggish, unresponsive, lacking in any motivation and dull-minded; it is as if the injury has completely slowed down the whole mechanism. The patient might even say how much they feel outside the body. This is exactly the picture of **Opium**. If it is there then nothing will shift the patient out of this state except this remedy – see your practitioner but if there is a delay do as advised with **Cicuta** (above) and take the patient to hospital as this is a potentially dangerous state!

Headaches, vertigo and nausea after a head injury that persist despite **Arnica** usually require a dose or two of **Natrum Sulphuricum** (1M is recommended in severe cases; follow advice as for **Cicuta** above). **Nat-sulph.** follows **Arnica** well so they will not quarrel.

Blows to the Back

The most common injuries to the back are the result of falls in which the patient either lands on the length of the back awkwardly and creates a torsion (a twist), or lands on the coccyx (the tail bone). Both are serious and have long-term implications if not treated promptly. **Take a severe back injury to Accident and Emergency!**

Arnica is usually the first remedy to think of in back injuries where the patient is winded and twisted. There will be bruising and shock. **Arnica** helps to release the spasm that is held in the diaphragm – which would have tensed up on the point of impact. This can cause palpitations and breathlessness as well as irritability. Because muscles have become involved (in the torsion) then **Arnica** will usually need to be complemented by **Rhus-tox.** which covers muscle spasm that causes stiffness, aching and restlessness. It is a good idea to use **Arnica** 200 (one twice per day for 3 days), followed by **Rhus-tox.** 30 (one every 3 – 4 hours till symptoms ease). In a case where the symptoms are severe it is justifiable to use **Arnica** 1M and **Rhus-tox.** 200 at the same rate. These two remedies are entirely complementary and work superbly well together. If pains continue despite these remedies it might be that the twisting that occurred during the injury has set up a torsion pattern throughout the system. This situation calls for professional treatment; the homoeopath may have to prescribe **Ayahuasca** to relieve the twist.

If you see a back-injured person get up and shuffle about restlessly trying to keep limber then this is an indication in itself for **Rhus-tox.** If this is strongly indicated then there is a third remedy that can complement both the **Rhus-tox.** and the **Arnica: Calc-c.** 30 is most useful in a situation like this if given last thing at night for 3 days while giving the other two as prescribed above. It settles the jangled nerves of the spinal cord while the other two remedies get on with their work.

Occasionally, in serious sudden injuries to the spine, **Arnica** is insufficient if there is spasm in the muscles that connect all the bones of the spine. **Arnica** does not relieve intense muscle spasm where there is also great sensitivity to the pain. In such cases alternating **Arnica** in a high potency with **Nux Vomica** 30 or 200 (at 20 – 30 minute intervals) is very helpful. It is not usually necessary to continue this prescription for more than 3 or 4 doses of both remedies. If the need for this prescription arises then it is essential to see the cranial osteopath as well. If nerve pain persists, give **Hypericum** 30 twice daily.

In cases of back injuries you should check the kidneys. These two organs are situated on either side of the spine below the ribcage, slightly higher than most people realise. If there is pain around the kidney area then an emergency appointment to see the cranial osteopath is recommended; phone your practitioner as well. **Arnica** might be indicated but if you have it use **Bellis Perennis** 30 or 200 instead. **If there is any blood in the urine then immediate hospital attention is necessary!**

One other remedy is worth considering in back injuries: **Oak**. This is invaluable when the patient is stoical about the pain, wants to try and carry on as normal but can't because of the spasms of pain that might even be bad enough to keep him on his back. **Oak** is a remedy for people who insist on keeping going, come what may. They recognise the severity of the injury (unlike **Arnica**) but fret because they can't continue as normal. It is also a remedy that can be used after **Arnica** has done its work on the bruised area; **Oak** helps people to feel sturdier after a severe accident. It is entirely complementary to **Arnica**. If it is given for an injury in its own right then use 1M. If it is given as a support remedy after **Aconite, Arnica, Rhus-tox.** then use 30.

Back Strains

Straining the back can also set up chronic injury patterns that can result in a whole raft of debilitating symptoms. Strains occur through lifting heavy objects awkwardly, through carrying heavy school, shoulder or shopping bags on one side of the body for too long and through sports injuries. The most common symptoms that arise are typically **Rhus-tox.** symptoms: stiffness and aching which is worse for resting in one posture for too long; better for a hot bath or shower; better for gently moving about; better for massage; worse on rising from bed in the morning. An acute **Rhus-tox.** picture might well include seeing the injured person lying flat on the floor, restless and with a pained expression on his face. To get up from this position or to turn over in bed, he has to roll over on his side and lift himself up very gingerly. For such a picture use **Rhus-tox.** 200, one every 4 hours till the symptoms become easier. Then slow down the rate of dosage. (In some severe cases the 200 is simply insufficient; your practitioner would then probably recommend using the 1M or even 10M.) There are occasions when alternating **Rhus-tox.** and **Calc-c.** is very helpful particularly if the patient is sensitive to pain and worried about the injury. (One twice daily of each.) The most useful tissue salt to support the action of indicated remedies after sprains is **Ferr-phos.** (take one twice daily).

If, after a back strain, there is pain that seems to be localised in the mid-back in addition to the aching and stiffness, then seek professional help because the injury might be the root of subsequent disturbances to the activity of the digestive tract. The same advice pertains with injury to the upper back as this can lead to chronic breathing or circulation symptoms.

Whiplash

Though whiplash is not caused by a direct blow to the spine it is an injury that still calls for either **Aconite** or **Arnica** or both. When there is stark fear from the incident then give **Aconite** 200, wait a few minutes for the emotion to subside and then give **Arnica** 200. The effect of the forward-backward-forward jolt to the upper spine is often deeply shocking. It can cause many concomitant symptoms or set up a chronic pattern of seemingly unrelated chronic symptoms. These include dizziness, nausea, dramatically lowered blood pressure, faintness, numbness and tingling in the arms, shallow or short breathing, disorientation, lethargy and various pains in the neck and shoulder area; these latter symptoms can be indications of serious damage to the spinal column and, if they occur, require hospital monitoring.

Occasionally these symptoms can come on suddenly, years after the injury as the result of coughing or a sudden jolting movement. What has happened is that the present exciting cause has 'reminded' the body of the accident of years before and it has adopted the pattern it went into in the accident. Unfortunately, whatever treatment was sought at the time was not thorough enough to eradicate for good this chronic pattern. This is definitely a moment to see the cranial osteopath as well as the homoeopath.

Blows to the Coccyx

This is such a common injury and one that is commonly neglected. Regard it as a rule: never underestimate an injury to the coccyx! Why? Because a blow to this vestigial tail bone can send shock waves up the entire length of the spine and into the head. It can result in the tensing up of the diaphragm of the pelvic floor (which controls the anal and urethral sphincters); the twisting out of alignment of the sacrum (which can result in anything from sciatica to menstrual difficulties – because of the displacement of abdominal organs); the tensing up of the thoracic diaphragm (which can cause breathlessness, palpitations and indigestion); coughing from tension in the fascial tissues of the chest and neck; chronic post-nasal catarrh with the shock triggering the membranes in the ethmoid sinus (above the bridge of the nose) into manufacturing mucus.

Usually the pain inflicted on the coccyx requires **Arnica** first. Use the 30 for a minor bump but use 200 if it is severe. You will need to repeat the dose at the rate of 2 or 3 times per day for several days unless the patient is particularly responsive. If there is sharp nerve pain then after the initial dose of **Arnica** give **Hypericum** 200; this can be given twice per day for 2 or 3 days. Sometimes it is necessary to alternate these two remedies till the patient becomes more comfortable.

In all cases of coccyx injury where you have had to give more than one day's worth of remedies it is essential to go for an appointment with a cranial osteopath or a practitioner who is well versed in correcting acute injuries. (McTimoney technique or Bowen technique should be considered.)

Eye Injuries

A 'black eye' is an injury to the flesh and orbital bone around the eye. As there is (or should be) bruising, the first remedy to think of is **Arnica** 30 or 200 (depending on severity). This not only makes sure that the trauma of the blow suffered is resolved but also ensures that all the bruising comes out onto the surface. Start with a single dose and then see what else needs to be done (see below).

Symphytum is the best-known remedy for a black eye especially if there is pain in the eyeball. After the **Arnica**, if there are no other complications, use the **Symphytum** 30: one dose twice per day till the eye is painless. **Symphytum** triggers the body to heal the injured periosteum (the covering layer of tissue on bone) and the bones themselves with both of which it has an affinity. It follows **Arnica** after the bruising has come out. It is the first remedy to think of for injuries which leave inflammation of the eye especially after a blow from a blunt instrument such as a ball or a fist. (**Symphytum** is also called for in cases of pain that remains long after all other symptoms of trauma to bone and periosteum have gone.)

Ledum is also well known for treating black eyes. It, too, is a remedy that has an affinity for injured bone and periosteum. It is useful when the patient has no particular injury to the eyeball. A chief characteristic of **Ledum** is that the injury feels better when a cold flannel is put on it. **Ledum** 30 is usually sufficient but in bad cases use the 200. Dosage: one 30 twice per day for 3 days or one dose of the 200 and repeat only if necessary.

If the injury is from a sharp object, **Aconite** is likely to be the first remedy. Use the 200 potency: one dose and wait for 15 minutes. If the surface of the eye is scratched then follow this with **Calendula** 30. **Calendula** is primarily a remedy to heal skin tissue; eyes are made from differentiated skin cells so **Calendula** has an affinity for the cornea. Repeat **Calendula** up to 3 times per day as needed till all the soreness and inflammation is gone. If there is a feeling that there is also nerve pain in the eye after the injury then consider using **Hypericum** as well. Don't hesitate to alternate two indicated remedies. **Calendula** and **Hypericum** 30 often do well together after injuries; give them at 4-hour intervals, first one then the other till the symptoms have cleared.

If there is any foreign object left in the eye after the injury, such as a splinter or a tiny sliver of glass it will be necessary to call on your practitioner. The number one remedy for foreign objects in the body is **Silica** which encourages the gradual and safe elimination of them, however deeply buried they may be. Though it may be necessary to go to the doctor with such an injury, you can still use **Silica** with confidence. Use the **Silica** 30 (3 times a day) unless your practitioner recommends otherwise.

After Eye Surgery

Healing of the eye after surgery calls for **Calendula**. It encourages the repair of damaged tissue after cataracts are removed. Use the 30 twice daily till the symptoms are relieved. If the surgery has left an acute and painful awareness of the surgeon's knife – a sense of the slice wound – then **Staphysagria** is the only remedy to consider. Use one dose of the 200. If this peculiar symptom is there then little else will heal till it is removed. This means that **Staphysagria** might be the first remedy to be given after surgery – but only if this sensation is decidedly felt.

One other remedy needs to be considered after eye injuries: **Euphrasia Ø**. This is a liquid herbal remedy that can support homoeopathic remedies working from the inside. **Euphrasia** helps relieve irritation and aching in the eye. Use one drop in a quarter cup of water and dab it on with cotton wool or use in an eyebath. It will not contribute to any infection in an injured eye as the tincture contains sterilising alcohol.

Injuries to the Nose

Use **Arnica** as the initial remedy unless there is the typical sudden shock state of **Aconite**. If the nose bleeds after a blow, **Arnica** is the first remedy to consider. Use the 30 or the 200. If the patient does not respond to **Arnica** and the nose continues to bleed profusely, even dramatically, and there is confusion and irritability then you may need to use **Millefolium**. This is an ancient wound healer and is occasionally needed when other remedies seem to fail. As it is not a common remedy you will need, if the bleeding persists, to contact your practitioner to get a few doses.

Injuries to Mouth and Teeth

Lips are rich in nerves and their surface skin is thin. Two remedies are outstanding here: **Hypericum** for nerve pain and **Calendula** for laceration. Topically, use **Hypercal** cream or ointment. If the cut is deep or the lip is badly torn then use **Calendula** 6 or 30 to work 'from the inside' to repair the surface skin. Even if stitches are needed still use the remedies.

For injuries to the inside of the mouth think of **Calendula** for torn or bleeding surfaces and **Hypericum** for nerve pains. Here you can use both a potency (such as 6 or 30 depending on severity) and **Hypercal Ø** as a mouthwash – 3 or 4 drops of the tincture in a quarter cup of water.

Damage to teeth usually calls for **Aconite**, **Arnica** and **Hypericum**. If there is sudden shock as a result of an injury to the teeth and mouth then start with **Aconite** 30. If there is soreness, bruising and tiredness after an injury (or once the shock has passed) then give **Arnica** 30. This stage does not always come up so be ready to give **Hypericum** 30 for the nerve pains of damaged teeth (one dose 2 or 3 times per day). A broken front tooth will probably need all three remedies as well as a trip to the dentist. If the pains from a broken or damaged tooth are unendurable and cause the patient to be extremely irritable and easily provoked to harsh words then use **Chamomilla** 200: one dose and wait; it is often followed well by **Arnica** or **Hypericum**.

After Dentistry

Nerve pains after dental treatment almost always respond well to **Hypericum**. (There is a good case for taking **Hypericum** 6 or 30 as a preventative just before the dentist sets to work.) Use the 30 or the 200 to suit the case. After an extraction, **Hypericum** is always useful but consider **Staphysagria** in older patients when there is regret at loss of the tooth for cosmetic reasons or if there is that 'memory' of the dental surgeon's 'invasion' of the mouth – use the 200 unless your practitioner would suggest otherwise.

After Wisdom Teeth Extraction

After the extraction of wisdom teeth it is almost always necessary to use **Arnica** (200 is best) and then **Hypericum** (30 or 200 depending on the severity of the pain) or to alternate the two remedies (twice each a day for a few days). Use **Hypercal Ø** as a mouthwash for as long as the socket is open and bleeding or raw.

Injuries to the Breasts

Any severe injury to the breasts **must be reported to your practitioner**. Though the breasts are made up of ducts and lymph vessels, glands and fatty tissue – so no vital organ is hurt – blows can have lasting and serious consequences including pain, swelling and, in some cases where there is susceptibility, tumours. In the case of injury take **Arnica** 200 at once and call your practitioner. If there is a delay in their returning your call then take **Bellis Perennis** 30 every 2 hours until you are given other advice appropriate to the condition. If the blow was the result of anger and abuse then give a single dose of **Staphysagria** 200 to deal with the emotional aspect.

(**Staphysagria**, **Bellis Perennis** and **Arnica** are entirely complementary.) If there is swelling in the glands that lead from the breast into the armpit and there is muscular stiffness and aching in the top of the arm then **Phytolacca** will be needed – use the 6 or 30. If the site of the injury starts to harden and, at the same time, the patient begins to be weak, chilly and trembly then it is likely that your practitioner would prescribe **Conium**. This is not a usual first-aid remedy and is mentioned here because a severe injury to a breast can become worrying quite quickly; use the indicated remedy until you can see the homoeopath.

Injuries to the Kidneys and Other Soft Organs

The best remedy to consider for damage to soft tissue of the abdomen and the vulnerable areas of the body such as the kidneys is **Bellis Perennis**. After blows to the sides of the back below the ribs (where the kidneys lie) and to the abdomen, where the stomach, liver, spleen, intestines, bladder and the reproductive organs are housed, give **Bellis Perennis** 30 or 200 (depending on severity). After any such injury you should contact your practitioner to ensure that the whole 'picture' is taken into account. **Never leave an injury to a vital organ unreported.**

Injuries to Muscles

The first remedy to use for injuries to muscles is **Arnica**. Wherever there is bruising then **Arnica** 30 or 200 should be given. Severe bruising seldom does well on a single dose; **Arnica** is a remedy that can be repeated quite frequently – the 30 can be repeated up to 3 times a day; the 200 up to twice a day for a few days.

Muscle injuries usually lead to inflammation of the muscle tissue and that then calls for other remedies. **Rhus-tox.** is the most common remedy for inflammation, stiffness and pain after injury. **Rhus-tox.** does little for bruising but it has characteristic symptoms: it is better for massage of the affected muscles; better for hot water (of the shower or a bath); worse on first moving from a resting position and there is restlessness of the injured part or generally. Use the 30 every 3 or 4 hours initially and soak in a hot bath.

Ruta is often needed to complement **Arnica** and **Rhus-tox.** as it has a strong affinity for the tendons and ligaments that are connected to the muscles. (See below in 'Injuries to Ligaments and Tendons'.) These three remedies are the sportsman's greatest aids on the pitch or the course.

Pulsatilla, **Sulphuric Acid** and **Symphytum** are all remedies that might be needed if **Arnica** and **Rhus-tox.** do not elicit a positive response.

Pulsatilla is indicated when the injury symptoms are accompanied by tearfulness and helplessness. (In men this is difficult to see; they become 'sorry for themselves' and accept help more willingly than usual.)

Sulphuric Acid follows **Arnica** when the marks do not go and there is still soreness and irritability.

Symphytum is indicated in the inflammation of tissue and bone after **Arnica** and **Rhus-tox.** have done their work or failed. It is characterised by tenderness of the affected part to touch even if the bruising has gone.

Injuries to Joints

Though **Arnica** may well be called for in an injury to a joint it is likely to be indicated mostly for the shock aspect. The tissues involved in a joint injury are bone and its covering, the periosteum. Here we need just three main remedies with an affinity for these tissues and the ligaments that attach them to muscle:

Bryonia follows both **Aconite** and **Arnica** well after a trauma and is needed for injuries where there is inflammation and the pain is < on the slightest movement (the opposite of **Rhus-tox.**). The patient is irritable.

Rhus-tox. has the characteristic symptoms of < initial movement; < staying still too long; < on rising in the morning; > rubbing and massage; > hot water or hot applications. The patient does not want to be too long in one position. They will be seen to rub the affected area or to do a lot of stretching.

Ruta is chiefly for bruising to the bone and specifically bruising to the periosteum. Where **Rhus-tox.** has done well for the muscles and the tendons, **Ruta** carries on the work and repairs damage to the bones and joints when bruising pain persists.

It can sometimes be helpful to rub **Ruta** cream onto the injured area.

Injuries to Ligaments and Tendons

Ligaments join bone to bone or anchor organs to structural tissue, and tendons join muscles to bone. They can be injured by a blow, by overuse (RSI: repetitive strain injury) or overstraining. (See page 267 for tennis elbow and housemaid's knee.)

The main remedies for injuries and strains to these tissues are **Rhus-tox.** and **Ruta.** Use **Rhus-tox.** where there is strain or injury resulting in stiffness, pain and > from movement; > rubbing the part; > hot bath; > from stretching; < keeping still for too long and < initial movement especially in the morning on waking. **Rhus-tox.** is more useful for strains and injuries to ligaments from too much lifting or awkward lifting of heavy loads. It is the main remedy after stretching upwards for things out of reach and causing arm strain. Use the 30 or 200. Use **Ruta** to complete the work of **Rhus-tox.** There will be bruised pains and soreness of the joints and tendons. **Ruta** is the main remedy for tenosynovitis (inflammation of the tendon and its protective sheath) after a strain or a trauma. If you are following **Rhus-tox.** with **Ruta** then start with the 30 twice or 3 times a day. If it is no better within 5 days then contact your practitioner. When **Rhus-tox.** and **Ruta** fail to relieve the symptoms of strain and soreness and when the part is better for being kept wrapped up and warm then your practitioner may consider using **Strontium Carbonate** in the 30th potency. This is a remedy with an affinity for ankle injuries that will not heal and that cause swelling around the part. One other remedy that might be needed is **Anacardium** which has a strong affinity for damaged ligaments; 2 daily doses of the 6 or 30 for 3 – 5 days should suffice. **Ferr-phos.**, the tissue salt, given twice daily, supports the action of the chosen remedy.

Injuries to Bones

Unless there is the characteristic picture of **Aconite** after a trauma to bone then start with **Arnica**. In severe injury – even when you suspect a break – give **Arnica** 200: one dose. If the bone is bruised and there is inflammation of the protective tissue (the periosteum) then give **Ruta** 30 every 6 hours till the pains ease; thereafter slow the rate of dosage.

If the bone pains do not respond to **Arnica** (even if the shock symptoms do) then you should consider taking the patient to hospital to have the limb checked in case of possible breaks. It is common for breaks to go undetected for some while; even for several days. This is even more common for fractures and hairline fractures. If there is persistent pain on using the limb and especially if pain arises from rotating the limb then call your practitioner and take the patient to the hospital for an X-ray. It is important not to prescribe more than **Arnica** for a break until the injury has been assessed by an orthopaedic doctor; remedies such as **Calc-phos.** and **Symphytum** are able to promote bone repair very quickly but this should not happen until the bones are set back in the right place.

Once bones are set in place then you can use:

Calc-phos. (6 twice per day) for irritation at the point of the break. It acts complementarily with **Symphytum**. **Calc-phos.** is the remedy for promoting the union of bones in children; it is very helpful to relieve the pains in greenstick fractures. Use 6 or 30 unless your practitioner has other advice.

Carbolic Acid is the main remedy to consider if the bone has been crushed. Use 30 daily till the doctor's follow-up and consult your practitioner.

Ruta (30 daily) can be used instead of the **Calc-phos.** if the break is near a joint. It works well with **Symphytum**.

Silica is sometimes a useful intercurrent remedy for delicate, slight children who have broken a bone. It not only supports the use of **Arnica, Calc-phos., Symphytum** and **Ruta** but it also acts on the general constitution. This is a remedy that your practitioner will advise on.

Symphytum (30 once per day) for sore, bruised and tender bones that are mending after a break. This can be continued till the follow-up visit to the hospital if there is a plaster.

If bones take a long time in healing then you should call on your practitioner as they would want to consider using a constitutional prescription; **Calc-C.**, **Pulsatilla**, **Lycopodium** or **Silica** might be required to galvanise the whole constitution. One tricky problem is when the collarbone is broken. This is a bone that cannot be set and plastered in the usual way. If you suspect that it has been broken after, say, a rugby game then take the patient to hospital for expert advice as the break can damage the adjacent lung. Only prescribe **Aconite** and/or **Arnica** and **Hypericum** if there is any pain from damaged nerves and wait for your practitioner's advice.

Injuries to Nerves

It is sometimes necessary to give an initial dose of **Aconite** (30 or 200) for shock when nerves have been damaged. The most important remedy for injured nerves is **Hypericum**. Whenever pains and observation suggest that nerves have been lacerated or crushed then give **Hypericum** 6, 30 or 200. The most common areas affected are fingertips, toes, knees, the coccyx, elbows and parts of the face and mouth.

If the affected part has a wound, swelling, redness and inflammation as well as nerve pain then use **Belladonna** 30 or 200 first, depending on the severity. If pains from nerve tissue damage are intolerable, keeping the patient awake in a heightened state of awareness of the injury, then consider **Coffea**. Ask your practitioner about this remedy as it can sometimes cut across any other current treatment. Use a 30 and repeat it only when the benefit of the last dose wears off.

Patients who are restless, anxious and demanding with pains in damaged nerve tissue need **Arsen-alb**. Use the 30th potency; it is most likely to be needed at night and can be repeated when the effects of the last dose begin to wear off. Recuperation can be assisted by using **Kali-phos.** and **Mag-phos.** tissue salts. **Kali-phos.** eases and repairs while **Mag-phos.** eases any spasms caused by nerve pain.

Cuts and Lacerations

For any ordinary cut first allow the wound to bleed a little (because this encourages the activation of lymphocytes in the area) then, if the wound is bleeding profusely, hold the part under the cold tap for a while (as this slows the blood loss unless it is particularly bad). Then, with clean hands, wash the part with warm water and dry with a clean towel. Apply lint that has **Hypercal Ø** drops soaked in (it will sting initially) and keep it in place with plaster that is made of fabric. Avoid using waterproof plasters as they prevent air getting at the wound. For healthy granulation (repair) the wound should be kept clean, warm and dry. The worse the cut, the more it should be kept covered till healing takes place. Redress a wound at least once a day.

The first *internal* remedy to think of for cuts and broken skin is **Calendula** unless there is an obvious picture of **Aconite** (or **Arnica**). For a clean wound use **Calendula** 6 or 30; give one dose of the 30 every 4 – 6 hours if the cut is deep. (**Calendula** helps to prevent scarring.) For serious, painful cuts **Calendula** and **Hypericum** may be alternated. If the wound and the surrounding tissue feel sore and bruised then use **Hamamelis** 30 rather than **Calendula**. **Hamamelis** follows **Aconite** and **Hypericum** very well. For a wound – particularly a slight one – that persistently bleeds in a patient who is pale and weak then give **Phosphorus** 30 intercurrently with **Calendula** and **Hypericum** as appropriate.

If the wound is from a knife or after being stabbed or after an operation then **Staphysagria** 200 (one dose) should be given.

If the wound becomes darker red or even bluish, swollen and tender and it bleeds more than it looks as though it should then give **Lachesis** 6 or 30: one dose every 4 hours for 3 doses.

Wounds that Go Septic

The usual culprit in septic wounds is staphylococcus which is a bacterium that is often found in the nose or on the skin. In those who are susceptible it can get into a wound and cause a pus-filled pocket, an abscess. If this continues without resolution the bacteria are able to migrate. If the infection is severe enough it can lead to septicaemia though, in healthy individuals, this is not likely. (Early signs are red streaks up the limb.) If pus forms in the wound there are a number of remedies to consider.

Apis: if the wound is red, swollen, puffy and has stinging pains.

Belladonna: the wound becomes swollen, hot and very red; the area might even feel as if it is throbbing. There may not be much pus evident. If the infection is severe enough then a red streak will travel up the limb. Use the 30th or 200th potency depending on severity. This dose might have to be repeated 4 – 6 hours later. If there is a red streak present then do not hesitate to contact your practitioner.

Calc-sulph.: this is for wounds that form pus, are slow to resolve and are not so intensely painful as **Hepar-sulph**. Usually a mass of pus forms, looks yellow or even yellow-green and then stays there. The patient is likely to be grumpy and complaining.

Hepar-sulph.: the part becomes extremely painful, red and swollen and there is obviously pus building up under the skin. The patient is extremely irritable and sensitive and can't bear the wound to be touched. Use the 30th or the 200th potency.

Myristica: this is an alternative to **Hepar-sulph.** though there is less sensitivity and irritability. This remedy is one of the best 'anti-septic' abscess remedies in homoeopathy.

Pyrogen: this is a remedy that your practitioner is likely to prescribe if the infection is bad enough to affect the whole constitution. The patient feels that 'flu is creeping on; there is lethargy and mental confusion with aching in the limbs. The face might even look a little dusky red with drooping eyelids.

Silica: this is for wounds that don't heal well while very slowly brewing pus. Unlike the other remedies above it covers infections that are not angry and hot but slow developing. Any pains are splinter-like.

In the case of each remedy use the 30 twice or 3 times a day till the problem resolves. If there is no improvement within 2 – 3 days then call your practitioner. **Calendula** is not included in the above list even though it is capable of resolving an infected wound in an otherwise healthy person. The reason is that **Calendula** can cause the surface skin to heal extremely quickly and sometimes this can have the effect of sealing the wound before the infection has cleared up thus creating an abscess. This happens in patients who do not have thoroughly strong and healthy constitutions. This is a situation best handled by your practitioner.

Shock from Loss of Blood

The most usual remedy for shock from loss of blood from a wound is **China Officinalis**. After a serious wound with a loss of blood that leaves the patient feeling light-headed, shaky and oversensitive to noise, draught and making any effort then **China** 30 can restore them to equilibrium quickly.

Puncture Wounds

Any wound that is caused by a pointed object – needle, pitchfork, drawing pin, splinter, bradawl, a rat's or a cat's teeth – is unlikely to bleed much, be more or less swollen and to be painful. A typical example occurs when a gardener puts a fork into the flesh of his foot. This calls for **Ledum**. Use **Ledum** 30 up to 3 times a day for 2 days. **Ledum** is one of the remedies acknowledged as dealing with tetany following an injury from a pointed object. Tetanus occurs when the tetanus spore (fungal bacterium), which lies dormant in soil especially in areas where cattle and horses have been kept, is introduced into the wound. Surrounding tissue dies off causing the bacteria to release a neurotoxin which brings about the characteristic symptom picture of a non-inflammatory swelling at the wound and pain that creeps up the affected limb. This then creates stiffness in the muscles eventually leading to the locking of the muscles of the jaw and spine.

Ledum is complemented by **Hypericum**. Not only is **Hypericum** another remedy that is capable of dealing with tetanus but it is also useful when wounds in parts that are rich in nerve tissue create excessive pain. If you have trodden on a rusty nail, for example, then **Ledum** 30 should be alternated with **Hypericum** 30 as the latter will help deal with the severe nerve pain that results while **Ledum** will cope with the muscle pain.

Ledum and **Hypericum** are also remedies that a homoeopath would consider if the patient needed to undergo a lumbar puncture as part of a medical investigation or before an epidural for a Caesarean operation. Despite the extraordinary skill of anaesthetists in administering this procedure, it is common enough for the patient to be left in considerable pain. If this is the case then a cranial osteopath should be consulted as well as the homoeopath. **No traumatic pain in the spine should ever be neglected**. Another remedy that should be considered for conditions arising from lumbar punctures is **Lumbricus**. It is best prescribed in the 30th potency once or twice a day for 5 days after an initial dose of **Hypericum** 200. It can also be used prophylactically in case of epidurals or lumbar puncture: one dose of 30 before the procedure.

Burns

There are various types of burn to be considered: from a hot object, scalding from steam or hot liquid, a burn from an exhaust pipe, chemicals or live electric wires and sunburn. With all serious burns it is essential to contact your practitioner! If the burnt area is widespread or concentrated over a large area (such as a leg or an arm or from a spill of boiling liquid down the front) then you **must** take the patient to hospital. **The combination of a deep burn and shock is dangerous!** If this is the case then give **Aconite** 200 if you have time and call your homoeopath once you get to the hospital. You can use the remedies listed below as soon as you see the appropriate indications. They will not interfere with anything the doctors may have to do.

There are three remedies that strongly feature for any type of burn: **Cantharis**, **Causticum** and **Urtica Urens**.

Cantharis covers burns and scalds where the skin feels raw, smarting and inflamed and is relieved by cold water or cloth; there is blistering of the wound and it has a tendency to burn when touched. It is especially indicated in burns which threaten to suppurate. The blistered skin begins to turn black and there are cutting or stitching pains. The patient feels very irritable and finds the pain extremely aggravating.

Causticum is useful in burns where the skin is affected over a wide area, feels raw and sore and is very slow to heal – typical of a burn from an exhaust pipe, for example. There is a sensation of tightening of the damaged skin with painful itching and the surface tends to ooze watery matter making it difficult to remove any covering lint.

Urtica Urens is useful for burns and scalds both as a tincture and in potency. It is indicated for skin that is blistering and feels sore, raw and painfully itchy; as if stung by nettles. Burning and prickling together is a prime symptom.

Tissue salts: Kali-mur. supports the action of indicated remedies in burns though if the skin is turning septic use **Calc-sulph**. instead. Sometimes **Calc-sulph**. is needed in a higher potency for suppuration; do not use the tissue salt in this case.

If any of the above fail to relieve within a few days then consider using **Carbolic Acid** 30.

As burns can cover a large surface area of skin, infection should be watched for. Using **Hypercal Ø** and/or **Urtica Urens Ø** topically in solution can considerably reduce the chances. Like any other wound, burns do better if they are lightly covered with gauze or lint that let the maximum amount of air circulate. Strap the covering on with micropore plaster. The covering can be damp with a weakened solution of the tinctures: 5 drops of the mixture to a quarter cup of water. Anything stronger can cause painful stinging initially.

Chemical burns may have similar symptoms to those caused by hot liquid or objects. **Causticum** 30 is the most likely remedy to be indicated though either of the other two may well be useful intercurrently. If **Causticum** fails then consider **Carbolic Acid** 30 especially if the area affected is extensive and the pains are burning, pricking like needles and come and go. If you are using **Carbolic Acid** it is sensible to be in touch with your homoeopath for support.

Though these remedies may be indicated, there is an even simpler way of treating acute burns to extremities (such as hands): as soon as the burn has happened, place the burnt area in bearable **hot water**. Very hot water (**not boiling**) matches the event of the burn and the body will react to it: like with like. This is useful to know in the case of hot oil splashes, for example. Putting the burn under the cold water tap is counterproductive.

Sunburn: this may call for any of these remedies: **Belladonna**, **Apis**, **Pulsatilla** or **Sol**.

Apis has skin that is puffy, either reddened or pale, burning and stinging. The patient may well feel drowsy and yet irritable. It is easily confused with **Belladonna**; **Apis** has more stinging and irritability while **Belladonna** has more heat (even general feverishness) and redness.

Belladonna has very red skin that feels burnt and hot and may even be throbbing. It may be accompanied by signs of sunstroke.

Pulsatilla may have the reddened skin and burning of the other two remedies but there is less irritability in the patient and more emotional distress with a tendency to weep and ask for help.

Sol is best for those who have great sensitivity to the sun; they tend to burn easily and get headaches if out in the bright sun too long. If there is sunburn then a few doses of the 6th potency will relieve.

For any burns that threaten to turn into ulcers with bluish or blackened skin and when the patient becomes anxious, restless and agitated then **Arsenicum Album** is indicated. This is a situation for the homoeopath to choose the potency.

Splinters

There are two basic remedies to remember for splinter wounds: **Ledum** and **Hypericum**. Splinters cause puncture wounds and do not bleed either much or at all. Therefore think of **Ledum** to begin with. If the part affected is very sensitive and painful then **Hypericum** can be given either after or in alternation with the **Ledum**. Use 30 unless the condition is very severely painful.

The most useful remedy to promote the expulsion of splinters and thorns and shards of glass is **Silica**. The body is capable of causing foreign objects to be expelled and it normally does this by surrounding the object with white blood cells which form a pocket of pus; the resulting debris gathers into a swelling that ejects both pus and object. **Silica** promotes this and usually does so painlessly. This is also true of fish bones caught in the throat. Sometimes **Silica** will encourage the body to throw the object or bone out without any pus. If there is any slow gathering around a splinter that is comparatively painless then use **Silica** 30 twice a day until the problem is resolved. This is also the case for thorns from gardening. Sometimes, with fish bones stuck in the throat, it is necessary to use a 200 or 1M. If there is acute pain, swelling, redness and extreme sensitivity in the part then use **Hepar-sulph.** 200: 2 per day till it really improves. The pus in **Hepar-sulph.** is more likely to be yellow or green and bloody while **Silica** tends to form paler pus that is slower in gathering. If **Hepar-sulph.** fails then use **Myristica** 200: twice daily for 3 days.

Bites

The bites of cats and dogs, rodents or horses all call for particular remedies. Cats and rodents leave deep stab wounds. Dogs (unless the patient has been savaged) and horses tend to leave shallower but heavily contused wounds. If there is shock then start with **Aconite** or **Arnica** depending on indications. If there is little blood but the teeth have made a puncture wound then use **Ledum**; if there is a lot of laceration then use **Ledum** for the punctures and **Hypericum** for the bleeding wounds as well as **Hypercal Ø** topically. Cats often make wounds that call for both remedies as they grab and tear with their claws and stab with their teeth. Dogs and horses tend to cause 'nip' wounds and don't so readily draw blood. This calls for **Arnica** for the bruising. If the dog or horse bite has damaged an area of soft flesh such as the breast then use **Bellis Perennis**. Use 30 or 200 depending on the severity of the damage.

Such animal bite wounds do not always resolve as quickly as might be expected. If the wound begins to suppurate then bacterial toxicity has found a susceptibility in the patient and will require swift professional attention. The following remedies are described in order to know when to call the homoeopath:

Acetic Acid (vinegar) is indicated very occasionally when the patient suffers a lacerated wound with swelling in the whole limb and gnawing pains.

Belladonna will be indicated if there is redness, swelling and throbbing around the wound and more especially if there are red streaks running up the limb from the wound. Use 200.

Echinacea Angustifolia should be used if the skin around the wound is irritated and itching and there is pus forming.

Lachesis is a common remedy for cat bites. The wound becomes bluish or purplish, feels tight and painful causing the area to feel full and even bursting; it might tend to bleed easily.

Lyssin, made from the saliva of a rabid dog, is a remedy that is sometimes needed after indicated remedies such as **Lachesis** and **Echinacea** fail to finish the job especially on animal bites. The wound is persistently painful, bluish and looks as if it could ulcerate or it simply responds to no other remedies. The patient may also complain of headache.

Pyrogen is indicated for swollen wounds that suppurate and cause the patient to develop more general symptoms. There is a feeling of malaise, soreness and aching in the limbs, dullness and lethargy. The pus may smell disgusting. The patient may say that they feel that 'flu is coming on. (**Pyrogen** is sometimes indicated when the wound is healed but the general state of lethargy, aching and soreness with depression remains. It is a remedy for long-held effects of toxicity – even after the infection itself has gone.)

Another aspect of animal bites is the emotional one; bites are often inflicted by family pets. The unexpectedness of the wound can cause emotional distress. If the patient feels abused by the animal; if trust is in some way affected then **Staphysagria** 200 may be required to resolve the trauma.

Flea and mosquito bites: these are puncture wounds and as such often call for **Ledum** 30. The site is lumpy, pale and very itchy. If there are a lot of bites and first one bite and then another itches so that different areas need scratching all the time then the remedy is **Staphysagria** 30.

Horsefly bites: consider **Cantharis** as it may well burn and feel blistered. If this does nothing then ask your homoeopath if it would be appropriate to use **Caladium**, not your average first-aid remedy but useful here. (30 is the most likely potency here.)

Spider bites: some people are so sensitive that these can cause both swelling and pain. All spiders are poisonous to some degree though in Britain there are few that can cause real hurt to anyone and the need for hospital attention is rare. Sometimes, however, if the bite is on a vulnerable area or one rich in nerves, such as an eyelid or a lip, then use **Ledum** and/or **Hypericum.** If the swelling is red and hot, use **Belladonna** 30. Occasionally, if there is a bluish swelling which starts to feel itchy and painful then it is best to contact your practitioner who will probably give **Latrodectus Mactans,** the black widow poison, in the 30th potency.

Snake bites: these are not common but can occur in spring when the venom is at its strongest, and summer especially to children and pets. The wound must be dealt with quickly to avoid very unpleasant symptoms. A viper's bite causes swelling and bursting pain with blueness of the skin as if it were contused. The pains move up the limb and suggest **Ledum** which would be indicated anyway for the puncturing of the skin. **Ledum** is not always suf-ficient. **Lachesis** is more indicated for the rest of the picture and it follows **Ledum** well. It may have to be given every 2 hours in the 30th potency. Alternating **Ledum** and **Lachesis** is also a reasonable course of action. **Snake bites should always be reported to the homoeopath and examined by the emergency staff at hospital.** This is not least because in the young and the weak breathing can be affected. There also may be chronic effects of the bite that persist after the emergency is over.

Stings

Wasps and bees account for most of the stings which need treatment. Hornets, much more vicious and threatening, are an increasing problem. For the average sting and the usual reaction it is only necessary to be familiar with **Apis.** **Apis** 30 covers a sting that leaves a red or pale puffy lump which is usually firm to hard at the centre, is painful and eventually itchy and stinging at the same time. The patient is often restless, tired and irritable. You will probably need to prescribe it 3 or 4 times a day for 2 or 3 days. If the itching becomes intense (especially with a wasp sting) then **Vespa Crabro,** the remedy made from a wasp's venom, may be called for. It is always a good idea to use vinegar as a topical salve; use cotton wool to dab it over the area.

There are other remedies that might be needed:

Acetic Acid: this is another remedy that is not part of the first-aid kit but is worth knowing about. The remedy is made from vinegar and acts when the part affected goes cold and waxy in appearance. There is also some oedematous swelling of the area. In a severe reaction to a sting the patient becomes thirsty, an indication that **Apis** does not have.

Carbolic Acid: this is not a usual first-aid remedy and if it is needed then you might want to talk to your practitioner about the symptoms. The stinging and itching will be very severe, the part affected will be weak and very painful. The site of the sting will probably be threatening to blister or break open. The patient will feel weak and even prostrated. This is a remedy for a very severe histamine reaction and one that does not respond quickly to other, equally well-indicated remedies.

Hypericum and **Ledum:** these two are always needed in puncture wounds with nerve pains. Use the 30 of both and alternate. These may come in useful if **Apis** is indicated but doesn't relieve as quickly as it should.

Lachesis is occasionally needed if the sting site goes dark red or even purplish and the part feels tense and tight, even bursting. Use the 30.

Tissue salts: alternating **Nat-mur.** and **Ferr-phos.** complements the indicated remedy. One of each twice daily.

Urtica Urens: if the sting causes raised blotches which sting and itch like a nettle sting then **Urtica** will help. **Urtica** is often useful when a histamine reaction develops. You can also use the tincture topically.

Severe reaction to stings must be dealt with promptly and when extreme the patient must be taken to hospital. Anaphylaxis is a condition in which the body releases chemicals including histamine into the system, causing dilation of the blood vessels and contraction of the airways. It can be extremely sudden, cause heat and difficulty breathing even to the point of suffocation. The blood pressure lowers dramatically leading to faintness and the heart may begin to beat erratically causing panic.

If you know that a member of your household has intense reactions to stings then make sure that as part of your first-aid kit you have **Apis** 10M,

Carbolic Acid 10M and **Acetic Acid** 10M. In the season for stings, ensure that the **Apis** is on hand or get the person to carry a 4-gram bottle of it just to be on the safe side. If the patient has difficulty breathing, feels sleepy, lethargic, irritable and has moments of fitful, angry restlessness as well as puffiness and heat which is all better for a cool flannel then you can be sure of **Apis**. The other two remedies should be kept as back-up. If difficulty breathing is the primary symptom then you may need to use **Carbolic Acid** if the **Apis** has not made any difference within 5 minutes. If the patient is very thirsty then go straight to **Acetic Acid**. Whatever remedy you give, take the person to hospital anyway so that they can be checked over. Take no chances where a patient might so easily collapse and go into anaphylactic shock.

Jellyfish stings: these are another kind of sting that you may need to minister to. There are two remedies to consider: **Urtica Urens** and **Medusa**. **Urtica Urens** deals with stings that leave a burning, red weal that looks and feels like nettle rash. (Use the 30 every 3 to 4 hours.) Practically identical in appearance is **Medusa**, the remedy made from the jellyfish itself. This is the remedy that is most likely to be of use if you run into trouble in Mediterranean or tropical waters while on holiday. Use the 200 every 4 to 6 hours.

Allergic Reactions

Allergic reactions can range from a few sneezes lasting five minutes to anaphylactic shock with consequent collapse. The list of causes is prodigious and includes dust, metals, chemicals, wheat, yeast, potatoes, pollen, peanuts, eggs and dairy products as well as insect bites and stings. Anyone suffering chronically from an allergy should seek professional help from a homoeopath. This is even truer of multiple allergies. There is always a considerable amount of treatment required not least because the origin of allergies such as hay fever and gluten intolerance lies in heredity. Skilled prescribing is necessary to effect relief. However, there are allergic reactions that you can do something about even if it is while you are waiting to see the homoeopath. The first thing that may be of help is **Aconite**; if the effects of the reaction come on suddenly and are shocking then a dose of **Aconite** 200 is a good start.

It is important to be able to differentiate **Aconite** and **Apis**; both remedies have great restlessness and sudden onset of symptoms. **Aconite** is far more obviously restless with anxiety and fright. It is clear that the restlessness is caused by the fear. With **Apis,** the restlessness and irritability are more from physical discomfort.

For extreme reactions use **Apis** 10M. This covers heat, puffy swelling, drowsiness with difficult or suffocative breathing, restlessness and extreme irritability when disturbed. Give this as you prepare to take the patient to hospital. If the reactions are similar to this description but not so severe that the patient needs to be monitored by the hospital then use a lower potency such as the 200.

The causes of needing **Apis** include stings, allopathic drugs, peanut allergy, chemical allergy and allergy to certain types of seafood such as prawns (this is a form of histamine poisoning). Some sensitive people can also have similar reactions to eggs.

Hives: various things can cause hives including food and drink additives and emotions. This is a condition of the skin where histamine is released into the tissues causing redness, swelling, itching and stinging. Weals and welts appear across the skin and the sensation is like that of stinging nettles.

- For this reason **Urtica Urens** is very often useful. Use the 30 (unless the case is severe and needs 200s). It might be necessary to repeat it several times over a 24-hour period. (If you do not have this or any other remedy for hives – whatever the causation – then you may fall back on a useful tip: get the patient to sit in a warm bath filled with nettles or nettle roots.)
- **Apis** is sometimes called for in hives. Symptoms include stinging pains and puffiness with irritability and > from a cool damp flannel.
- If the patient becomes restless, anxious and thirsty for small amounts of water (sipped) then use **Arsen-alb.** 30.
- If the eruptions start to break open and threaten to become infected then give your practitioner a call as they may well prescribe **Carbolic Acid** 30.
- If the patient's skin becomes generally pale and the hives are widespread (even in blotches over the whole body) and there is a tearful mood then use **Pulsatilla** 200.
- If the skin is generally dry and the patient is withdrawn or hard to get symptoms out of; if the hives are caused by exposure to the sun then

Nat-mur. 30 will give relief. A **Nat-mur.** patient is often very thirsty.
- If the cause of the hives is a meal of shellfish then use **Astacus Fluviatilis** 30. This is a remedy that your homoeopath will need to supply. There is usually a general nettle rash over the whole body, the glands may swell and the patient probably feels rather bilious.
- If no other indicated remedy seems to help within a few hours of prescribing then consider using **Sulphur** especially if the patient is hot, tired and thirsty.
- **Tissue Salts:** alternating **Nat-mur.** and **Calc-phos.** supports **Apis, Pulsatilla, Sulphur** and **Arsen-alb.** in this condition. One of each daily.

Allergic asthma and lung conditions: (see Hay Fever) dust and dust mite, bacteria or chemicals when inhaled can cause pneumonitis, a condition characterised by shortness of breath, coughing and sometimes sneezing. (See below: **Arsen-alb., Allium Cepa, Carbo-veg.** and **Nux-vom.**) Occasionally the coughing can lead to retching and even vomiting. If it is persistent it is likely to be misdiagnosed as asthma and inhalers of Ventolin and steroids are prescribed. If these are prescribed too soon with a consequent suppression of the symptoms then it is likely that the opportunity to investigate the possible causative allergen(s) will be missed. Elimination of the cause is always better than the removal of symptoms.

Asthmatic breathing is also a common reaction to fungal spores that are found in hay and straw and growing in damp buildings. (The black fungus that is sometimes left to grow on the inside of window panes might be suspect!) The same mistaken diagnosis can be made; asthma is a condition based primarily on suppressed and unexpressed emotions. In allergic asthmatic breathing there may be wheezing, rattling, coughing and retching; it may be easy or difficult to bring up mucus formed in the lung, bronchus or larynx. The nose may stream with various shades of mucus and the eyes might be itchy, swollen, puffy, reddened and watery or excessively dry and itchy. In any serious attack you should inform your practitioner or, if there is obviously obstructed breathing, **take the patient to hospital immediately.** If the indications of the acute reactions are clear, use the appropriate remedy in the 30, one dose every 2 hours. If no improvement is obvious within 24 hours then call your homoeopath.

Allium Cepa has a lot of sneezing and coughing; there is oppressed breathing with a sense of pressure in the middle of the chest. There is tickling in the larynx with a lot of mucus in the throat. The voice sounds hoarse. The nose produces a lot of watery discharge which makes the nose and the top lip sore. The eyes may burn and cause a lot of rubbing. This remedy is made from the onion; the symptoms are not dissimilar to the irritation caused by peeling and cutting onions. (Often needed in August or early autumn.)

Arsen-alb. covers wheezing, whistling breathing which is < lying down; > sitting up at 45º; the mucus is often like white of egg and frothy though it can be yellowish. The condition is < around midnight to 1 a.m. and the usual modalities (see part III) apply. The face sometimes has a pinched look and the patient wants to wrap up well but hang their head out of the window. If the patient seems to have all these symptoms but also a lot of deeper coloured nasal mucus and a sore nose and top lip then use **Arsen-iod.** 30 instead. One possible causation is the reaction to pesticides.

Carbo-veg. is a remedy commonly needed by the old and the very young though anyone with its symptom picture will respond to it. There is a lot of rattling of mucus on the chest, there is exhaustion, feebleness and a bluish tinge around the mouth. The breathing is audible and laboured. The patient may sneeze, gag and retch and have a spasmodic cough. An obvious feature is wanting to belch with breathing difficulties. Symptoms can be brought on from car fumes, eating fish (this would also bring on bowel symptoms) or from alcohol.

Nux Vomica has a reputation for dealing with reactions to many forms of toxicity; it covers symptoms of asthmatic breathing resulting from eating food enhanced by monosodium glutamate (see **Phos**. below). The asthmatic breathing will be present with fullness in the stomach, uneasiness in the bowels and a possible congestive headache. It is sometimes needed for difficult breathing and nasal congestion after becoming oversensitised to scented plants. (**Nux-vom.** has a more stuffed up, snuffly nose than **Sabadilla** whose nose is much runnier.)

Phosphorus is sometimes needed for those who have been affected by industrial chemicals or food enhanced with monosodium glutamate (so-called 'Chinese Restaurant syndrome'). There is an asthmatic reaction with anxiety and palpitations as well as possible burning sensation throughout the body and pressure sensations in the face. The chest feels tight and constricted; there is a feeling of weight and heaviness. The patient is likely to be weakened and listless.

Sabadilla is indicated in those who are particularly sensitive to scented garden flowers; after pollen is inhaled and causes intense itching, sneezing and profuse watery nasal discharge. The patient wants to rub the nose furiously for relief. A severe reaction can start wheezing and shortness of breath.

Tissue salts: Kali-mur. and **Ferr-Phos.** can be alternated in any inflammatory condition of the ear, nose, throat and chest. One of each twice a day (4 pills) for a few days can complement the indicated remedy.

Electric Shock

The first remedy in electric shock is **Phosphorus**. Give this remedy as soon as possible and if symptoms are severe or persistent then you should contact your practitioner for advice. Use the highest potency you have to hand but if you only have the 30 then consult your homoeopath in case a deeper acting potency is required. If the patient is more obviously showing signs of **Arnica** then give this remedy instead (see page 339). Give the 200th potency: one dose.

If neither of these remedies is indicated or neither appears to make any impression on the symptoms then call your homoeopath as soon as possible; more precise case-taking may be required. **If there is loss of consciousness or a persistent state of shock with confusion, take the patient to hospital.**

Sunstroke and Heat Exhaustion

Lying in the sun too long, exertion for a long time in hot conditions (especially humid ones) and the loss of fluid from the system through sweating leads to heat exhaustion. The electrolyte balance is disturbed (i.e. the loss of the body's salts disturbs the circulation and brain function) and leads to fatigue, muscular weakness and changes in body temperature with the skin feeling cold and clammy while blood pressure drops and the patient feels faint. Get the patient to lie down with head low while you make a drink of Bovril or Marmite or some salty drink which will restore the electrolyte balance. Those most susceptible to this problem are the old, the overweight and alcoholics. The chief remedies include:

China is useful when there is debility, trembling and sensitive irritability with a feeling of being drained after being in the sun. The patient cannot make any mental effort.

Gelsemium which is identified by the patient becoming drowsy, droopy, light-headed and unable to think properly. The eyelids droop and the patient might appear to be almost drunk. The face might look flushed but not red; more a dusky colour. If you take the pulse (hold your fingers on the thumb-side of the inside wrist) you will notice a weak, soft beat. If you ask about the patient's temperature, they are likely to say that there are chills running up and down the spine from time to time.

Pulsatilla easily suffers from the heat; either of the sun or in a hot room. This remedy is the most important one to consider when a patient complains of 'air hunger', weakness, light-headedness and feeling 'sorry for themselves'. The **Pulsatilla** patient is likely to be dependent and rather tearful; they need looking after.

Two other remedies are useful though they are not in the average first-aid kit: **Selenium** and **Natrum Carbonicum**. **Selenium** is particularly indicated in older people who suffer from exhaustion, sleepiness and debility after a period in the heat or under the sun. The patient is likely to know that the sun is bad for them and to ascribe their symptoms to this cause. The weaker the patient is, the more likely **Selenium** will help resolve the situation. However, you may need to ask your practitioner to supply the remedy unless you know that someone in your care would benefit from your keeping it. **Nat-carb.** is not as weakened by the sun as **Selenium** but suffers much more from headaches. If a patient has a headache in hot or sunny weather but does not have the typical picture of feverishness with it (like **Belladonna**) then **Nat-carb.** should be considered. With this remedy you might see puffiness of the face or around the eyes when they are suffering from heat. As **Nat-carb**. is a deep-acting remedy it is a good idea to let your practitioner know when it has worked well as there is probably an underlying chronic state that might benefit from constitutional prescribing.

Sunstroke or **heatstroke:** this is more serious. The symptoms include a fever state with the temperature reaching sometimes alarming levels, even 104°F. or more, dehydration, rapid breathing and increasing risk of delirium. For the old, the very young, alcoholics and those with poor ability to sweat, the situation is potentially dangerous. These patients need to be treated pro- fessionally. **Do not hesitate to take the patient straight to hospital!** The usual conventional treatment is to wrap the patient in a cooling wet blanket or to pack them in ice. This may be lifesaving but it is potentially a serious shock to the system and can cause long-term side effects. Once the emergency is over, the patient must be seen by their homoeopath for treatment to deal with any lingering symptoms and the after effects of hospitalisation.

The first remedy to consider for sunstroke is **Belladonna**. The usual picture of radiant heat coming off the upper body, redness of the face, headache, throbbing arteries in the neck and glassy eyes will be present for **Belladonna**. If the fever is up as far as 102°F. or 103°F. then use a 200 as you need a fast acting potency that goes deep enough to bring about a lasting effect. (If the fever is higher then use a 10M if you have it.) If symptoms persist then either the 200 is not deep enough or the patient needs a remedy that looks very similar to **Belladonna: Glonoin**. The symptom picture of **Glonoin** has an internal sensation of blood rushing up into the head and causing a bursting, throbbing headache. The veins on the temple stand out and the pounding in the head will be the chief characteristic. **Belladonna** can have this headache too but the difference is that **Glonoin** patients are << for any movement, jar or motion and reassured by help while **Belladonna** patients can be irritable and want to be left alone in the dark. Patients needing **Glonoin** might well have their jaws clenched in an effort to maintain absolute stillness. When indicated and given early enough, hospital treatment can be averted. Always let your homoeopath know that you have had to use a high potency.

Occasionally **Arnica** will be needed. If the patient has been working in the sun for any length of time, has sweated profusely and looks prostrated, flushed dark red in the face, strained and morose then consider giving **Arnica**. The patient is likely to be of a heavy set and have ruddy cheeks; **Arnica** does less well on those who are spare of flesh. Use the 200th potency.

Poisoning

In the average household the most common causes of poisoning are allopathic drugs, household cleaning products, industrial chemicals, hallucinogenic drugs, garden plants and contaminated food. Some of these may cause internal symptoms and others may bring on skin reactions. Initially, the most important thing to do is to identify the source of the poison. If the patient has swallowed a drug meant for someone else or is suffering from the effects of a toxic chemical cleaner or a hallucinogenic drug then it is **absolutely imperative** to seek expert help. **Dial 999 or take the patient to hospital and ring your practitioner as soon as you can!** The more you can tell the doctor about the poison the better he or she will be able to assess the extent of the damage and how to treat the problem. If the patient is suffering from reactions to a plant, the symptoms are most likely to be on the skin in which case get onto your practitioner at once. You may be advised to use one of your first-aid remedies such as **Rhus-tox.** and to bring the patient in for an examination.

There are certain things that you can do in an emergency. Ensure that the patient is lying on their side so that the tongue cannot drop back. In the case of chemical or drug poisoning check whether the substance swallowed is one likely to cause more damage if vomited; if it is an acid or a petroleum product then it might. The British National Formulary advises against inducing vomiting of swallowed toxins. **Dial 999**; the operator will put you through to someone who will talk you through what you need to do. If the patient is cold then cover them with a blanket. There are various remedies that might be useful and would not interfere with any emergency treatment.

Allopathic drugs: drug side effects include drowsiness, dizziness, faintness, clouded thinking, clumsiness, nausea, thirst, deranged taste, visual disturbances and photosensitivity. These symptoms are common to many of the sedative (anxiolytic) and hypnotic drugs such as the benzodiazepines. Other drugs, such as the non-steroidal anti-inflammatories, can bring on gastro-intestinal symptoms such as nausea, vomiting, diarrhoea, bleeding and ulceration. They can also cause skin rashes, hypersensitivity, vertigo, headache, depression, nervousness, tinnitus, photosensitivity and raised blood pressure. If a patient has been prescribed a drug that has any of these reactions recorded on the blurb that comes with the packet then they should return to the doctor and report the side effects. It is not advisable to prescribe any homoeopathic remedies to remove these symptoms. The relief of side effect symptoms after a prescription from a doctor requires expert professional prescribing from your homoeopath who needs to be well aware of the niceties of professional etiquette. However, if someone should inadvertently swallow any drug and such side effects appear then you do need to contact your homoeopath. The very young and the elderly, because of any confusion, are the most likely to require treatment for this situation. You may be advised to give one of several remedies that are in the first-aid kit. The most common remedy is **Nux-vom.** and it can cover any of the list of symptoms above. This remedy, when given in the 30th potency over a few days, can relieve most drug-induced symptoms. It is best given at night or, if prescribed twice daily, at midday and at bedtime. **Nux-vom.** is a liver remedy and is superb at detoxifying this organ which is so crucial to the process of dealing with chemicals from outside the body. The second remedy that might be indicated here is **Sulphur** which covers heat, prostration, increased thirst and diarrhoea as side effects. Sometimes, the homoeopath will recommend that you should alternate **Nux-vom.** and **Sulphur** 30 over a few days as the action of these two will cause the liver to open up its storage cells and initiate the speedy excretion of any drug toxicity. One further remedy might need to be considered: **Pulsatilla**. This is useful when the other two are not indicated but the patient is dependent, tearful, with a skin rash or has vertigo that comes on when they get up or look up. **Pulsatilla** patients are seldom thirsty though they may drink from habit or from an inherent understanding that they need to. Sometimes practitioners will recommend that you should alternate **Nux-vom.** and **Pulsatilla** rather than **Sulphur**; **Pulsatilla** has the reputation for being better for sensitive people.

Chemicals: the toxic chemicals available in most households include ammonia, bleach, detergents, glue, solvents and pesticides. Those most at risk are very young children and the elderly though teenagers may succumb to the temptation of sniffing glue. Symptoms that are likely to be experienced are skin burns, dizziness, weakness, disorientation, burning and watering of the eyes, burning in the oesophagus and lung area, breathing difficulties, nausea, diarrhoea and changes in rhythm of the heartbeat. There are two remedies that are useful here: **Arsen-alb.** and **Phosphorus**. There is no mistaking **Arsen-alb.**: burning pains in the throat, oesophagus, stomach or gut which are often accompanied by dryness of the mouth and throat, thirst for cold water (in sips very often) and anxiety with great restlessness and nausea. If there are **Arsen-alb.** lesions or rashes on the skin (possibly as a reaction to a pesticide) then they are going to be itching, burning and swollen, even blistering; they may, oddly, be better for hot water. **Phosphorus** also has burning pains but the skin reactions are less aggressive (though contact eruptions might bleed readily) while the internal symptoms from chemical poisoning are likely to leave the patient feeling weak, light-headed, disorientated and oversensitive. The five special senses can be markedly affected with sight and hearing being particularly damaged. There might be palpitations or a raised heartbeat as well. Your practitioner would be most likely to prescribe the 30th potency over the phone though severe cases would need the 200. **The patient should be taken to A & E.**

Carbon monoxide poisoning: this is rare and requires expert treatment. However, the most likely remedy needed would be **Carbo-veg.** This remedy is important for anyone in a state of collapse with breathing difficulties and who is turning glowing red in the face. Use the 200 and **dial 999**. (The question arises of how to administer remedies when the patient's breathing is severely compromised. Drop the remedy into a glass half full of water and wet the patient's lips or dab it onto the wrist just where you would look for the pulse: inside wrist on the thumb-side.)

Animal poisons: see page 38 for the entry on Bites and Puncture Wounds.

Vegetable poisons: the most usual reaction to poisonous plants is on the skin. They can bring up rashes, blisters, oedematous swellings and itching or burning sensations on any part of the body, even on the lips and into the mouth or eyes (see Hives). The patient may not know which plant has caused the problem; some are affected by plants that are innocuous to most people.

The best-known plant to cause symptoms is Rhus Toxicodendron which provides one of the most frequently used of first-aid remedies and which covers far more than just skin symptoms. It is a member of the sumach family, all of which might cause symptoms though it is Rhus Toxicodendron that is most virulent; it is even able to provoke symptoms in the most susceptible without actual contact. However, the most usual plants to cause trouble are the hairy-leaved ones; an example is the Fremontodendron, a tall shrub with waxy yellow flowers. The most common remedies are **Rhus-tox.**, **Urtica Urens**, **Arsen-alb.** and occasionally **Clematis Erecta**. **Rhus-tox.** symptoms are intense: itching, swelling, dry and hot. There is redness; the part can look and feel burnt. The surface skin may take on the appearance of eczema. Generally the patient becomes restless and very irritable; glands near the affected part might swell. The muscles near the site often become stiff and achy. **Urtica Urens** is the remedy for a skin reaction that most resembles nettlerash with its characteristic itching and burning with raised pale bumps on the surface with a background redness. (**Urtica** is also useful as a tincture; in a solution of 4 drops to a quarter cup of water it can be applied topically.) **Arsen-alb.** has burning, itching and heat too but the patient is restless and anxious; the more anxious, the more likely that **Arsen-alb.** is needed. One oddity is that **Arsen-alb.** pains, even on the surface, are > heat or hot applications. **Clematis Erecta**, not a usual first-aid remedy, has been known to affect the eyes: burning sensations with profuse watering and photophobia though, paradoxically, it is worse on closing the eyes. The plant itself can be the culprit in those who are sensitive to it. A very common wild plant to watch out for is ragwort which can cause sore, red skin for which **Urtica** and **Arsen-alb.** are useful.

Alcohol poisoning: acute alcohol poisoning can range from the distressing to the dangerous. Children and older people who take drugs for insomnia and anxiety are most at risk. The organs most affected by large amounts of alcohol are the liver, heart and brain. It is essential to seek advice if the patient is in any way uncontrolled or uncontrollable. For an older person with a tendency to drink too much alcohol to become confused, sleepy, incoherent and with a tremor and flapping of the hands, **it is imperative to seek medical assistance!** The range of possible symptom reactions can be broad; some patients will be aggressive, some will be sleepy, others will feel sick and vomit.

There is usually a need for fresh air and plenty of water to drink. (For those who vomit copiously and become dehydrated, there is a need to restore electrolyte balance. This is particularly true of older people who may not be naturally thirsty anyway.) If the patient is paralytic then watch carefully in case of suffocation from vomit. If possible, keep the patient walking around. The most useful remedy is **Nux-vom**. This covers the toxicity in the liver and blood as well as the typical mood characteristics – even when the patient displays placid good humour, not usually associated with **Nux-vom**. (a generally irritable medicine) but, nevertheless, part of the picture in some who need it; usually those who are peppery tempered and 'driven' when sober. **Nux-vom.** is also well known as the remedy for hangover. Some people will take **Nux-vom.** before they go out for a binge; others will take it before getting into bed after a night out so that when they wake they will not suffer headaches and nausea. Both methods can work well, but beware! **Nux-vom.** is a remedy that is uncompromising and it can easily antidote other remedies that might have been taken recently. Before using **Nux-vom.** in this cavalier fashion, ask your practitioner about the advisability of doing so. There are other remedies that are needed if the picture is more particular. Older people, especially those with a reputation for liking alcohol, who become maudlin, weepy and cloudy-minded will need **Crotalus Horridus** 30 which is not a usual first-aid remedy unless there is a particular need within the household. The patient tends to be sleepy and bilious when 'in their cups'. **Arsen-alb.** is useful when the patient becomes exacting, precise in choice of words and anxious with a nervous restlessness probably due to nausea. They can be bossy but do not be intimidated by this. Simply give the patient **Arsen-alb.** 30 and make a drink of hot water for them to sip. **Arsen-alb.** or **Pulsatilla** might be needed when someone has drunk cheap wine that has a lot of chemicals in it; sulphur dioxide is often used as a preservative and causes symptoms that might call for either. **Pulsatilla** would show signs of overheating and wanting fresh air. The patient would have a distressed, rather helpless expression, might become weepy and would refuse any food or drink. Those who become hot (especially in the face with reddened lips), sleepy, mildly abusive and dishevelled usually respond well to **Sulphur**. (This is the remedy for those who, when drunk, tell long, rambling, possibly obscene stories.) Those who become evil-tempered, foul-mouthed and suspicious of everyone else's motivation need **Lachesis**. This is a remedy state that you might feel more comfortable about if you seek back-up from the practitioner even if you have the remedy. For those who become wildly excitable and over the top with silly behaviour and who seem to be in a heightened state of adrenal rush (often because they haven't eaten before drinking), give **Coffea** 30. The result should be that they become drowsy and in need of sleep. **Ranunculus Bulbosus,** the common buttercup, is a curious remedy picture in alcohol poisoning: the patient tries to take deep breaths but is prevented by hiccoughs. They want to appear sober and when they speak they try extremely hard to enunciate every word properly – it often appears to be comical. This is not a usual first-aid remedy so you may have to call the practitioner. In any of the above cases use the 30th potency unless advised otherwise by the practitioner. The remedy can be repeated quite frequently; up to one every 20 to 40 minutes if need be. There are other scenarios for alcohol poisoning but they really require expert treatment. Phone for back-up and give the remedy most similar while making sure the patient is safe from their symptoms.

Hallucinogenic poisoning: the most common hallucinogenic drugs that create symptoms are cannabis, cocaine and Ecstasy. Others include amphetamines, magic mushrooms and heroin. The most likely to cause acute symptoms of poisoning are Ecstacy, LSD and heroin: headache, nausea, vomiting, , hallucinating, trembling and convulsions. Call the homoeopath and **take the patient to hospital**. See pages 326–9 for further information.

Fainting

Fainting is a temporary loss of consciousness due to a lack of oxygen to the brain as a result of reduced blood flow. It can result from a traumatic psychological shock, anxiety, overheating, pain, hypoglycaemia (low blood sugar) or anaemia. By falling a patient is often causing their own recovery by being horizontal, the quickest way to restore blood to the brain. Transient faint feelings can be caused by getting up too soon from lying or sitting. This is common in those who have low blood pressure, tachycardia or heart fibrillation. If fainting becomes more than an unusual occurrence it is essential to seek professional advice. The main remedies to consider in an acute fainting attack are **Aconite, Arsenicum Album, Ignatia, Nux Vomica, Pulsatilla, Phosphorus** and **Sepia**.

Aconite is useful when fainting occurs from constriction of the chest with difficult breathing. This can happen after a fright or with severely restricted breathing as with an asthma attack. This is when the attack is of sudden onset. (Use the 200.)

Arsenicum Album covers fainting with the effort to cough; during a fever; during nausea; from pain. It is always indicated with the usual symptoms of anxiety, restlessness and dry mouth with a desire for sips of water. (Use the 30.)

Ignatia is the first remedy to consider for fainting from grief. (Use a high potency such as 200 or 1M.)

Nux Vomica is useful for fainting from anger, from fright or from smelling foul odours. It is also useful in those who suffer menstrual pains and irritability in the menstrual cycle. Fainting with nausea is common as well. Occasionally, **Nux-vom.** is indicated in fainting after copious diarrhoea. (Use the 30.)

Phosphorus covers fainting from loss of blood (i.e. from a nose bleed) or from strong scent. (Use the 30.)

Pulsatilla is the most common remedy for fainting in any domestic situation. It is most useful for fainting from becoming overheated in a stuffy, crowded room. This can be aggravated during a period. The patient might well be a bit dehydrated having forgotten to drink enough. (Use the 30, 200 or 1M depending on how well you know the person and how severe the symptoms.)

Sepia is indicated in those who feel faint when they stand in queues or at the sink too long (or standing in church!). It is also called for in faint feelings after exertion and during feverishness. The patient is often exhausted anyway and it is commonly needed as a support remedy in those who are going through the menopause – in which case it is necessary to ask your practitioner's advice. If a patient has been given a high potency dose of **Sepia** by the homoeopath for constitutional reasons then it is a mistake to take **Sepia** as a first-aid remedy.

Transient Ischaemic Attack and Stroke

A TIA is a short episode of disturbed brain function due to reduced blood supply to the brain. The cause is a small blood clot that has migrated towards the brain from a larger blood vessel. The clot slows the blood supply and the brain cells affected become unable to perform their task. It is a situation more common to those in middle and old age who have raised blood pressure or hardening of the arteries. Symptoms include dizziness, feeling faint, slurred speech, clumsiness, disturbance of vision, hearing or feeling, forgetfulness and weakness or sensations of numbness and tingling. All these symptoms may also be found in those who suffer a stroke but they are transient and will pass after a TIA. It is important to report a suspected TIA to your practitioner and to the doctor because it can be a precursor to a stroke. The homoeopath needs to prescribe remedies indicated by the local effects and by the constitution as a whole. The doctor needs to know so that all the relevant tests (MRI, ultrasound and CT scans) can be arranged. These tests can determine just where the problem might lie and whether there is any other hidden cause. Always inform your homoeopath of any medical tests as it is imperative that patients are given remedies to deal with the side effects of MRIs and X-rays etc.

A stroke is the result of the death of brain tissue after the blood supply to a part of the brain has been blocked. This can be caused by either an embolism (a clot that has travelled from a larger artery to the smaller arteries of the brain) or a haemorrhage (as the result of a burst blood vessel in the brain). The effect of a blockage is to cause local brain damage; the functions that are affected by this depend on which part of the brain is involved. The usual result is to cause one-sided weakness, loss of sensation or paralysis.

The main remedy to consider in an emergency TIA or stroke situation is **Arnica** 200. Give this remedy at once and call for professional assistance. You will not be undermining any necessary treatment that will be given by paramedics or by the hospital. **Arnica** is the first remedy to consider to encourage the body to remove damaged or dead blood cells swiftly. It can only promote the best possible outcome. There are other remedies indicated by the various different after-effects of stroke but they should be handled by your practitioner. As homoeopathic remedies can do wonders for patients who have had emergency treatment but are not fully back to normal, don't delay in consulting your practitioner. For example, **Baryta Carbonicum** and **Bufo** are capable of restoring to health those with mental symptoms such as withdrawal, irritability, childish behaviour, perpetual moaning, reluctance to meet people, poor memory for words or faces and fearful anxiety; **Lachesis** can be useful in encouraging recovery from one-sided paralysis. It is not always necessary to believe those who say, 'It is something that you'll have to learn to live with'. These last three remedies are mentioned to encourage sufferers to seek professional help.

Collapse

Sudden collapse requires a quick response. Knowing what to do therapeutically becomes most useful for those looking after the old, children with poor health and those with a chronic debilitating condition such as asthma or Parkinson's. You need professional help even if you have a comprehensive remedy kit. The main remedies to keep in mind are **Arsenicum Album, Camphor, Carbo Vegetabilis** and **Veratrum Album**.

Arsenicum Album is most indicated in collapse from diarrhoea and vomiting or sudden collapse with anxiety and restlessness. The patient will have a pinched and frowning expression and may ask for a little water. (Use the 200.)

Camphor is less commonly indicated but is useful for old people who are brewing an infection such as a cold or 'flu which leaves them extremely cold, weak and yet intolerant of too much applied heat. The patient's face will have a very pinched look and they will not want to be left alone – both symptoms are very similar to **Arsen-alb.** (Use the 30 unless you consult your practitioner.)

Carbo-veg. is more indicated for those who collapse from exhaustion and breathing difficulties. The patient appears gasping for breath, bluish round the face and in need of fresh air. (Use the 200 unless the practitioner advises otherwise.)

Veratrum Album is also indicated in collapse from diarrhoea and vomiting but it comes with other symptoms: sweat with extreme thirst and total exhaustion. (Use the highest potency available.)

Unexplained Symptoms of Injury or Trauma

There are times when symptoms of an injury seem to appear spontaneously without any obvious cause. The most common is bruising. Spontaneous bruising is the result of broken capillaries (small blood vessels near the surface of the skin). The cause can be one of several: heredity, excessive exposure to the sun, diabetes, old age, a blood clotting problem and prolonged use of steroid drugs or aspirin. Women are more prone to bruising from small injuries than men. Spontaneous bruising is important to mention to the homoeopath as it will form part of the overall picture that is necessary for the formulation of a constitutional prescription.

Another symptom that can appear to be the result of an injury is pain in a large joint with associated muscle weakness and strain. This is exemplified by a frozen shoulder. This condition can be the result of an old injury pattern, forgotten since an earlier treatment but now resurfaced as the result of another trauma. It can also be the result of a problem in the liver. Toxicity in the liver and stones forming in the gall bladder are very common indeed and can cause a number of conditions that are not immediately recognisable as liver trouble, one being a frozen shoulder: pain and stiffness with reduced range of movement in the joint which sometimes extends to the shoulder blade. This is an important symptom to take to your practitioner as, apart from prescribing the indicated remedy for the shoulder, they would be likely to give remedies to clear the toxicity from the liver. The most commonly useful supplement from the health food shop is milk thistle which comes in either capsule or liquid form. Similarly, a pain under the bottom corner of the right shoulder blade should be reported to your practitioner. This symptom can feel like a pulled muscle but is in fact a referred pain from the liver or gall bladder and can be indicative of gall stones.

Pains in the soles of the feet worse for initial walking in the morning on rising can start for no apparent reason. So can a pain in the heel on stepping. These are symptoms that on their own make little sense to anyone but a homoeopath. They can be signs of an inherited disease pattern, old injury patterns in other parts that have at last emerged in the extremities even years after the original trauma, or they can be early signs of rheumatism, often the result of an earlier suppression of some constitutional condition that has been long forgotten. This is also true of headaches of unknown origin; these can be associated with birth trauma even if that event was decades earlier. Consult the homoeopath first but be prepared to see a cranial osteopath as well if it proves that an old injury pattern is involved.

Sudden sensations of jumped or missed heartbeats can be alarming. These are not uncommon and not necessarily a cause for alarm. A sensation of a missed heartbeat (ectopic beat) can be a manifestation of stress and a sign that one needs to slow down or give oneself a break from attending to others. It is not the heart that is causing the problem but the vagus nerve, the nerve that tells the heart how to beat. In stress from overworking and from tension held in the cervical spine (between the shoulders) the vagus nerve can 'trip'. An old whiplash pattern that was never fully resolved can be the main-taining cause. See the homoeopath and/or go to the osteopath.

Clinical Shock

The symptoms of clinical shock are debility, mental confusion, rapid pulse, cold clammy skin and a bluish pallor. Bowels and bladder may also have stopped functioning. It can occur in various kinds of pathology, particularly where there is a considerable loss of body fluid (excessive haemorrhage or vomiting or diarrhoea), a condition of low blood pressure (which can result from head injuries, infection which causes septic or toxic shock, overdosing on certain drugs, liver failure as might occur in alcoholics) or feeble heart pump action. **Don't give fluids to drink. If you suspect clinical shock take the patient to hospital immediately!**

2   EMOTIONAL TRAUMA

Grief

For the bereaved there are two main remedies to consider: **Ignatia** and **Pulsatilla**.

> **Ignatia** covers a range of states from episodes of weeping to hysterical sobbing. The main telling symptoms are a sensation of a lump in the throat (or a fist in the chest) and quick changes of demeanour. There is likely to be loss of appetite as well. It is the main remedy to have on hand at funerals but it is also invaluable for less momentous occasions: parting from loved ones, the death of a pet animal, overreaction to tragic news. It will not suppress the natural expression of grief but it will help the patient to function during the moments when they are needed to hold things together. Use the 1M or the 10M.

> **Pulsatilla** is for those who become tearful and dependent. There can be a loss of appetite as well but the chief symptom is the weeping with the need for company. The 200 or the 1M can be safely used.

For some it will seem a surprise not to find **Natrum Muriaticum** listed here. This remedy is more for grief that has already taken root and is by now a chronic pattern. It can indeed be useful for those who are grieving afresh; perhaps at an anniversary of a loved one's passing or an event that reminds them of an original cause for grief. **Nat-mur.** is a deep remedy and often has its depths well hidden in the past. It is best to consult the homoeopath about this aspect.

Two other remedies that have proven to be extremely helpful in acute situations of grief are **Sandalwood** and **Buddleia Davidii**. Neither are usual first-aid remedies but they are worth mentioning as they are new additions to the materia medica and not all practitioners know of their existence. **Sandalwood** is indicated in those who cannot 'let go' of loved ones who have recently passed away. It has been effective when given to those officiating at funerals who would otherwise be unable to carry out their responsibilities because of emotional upset. The 1M or the 10M (ask the advice of your practitioner) is most useful here. It is entirely complementary with **Ignatia**. **Buddleia** is of great service for those who feel devastated by an event; they feel as if their lives have been blighted. It was of tremendous benefit when people were so affected by the news of the Twin Towers tragedy in New York. Buddleia, the plant, is usually the first plant to colonise bomb sites. (A note for practitioners: **Buddleia** is often indicated for those who have had a cough ever since receiving traumatic news.)

    Rescue Remedy is also helpful in any grief-laden situation. Sometimes, the feelings of grief are so overwhelming that even high potency **Ignatia** is insufficient to hold the patient 'together' especially if the emotions have drained them of all energy. In such cases inventive prescribing can be of value. For example, combining several of the most indicated Bach Flower remedies with a drop of **Lotus** 30 has been found to be very supportive: **Lotus** 30 + **Sweet Chestnut** + **Star of Bethlehem** is an example of a prescription that is very calming and supportive – one drop 3 times per day during periods of grieving. (**Lotus** is not indicated in people who are calm and stress free.) Another combination might be of service where a person must remain strong and responsible even though grieving themselves: **Chalice Well** 30 + **Elm** + **Red Chestnut** + **Oak**. **Chalice Well** is a remedy made from the water of the Chalice Well garden in Glastonbury and has been found to cover acute states of grief and stress which threaten to overwhelm the patient and interfere with normal responsibilities. (If your practitioner agrees with this supportive treatment then ask for a 4-ml bottle of either of these combinations to be made up for you at the homoeopathic pharmacy.)

Bad News

Bad news can bring on a range of different symptoms including anxiety, trembling, a lump in the throat, histamine reactions, sleeplessness, feverishness, hysteria or even catalepsy. Of all the remedies to consider think first of **Arnica** (see page 339). Others include **Ignatia**, **Calc-c.**, **Gelsemium**, **Apis**,

Pulsatilla and **Aurum** (and see above on **Buddleia**).

Apis is useful when any bad news causes a sudden histamine reaction so that the patient produces raised red lumps and weals. They become listless and irritable when disturbed. **Apis** is a very 'jealous' remedy so it is of use in those who have found out some news that relates to a relationship in difficulties. (In severe reactions use the 200 but otherwise 30 should be sufficient.)

Aurum is required when the bad news is of financial loss. The patient feels that everything is lost and that all their efforts were useless; there is little or no point in carrying on. The news can cause them to think of suicide. **Aurum** is not a first-aid remedy and is included here to encourage those affected to seek professional help rather than sliding into depression.

Calc-c. is useful in those who become anxious and sleepless from worry as a result of bad news. (Use a 30 and consider repeating it daily for 3 days. **Calc-c.** is a very deep remedy so ask your practitioner if in doubt.)

Gelsemium is indicated when the person is filled with dread, becomes weak and timid and yet is apathetic and brooding. They appear to be dulled intellectually and their reactions are slow. **Gelsemium** is indicated for those who fear hospitals and doctors so it covers distress from hearing bad medical news. (The 30 is often sufficient.)

Ignatia will be needed for those who develop a lump in the throat, who weep and who become unpredictable in their reactions. Frequently needed by those who are going through relationship problems. (Use a 200 or a 1M.)

Pulsatilla is called for in those who break down and weep pathetically when told any bad news. They are timid and needy. Initially they can excite lots of sympathy from others but can cause despair in equal measure if not encouraged to come out of their condition. (Use the 200 or the 1M depending on the level of effect of the news.)

Fright

The results of a fright are varied and require different remedies. Chief of all fright remedies is **Aconite**. It can be given before anything else based on just the fact that the patient has had a fright. Sometimes a fright is the main emotional element of a traumatic physical accident. If this is missed then **Arnica**, if chosen as the remedy to deal with the shock, will not do much. **Aconite** should be given first to remove the fear; **Arnica** can then be given even within a few minutes. If **Aconite** is inappropriate it will do nothing but as the result of giving it should be obvious within 10 minutes there is little to lose by giving it first while you are observing what else might need to be done.

Gelsemium, **Ignatia** and **Pulsatilla** are all indicated for fright for their various reasons. (See above under 'Bad News' for the indications of each of these.) One other remedy is outstanding in ailments from fright even though it is not really regarded as a first-aid remedy: **Opium**. If it is suspected that the results of a severe fright are lingering on the patient's mind; that the patient is unable to get the image of the fright out of his head then **Opium** is invaluable. If there is a delay in getting to the homoeopath then **Opium** 200 or 1M given for the indications may save distress. If the patient has not responded to the remedies described then consult the homoeopath because it may be necessary to look deeper into the 'picture' to differentiate between other remedies not so commonly required. Occasionally, a patient will need several remedies to resolve the issues that arise from fright. It is only with hindsight that patient and practitioner can see that the remedies in the sequence needed were all indicated but required for their individual reasons to unlock layers of chronically held patterns of emotional history. This is the stuff of constitutional prescribing that demands the expert attention of a qualified practitioner. Homoeopaths never underestimate fright as a causation of future conditions even if they arise years after the event and in unexpected ways. This is true of much emotional trauma.

Rescue Remedy should also be considered. It is a very good way of supporting a patient while you are waiting for the homoeopath to answer your call and you can't overdose on it.

Humiliation and Abuse

Humiliation can come in many guises: through bullying at school, being made redundant or sacked, being unfairly criticised or held up to scorn especially publicly, and physical, emotional and sexual abuse. The effect of humiliation on the emotional body can be devastating in the long term and it can set up patterns of reaction and behaviour (often kept hidden) that must sooner or later be resolved or they will result in pathology that will demand radical (and usually suppressive) treatment. For this reason, prevention is always better than cure; if parents are able to step in to control a potentially traumatic situation then they should. For example, if a child is being bullied at school it is imperative that the situation is not allowed to persist; better to remove the child from school until the issue is resolved than allow it to continue. One of the worst aspects for children who are victims of abuse is to feel that their parents are not supporting them and schools are not always quick enough (and sometimes reluctant) to notice individual cases of such stress.

If you think that your child is the victim of bullying or worse then you do need to consult the homoeopath, not least for yourself! If the circumstances require it you may also need to contact the appropriate authorities. Remedies for various different scenarios (and there are more than can be described here) are not difficult to spot and make such an important difference to the whole future of the patient. The same goes for someone who has suffered the indignity of redundancy or ridicule or the devastation of physical or sexual abuse. Homoeopaths do not necessarily need to be trained psychiatrists or counsellors to know what to do in the following circumstances:

Colocynth is not a first-aid remedy in the same degree as **Ignatia** or **Staphysagria** but when it is indicated it is vital that the patient is treated. The symptoms of **Colocynth** can be so severe that they might seem to call for drastic measures, usually suppressive. When abuse and humiliation or loss of dignity and pride are followed by anger and rage, the **Colocynth** patient will feel excruciating pain in the gut. It can be as if knives are cutting through the intestines and it makes the patient double up in agony and try to stop the pain by putting pressure over the painful area. With the pain, nausea and sweat can come on. In such circumstances **Colocynth** can remove the need for fruitless and worrying tests at the hospital. (Your practitioner would be likely to use a 200 or higher though a 30 might be all that is needed in a patient with abdominal cramps after bullying.)

Ignatia is often indicated after a loss of dignity and pride especially if the patient is left with swinging emotional states: one moment they are sobbing, the next they are furious or anxious and restless and the next, quite quiet and distant. The characteristic symptom of a lump in the throat or a sense of obstruction and pressure in the middle of the chest is more than likely to be there.

Staphysagria is the most usually prescribed remedy for acute humiliation when the patient is left after the event feeling utterly disempowered, as if unable to express how wretched they feel about the indignity or shame. They can be seething with righteous anger even if this emotion has no obvious outlet. This is the person who might, afterwards, be so angry that they throw things about the room, smashing them. They are left feeling inadequate and downtrodden. **Staphysagria** is sometimes known as the 'mother-in-law's remedy' because it is needed by the daughter-in-law who feels criticised and shamed by inadequacy over her inability to come up to her husband's mother's standards. It is also the remedy that is most indicated after physical and sexual abuse; so much so that it is often routinely prescribed. It is capable of encouraging the patient to release much of the terrible pent-up feelings that would otherwise fester for years until pathology became the only way the body could use to seek resolution. (**Staphysagria** is often given too late in the day, years after the event and when the buried emotions have established a strong root-hold. It frequently has a wonderful but temporary effect. It is not a deep enough acting remedy to do more than prune the problem planted so long before. Other remedies are almost always needed to dig out the plant of abuse; **White Chestnut Flower** in homoeopathic potency is one of those most useful to deal with a chronically held **Staphysagria** problem. **WCF** is not a first-aid remedy. Such 'deep' constitutional prescribing needs to be in the hands of an experienced practitioner. Do not be surprised if your homoeopath uses a 1M or 10M even on quite a young patient.)

For patients who become unaccountably withdrawn, rude and irritable even showing a tendency to be arrogant and dictatorial one moment and dissembling and furtive the next, suspect that there is an unexpressed emotional conflict going on that needs homoeopathic help. The usual remedy for this state is **Anacardium**, one that is very useful for those who have lived or worked in a humiliating situation for a long time and are made to feel out of their depth or out of their league. For those who are withdrawn and become extremely emotionally sensitive without any inclination to show this by crying then the remedy is likely to be **Nat-mur**. It is really important that such pictures are prescribed for professionally. There are many other remedies for this category of emotional turmoil and it often requires a practised eye to differentiate between them. Furthermore, it will take experience to know how to deal with the healing results of these remedies; despite the deep work they can do, neither of them is going to be all that will be needed. They are 'layer' remedies: beneath one remedy layer there is often another waiting to be exposed.

Rage

Rage can be a powerful enough energy to cause pathology. Usually it is just a symptom that we witness as part of a childish tantrum. Tantrums, whether they are thrown by 2-year-olds or teenagers, menopausal women or tyrannical managing directors, are a better expression (because nearer the surface) of emotions than frequent tears or bouts of depression. Childhood tantrums that persist should be taken to the homoeopath; they are often deeply ingrained in the psyche from a hereditary, miasmatic origin. The same is often true in menopause (in men just as much as women). However, a fit of rage can cause distressing symptoms in the person who is angry and those who bear the brunt. The latter might need one of the remedies listed above under 'Humiliation'. Rage can be brought on by frustration, pain, grief, alcohol, bad diet, drugs, incipient heart disease and malice. Usually it is advisable to see the homoeopath over a lengthy period to resolve all the issues that underlie the problem; if not, it is likely that the patient will end up with a serious pathology that will have to be dealt with by drugs and surgery.

For those who suffer symptoms from a bout of rage the following are useful:

Apis covers hives after rage. The skin becomes puffy, angry and stinging. The patient is likely to be very irritable, peevish and wanting to be left severely alone. (If the 30 does not shift the skin symptoms at least then call for advice.)

Arnica is often needed after a bout of rage when the patient is exhausted, looks battered and says that he is 'fine'. Use the 30.

Nux Vomica is the prime remedy to consider when the patient finishes the rage in tears. This is especially true of those who are frequently sensitive, driven and overwrought. Even more so if they seek to drown the moment of fury in a glass of wine or whisky. The 30 is usually sufficient.

Rescue Remedy can be helpful in the aftermath of a family row or an office crisis. Consider the Bach Remedies **Rock Rose** and **Mimulus** if the patient is intimidated by more powerful forces that frequently threaten to erupt.

Staphysagria covers trembling, sadness, crying and self-recrimination after fury. It also covers toothache (gums feel spongy and tend to bleed), headache (patient wants to lean head against something hard), menstrual cramps (or the period stops altogether) and cystitis (frequent need to pass water with burning when not passing water) after rage. If the 30 is insufficient to relieve the acute symptoms call the homoeopath for further advice.

Sustained Tension in Difficult Situations

There are many situations in which people are obliged to continue living that make it hard to sustain one's equilibrium. For example: working permanently overtime in crisis mode; waiting for and then attending court sessions; hospital visiting for any length of time when the patient is a loved one and in danger; caring for the handicapped or terminally ill at home. For some people, lesser sustained traumatic circumstances are enough: buying and selling a house; waiting for the results of examinations and interviews; making wedding arrangements. Whatever it is that causes someone to struggle with their focus, stamina and ability to respond to fast-changing situations, it is enough for them to need remedial help. There are a number of ways in which one can help oneself:

Oak is both a Bach Flower Remedy and a homoeopathic potency. It can be used here in both formats: the flower essence is supportive on the level of the psyche while **Oak** in potency works on both the emotional and the physical body. It can help to maintain stamina and an ability to judge one's capability; knowing when to stop, sit down and take stock becomes part of one's ability to manage. Typical symptoms of needing **Oak** in potency include tension in and across the shoulders, backache and a refusal to give in to common sense advice. **Oak** 30 daily during a crisis makes a good support.

Bach Flower Remedies A useful combination of Bach Flower Remedies is **Oak + Hornbeam + Olive + Red Chestnut**. One drop 4 times a day; the combination can be made up by the pharmacy if you are unable to find the individual bottles in the health food shop. Adding these to a bottle of liquid **Lotus** 30 can deepen the calming effects.

Fears

Phobias should be dealt with by a professional homoeopath. They are part of a psychological picture that requires experienced prescribing. They are important to mention in consultation even if the patient is not seeking specific help for them. Different phobias are covered by different remedies so someone's overwhelming fear of heights, for example, would help to differentiate between one remedy and another which might have other similar characteristics but no phobia about standing on a ladder. However, there are certain fears that can be alleviated in the short term by looking in the first-aid box.

Fear of seeing the doctor, dentist or going to the hospital: **Gelsemium** (feeling of dread which makes the patient go quiet, dull, weak, tired and wanting to be left alone); **Aconite** (sheer terror); **Arg-nit.** (restless, anxious, wants to be cool or outside, trembling, feels rushed but time seems to pass slowly, might pace up and down, could suffer diarrhoea with the anxiety, fears losing control).

Fear of aeroplanes and flying: Arg-nit. (see above); **Calc-c.** (becomes forgetful and confused with worrying long before the event; worries more in the evening and wakes at night with worry); **Gelsemium** (see above); **Opium** (abject terror of flying which causes a feeling of shutting off from everything); **Aconite** (see above).

Fear of failure in an examination: Arg-nit. (see above); **Gelsemium** (see above); **Aethusa** (when faced with the test, knowledge is blocked and memory fails; person goes blank).

Trembling with acute fear: Gelsemium (see above for fuller description); **Pulsatilla** (with anxiety, tearfulness, timidity and clinginess); **Arsen-alb.** (restless, anxious, impatient and inclined to be demanding – for attacks of fear for no apparent reason).

Agoraphobia and claustrophobia are both fears that are likely to require constitutional treatment over an extended period.

When fearfulness and stress causes a loss of energy a suggested combination of Bach Flower essences and the homoeopathic remedy **Lotus** 30 can be useful. **Lotus** acts in a similar manner to **Rescue Remedy** but also works to relieve stress on the physical and emotional bodies while maintaining physical energy. **Lotus** 30 + **Mimulus** + **Larch** + **White Chestnut** will act as a subtle support in difficult situations. Ask the pharmacy to make up a 4-ml bottle of drops and take one drop up to 3 times per day.

Depression

Depression is an illness and when it is manifest it requires long-term homoeopathic help. Even in severe cases, homoeopathy is capable of fostering self-healing. This is important as, so often, patients feel that they have no other option but to accept antidepressants, drugs that mask the symptoms but suppress the causes of depression. However, being on antidepressants is not a reason for not seeking help from a professional homoeopath as remedies are helpful in coming off antidepressants safely and without the backlash of going 'cold turkey'. Very often depression has its roots in a hereditary disposition which always needs expert and respectful handling; finding a practitioner who engenders trust is a prerequisite to successful treatment.

3 CHILDHOOD INFECTIONS AND CONTAGIOUS DISEASES

Despite widespread vaccination childhood diseases have not disappeared. Children still contract measles, mumps, chickenpox, whooping cough and even scarlet fever though the incidence of all these (except chickenpox) is less often reported because the symptom picture of each has been altered over the last few generations by artificial immunisation; viruses, faced with strong opposition, have had to adapt. Nowadays it can be unclear whether the patient is suffering from measles, German measles or what has become known as 'slap-face', a viral condition that causes bright red cheeks and a general mild malaise. Whooping cough is frequently only evident in a child who develops a chronic croupy-sounding cough with intermittent mild fevers and colds with sore throats; such children are often erroneously diagnosed as suffering from asthma and put on inhalers which suppress the original disease and induce lifelong susceptibility to lung problems. Mumps is missed out by younger children but occurs in short epidemics in older children or late teenagers. Because of this situation, knowing how to treat childhood diseases can be extremely important. Even if you are unsure precisely of the nature of the childhood complaint, the description of the remedy picture is what is important as it will cover the disease state whatever the name of the condition. Thus **Pulsatilla** will be required in any of the above named diseases if the core symptoms of medium fever, dryness yet lacking thirst, tearfulness and clinging behaviour are present; **Belladonna** will be indicated with hot head, red face, pulsating carotid arteries, high fever, glazed eyes and cold extremities. Treating children in their acute diseases is straightforward, for the most part, if you remember that you are *not* treating a disease but a *child with a symptom picture!*

Chickenpox

Chickenpox is a viral infection that has characteristic spots that form as itchy, fluid-filled vesicles that usually cluster around the neck, the scalp and hairline and the groin though the disease can be so mild that only a few flat, red spots appear or so virulent that the whole body is covered. (Sometimes, spots can form in the mouth and vagina as well.) The spots appear in clusters and, if left alone, tend to form a crust and then dry up. If they are scratched then a crater can result which will leave pitted scarring. The fluid in the usual spots is clear or yellowish serum but sometimes the spots become inflamed and filled with pus. The infection takes 10 to 14 days to incubate and as the patient is infectious before any symptoms appear it will make little difference whether you keep other children away. If a person is susceptible to the infection then it will occur; if not then it won't. Once the spots are fully out on the surface infectivity is reduced. Older patients will suffer more severely than younger ones.

There are cases when the child becomes ill with weakness, a malaise with cold symptoms, a cough and lots of mucus. There is no evidence of spots and little more than a possible contact with other affected children to suggest that the disease might be the cause. In this case, the child's immune system is too compromised to produce the frank evidence of the spots and **Antimonium Tartaricum** should be prescribed. Give the 30th potency: one every 2 hours for 3 doses. This should bring out the spots and lead to a resolution though the symptoms of one of the other remedies below may well come up.

Rhus-tox. is the main remedy. It is characterised by spots coming out on the scalp and in the groin (though in severe cases they can be everywhere). The skin is hot and dry and the glands below the surface of the clusters might be swollen. The spots are very itchy and scratching can be irresistible. The patient is generally restless and complains of achiness in the muscles or joints or, if too young to make verbal complaints, simply fractious and petulant with obvious discomfort from being confined to bed. Use the 30 up to 3 or 4 times per day.

Pulsatilla is often needed at the beginning. There is a mild, low-grade fever with dryness of the skin, lack of thirst, tearfulness and clinginess. The rash in this remedy can be widespread and have irregularly distributed spots. It is not uncommon for a child to need **Pulsatilla** and then **Rhus-tox.** to complete the cure. If the **Pulsatilla** picture is very evident then use the 200 or 1M and follow on with **Rhus-tox.** 30.

Belladonna is sometimes needed when there is a high fever with the eruptions. The child becomes red in the face or on the ears with radiant heat of the head, pulsating arteries in the neck and glazed eyes. The eruptions are likely to be very red while this remedy is indicated which should become less aggressive after the dose. Depending on the fierceness of the fever use 200 or 1M.

Sulphur is indicated by a red rash with the spots with general heat of the body, thirst and a characteristic unkempt condition generally. You'll find the patient slumped on the sofa, lacking all energy. **Sulphur** is often needed in chickenpox when other remedies that are well indicated do not work or at the end of the disease when the patient seems not to be able to recover fully despite the fever, mucus and spots going. The 30 is usually sufficient.

Merc-sol. is usually indicated when the spots suppurate and become pustular. **Merc-sol.** covers spots full of pus that exude yellow or green matter. There is usually an unpleasant sweating and swings of temperature as well: one minute hot and the next chilly. The patient is likely to be very thirsty despite salivating copiously; there might even be dribbling onto the pillow. The breath is likely to smell foul.

Ant-crudum is only indicated if the spots are thick and crusted and look honey-coloured with a bluish tinge to the surrounding skin. The patient is likely to be disagreeable; the child can't bear to be touched or even looked at. The tongue is usually coated white. There is more than likely to be a cough that is persistent and even continues after the spots are gone. Use the 30 which you may need to repeat up to 2 or 3 times a day for a few days. If it is indicated and does nothing after a few doses then give **Sulphur** 30.

It is highly likely that after a bout of chickenpox the child patient will put on a growth spurt or make a developmental advance. This is just one reason why successfully coming through chickenpox should be a cause for being pleased.

It is not a good idea to use calamine lotion. Spots are always best left uncovered. The only time to consider using a cream is if spots are threatening to cause scars. You can get 'scar cream' from the pharmacy to deal with this problem. Nor is it a good idea to use paracetamol or Calpol. These drugs only delay the natural healing process by interfering with body chemistry. Treating chickenpox with remedies also helps prevent the likelihood of a later bout of shingles (see 'Shingles') which results from the chickenpox virus migrating to the nerve tissue in the spinal column to lie dormant,until some later stress encourages it to mature and then travel out along the nerve lines causing the severe pain characteristic of this unpleasant condition. It is useful to give **Nat-mur.** tissue salts after the initial fever has gone as this helps prevent the virus migrating to the spinal column (one dose twice daily for 10 days).

Measles

Measles is an infectious viral disease that is characterised by a red rash that covers the torso and sometimes the extremities which is mildly itchy. During the incubation period, which lasts about a week to 10 days, there is a fever, cold symptoms with a runny nose and sore throat, red and watery eyes and white spots in the mouth on the inside of the cheeks (known as 'Koplick spots'). This is not so common a picture nowadays as artificial immunisation has meant that patients' symptom patterns have had to change; it is more usual to have a longer drawn-out state of malaise with no rash but headache and abdominal pains instead. Sometimes a fleeting rash will appear on the face or chest. It is rare that anything worse happens though it is important to recognise signs that might betray more serious complications. Occasionally, and because a person with measles can be susceptible to harbouring the streptococcus bacterium, persistent sore throat or kidney infection can brew trouble. In others there are the more alarming symptoms of encephalitis or meningitis. These are almost always heralded with a very high fever which requires high doses of **Belladonna** or, more rarely, **Apis**. This is one of the reasons for people who have decided not to have their children vaccinated against MMR to keep **Belladonna** is various potencies even up to the 10M. Notwithstanding the current orthodox belief that it is best to prevent measles, remember that this disease, when experienced, treated and resolved thoroughly, is part of a child's development, not least as it strengthens the immune system against later chronic ill health (especially of the syphilitic miasm).

Aconite is often called for when there is a sudden onset of high fever with dry skin, dry hacking cough (sometimes croupy), restlessness, agitation and anxiety and moaning. This is all the more indicated if the fever symptoms come on at midnight or midday.

Apis is indicated when the rash covers an extensive area and causes puffiness of the skin beneath. The eyes become puffy and inflamed. There is a croupy cough which may even remind you of whooping cough. The patient is likely to be drowsy and irritable when disturbed.

Belladonna is unmistakable if there is a high fever, red face or ears, cold extremities, glazed sometimes bloodshot eyes, photophobia, drowsiness, dry cough and thirst. The peak time of **Belladonna's** fever is 3 p.m. or 3 a.m. Sometimes a child will go into delirium and say that they are seeing curious things such as animals marching across the bedroom wall or soldiers coming out of the lavatory pan. **If the child is crying with head pain (especially in the back of the head) and rolling the head into the pillow from side to side then you should be on your way to hospital,** in touch with the homoeopath and administering **Belladonna** 10M. This is the scenario for meningitis.

Bryonia is always indicated by strong thirst, fever (usually not more than 101°F. or 102°F.), dryness of the skin and irritability. The mood is anxious and cross when asked to move – all movement is worse for the patient. It is likely that a **Bryonia** patient feels uncomfortable from aches in the limbs. All this may be because the body does not have the energy to put the rash out onto the skin.

Euphrasia covers the measles type most likely to affect the eyes adversely. There are hot tears and photophobia. The nose runs with watery mucus and there is a pressure headache before the rash appears. There may be conjunctivitis as well.

Ferr-phos. is a remedy often indicated in the early stage. There is a low fever with alternating flushing and pallor of the face. The patient is sleepless, restless and feeble. They appear to be brewing a fever but don't have the strength to go into a full-blown **Belladonna** state. There is likely to be a cough with runny nose. It is of no service after the initial stages of the condition.

Gelsemium starts the infection with chilliness and shivers in the spine with a watery discharge from the nose and a sore throat. The patient appears dull and lifeless; they don't want to drink or eat and want to lie torpid on a sofa or in bed. There is often a white tongue. The voice might be hoarse and there is usually a harsh cough with a sore feeling in the chest. After **Gelsemium** the rash is likely to come out onto the skin in full.

Pulsatilla is indicated by low-grade fever, a measly rash, a lack of thirst, a dry cough in the daytime (looser at night) with a nose runny with thick, yellow or greenish mucus and watery eyes (though this symptom may take time to come out). The mood is typically weepy and clingy. There may be a headache but more likely there is an earache in the left ear and some have conjunctivitis.

Generally use the 30 or 200 depending on the severity of the symptoms unless **Belladonna** or **Apis** are called for; in which case call the homoeopath and ask for back-up. Frequency of dosage: one 30 every 2 – 3 hours till symptoms abate or one 200, wait and watch for change then repeat if the progress slows or halts. There are other remedies that cover measles but these are the most usual. However, if the sequelae (symptoms that persist or follow on after a disease) do not resolve then you must contact your practitioner. It is likely that there is need of a constitutional prescription or a dose of **Morbillinum**, a remedy made from the blood of a patient suffering from measles. Don't let this description put you off; remember there is no material substance left in a potentised homoeopathic remedy. If symptoms suddenly get worse when you thought the patient was on the road to recovery, don't waste any time: call your homoeopath. Finally, it is not unusual for measles to need a dose of **Sulphur** to clear up the last symptoms.

Mumps

Mumps is another infectious viral disease but this one affects the glands in the neck especially the parotid glands which are just below the ear and behind the jaw. In children before puberty it is usually very mild and sometimes affects only one side of the head (and *which* side is important to notice!). After puberty, mumps can affect other glands, notably the breasts, ovaries and testicles. The incubation period is two to three weeks long. It often begins with chills, headache and a low-grade fever though with some patients the first signs are of pain on consuming certain types of acidic food or drink: citrus fruit, fruit drinks, flavoured ice cream, apples, etc. (Acid foods cause the salivary glands to secrete saliva.) The swollen glands are tender to touch and the fever can climb to 102° F. or more. If, usually around the end of the first week, the patient starts to feel nauseous and then vomits and suffers abdominal pains then it is likely that there is inflammation of the pancreas, a very uncomfortable but not a threatening complication though it does need your practitioner's attention; immediately if there is a raised fever and shock-like symptoms. Occasionally meningitis or encephalitis can result. **These are both conditions that must have expert help, especially the latter, as they can leave nerve damage.** (See above under **Belladonna** in 'Measles'.) If the ovaries or testicles are affected, sterility is not by any means inevitable though treatment often takes a little longer and must be directed by the homoeopath.

Aconite is for sudden onset of symptoms: hot, dry, burning skin with chills. Not usually of any use after the swelling comes on.

Arsen-alb. is called for when the patient becomes restless, anxious and thirsty for sips of water. They are chilly but want fresh air circulating round the head; they wrap up very well and want to put the head out of the window. Motions may become loose and there could be nausea. This is one of the remedies for metastasis to the generative organs or to the pancreas. This patient suffers the worst pains at night between midnight and 2 a.m.

Belladonna covers the fever: hot head, red face and ears, cold extremities, glazed eyes and thirst with a temperature of 101°–104° F. or more. It is common these days to need high potencies of **Belladonna** so use a 200 to start with and only move up to a 1M if there is little or no response. (It is occasionally called for when pancreatitis comes on.)

Occasionally, **Calc-c.** is indicated in cases where you think you can see **Belladonna** but this doesn't do anything. **Calc-c.** is mostly a right-sided remedy but it also covers metastasis to the other glands. You are most likely to need expert help if this situation arises.

Jaborandi or **Pilocarpine** as it is sometimes known, is often given as a first remedy, regardless of the symptom picture as a whole, simply because of its affinity for this particular condition. It is, however, indicated in cases when profuse salivation and excessive sweating (especially at night) are prominent. This is easily confused with **Merc-sol.** though there is less thirst in **Jaborandi** and the alternation of heat and chills is not nearly so marked. The foulness of body smells is not apparent either. The area of the swollen glands and even the face is likely to be quite flushed. The patient might complain of feeling eye strain which can lead to light-headedness and nausea. This is a remedy for metastasis of the mumps from the parotids to the breasts and the generative organs.

Lycopodium is called for when the mumps start on the right and move to the left and are accompanied by flatulence and a very snuffly nose.

In **Merc-sol.** the patient see-saws between hot and chilly especially at night when heat is followed by profuse sweats. There is a strong thirst for cold water (sometimes a craving for ice). The breath smells foul and there is a lot of salivation even enough to cause dribbling. This makes **Merc-sol.** the most painful mumps remedy as the swollen glands work overtime. **Merc-sol.** is mostly a right-sided remedy so might be indicated in a case of swelling of the right parotid gland. However, occasionally one of the other mercury remedies might be needed. **Merc-iod-flav.** is also chiefly right-sided but is accompanied by characteristic light-headedness (particularly on rising), fullness and windiness of the abdomen and a tongue that has a thick yellow film at the back. **Merc-iod-rub.** is left-sided (though pains and swelling can shift over to the right) and covers a stiff neck (hard to turn to the left), rheumatic pains in the muscles and dark red tonsils in the throat. Both remedies have a thirst and foul breath, chills and heat.

Pulsatilla is useful in cases when there is the usual picture of helplessness and tearfulness with clinginess and no thirst despite the dryness. This might come at the beginning before the glands swell; if given for this picture alone then it will call for another remedy shortly after to deal with the mumps symptoms. However, **Pulsatilla** is also indicated when other glands such as the breasts (in boys as well as girls) and generative organs are affected. There is almost always likely to be the typical lack of thirst and intolerance to stuffy atmospheres.

Rhus-tox. is sometimes needed when the mumps are mainly on the left side and there is a sore throat with aching and stiffness in the limbs with restlessness and a need to keep moving about gently. The patient wants to stretch the limbs to prevent the stiffness.

Use the 30 or 200 potencies depending on the severity of the symptoms. The 30 can be given up to 4 times a day while the 200 might be needed twice in a day. If a **Belladonna** fever comes on then prescribe the 200 or 1M but call the homoeopath if the remedy fails to achieve a lowering of the temperature within 4 hours.

Rubella or German Measles

Rubella is a mild, infectious viral disease characterised by a body rash and joint pains. The incubation period is between 2 and 3 weeks and results in a mild malaise, swollen neck glands (in the nape of the neck, very often) and red discoloration of the throat. Joint pains usually follow with a rash that starts on the head and works down the body. Sometimes the symptoms are mild enough to be missed while others might have it so severely that glandular fever is suspected. Indeed, it is not unlikely that one of the results of artificially immunising against Rubella is to make some people more susceptible to the more serious condition. The reason for orthodox medicine's attempt to eradicate Rubella by vaccination is that if a woman contracts the disease within the first three months of pregnancy there is a considerable risk of having a handicapped child. For those who choose not to opt for the vaccine programme it behoves them to consider this aspect of Rubella. It is a subject worth talking over with your practitioner if you have never had the disease and wish to become pregnant or if you have a daughter who needs to be fully informed. Some homoeopaths might recommend the jab while others, calling on the experience of previous generations of practitioners, would recommend homoeopathic prophylaxis.

Pulsatilla is the most usual remedy. There are the typical characteristics of this remedy: mild fever, lack of thirst, weakness, tearfulness and clinginess. The joint pains are most likely transient and wandering from one part of the body to another. In older boys and young men the tearfulness may not be there; what you will see is a state of feeling sorry for himself, grumpy but easily mollified when help is offered. Usually the patient will respond quickly to a dose of the 200th potency.

Belladonna is sometimes needed if the fever is a bit high (101–102°F.) and the face and neck are red.

Rhus-tox. is needed when the rash is markedly accompanied by joint pains with stiffness and a need to keep moving about restlessly and stretching. The pains of **Rhus-tox.** wander far less than those of **Pulsatilla**.

Whooping Cough

Whooping cough is sometimes referred to as pertussis (the 'P' part of the DPT inoculation). It is a highly infectious bacterial disease that causes a cough characterised by a 'whoop' sounding intake of breath at the end of every spasm of coughing. Despite the fact that pertussis has been immunised against since the 1940s the disease has never been threatened with eradication though its behaviour has been altered. Local attacks (rather than widespread epidemics) have been common since the 1980s and sometimes are misdiag-nosed as asthma attacks as the most prominent symptom is the cough with compromised breathing. This is regarded by most homoeopaths as one of the long-term results of artificial immunisation and usually successfully treated as such.

The symptoms of straightforward whooping cough include an accumu-lation of increasingly thick, sticky mucus in the throat which leads to progressively more severe coughing fits. Sometimes the symptoms amount to no more than one might have in a heavy cold but if it is a bad case then it is important to monitor progress very carefully as the cough can be so violent as to cause damage to the lungs. It can also cause hernia in the navel or even bowel prolapse in the very young. The chief long-term side effect is bronchiectasis which is a condition in which the lung tubes are damaged with the result that more mucus secretion is created and inflammation happens more readily thus predisposing the patient to chest infection and pneumonia.

The incubation period of whooping cough is around 7 to 10 days. There could be sneezing and 'flu-like symptoms followed by listlessness, loss of appetite and watery eyes; otitis media is a common concomitant. (Frequent bouts of middle ear infection that lead to 'glue ear' and catarrhal deafness are among the common results of the pertussin vaccine.) There are many remedies for the cough of whooping cough and it is not unusual for a patient to need a sequence of more than two of them. The most usual ones include: **Ant-tart., Bryonia, Carbo-veg., Coccus Cacti, Corallium Rubrum, Cuprum, Drosera, Ipecac., Lycopodium, Nux Vomica, Phosphorus** and **Spongia.** (See the section on 'Coughs' on pages 167–73 for a description of each.) Fever is not particularly a feature of whooping cough but it is worth considering **Belladonna** if there is a rise in temperature with red face and radiant heat from the head and the other characteristics of the **Belladonna** cough. Caring for a person with whooping cough or a cough with this disease's characteristics requires patient observation; remedy pictures can change unexpectedly and it is best to have expert help if the coughing persists. Plenty of fluids are important and steam inhalations can be helpful. (It is not a good idea to use eucalyptus or any other inhalant nor any vapour rub as they antidote remedies.) Hard coughing can result in bloodshot eyes, bringing up blood with the sputum and umbilical hernia. **If the child persistently cries after coughing or a sudden fever develops then you must seek expert help.** Even if you recognise the **Belladonna** picture and give this remedy, don't hesitate to call your practitioner as well. Complications can include pneumothorax (collapsed lung) **which needs emergency hospital treatment** (see page 179), pleurisy (inflammation of the lining of the lung) or pneumonia.

Slap Face

This is a new addition to the list of childhood complaints but it is a mild one. It is characterised by reddened cheeks and slight malaise. Many parents don't even notice it and send their children off to school with it. Very often nothing needs to be done about it except to make sure that the patient has plenty of refreshing sleep and keeps up fluid intake. Sometimes, if there is a slightly raised temperature as well, it is worth giving a dose of **Belladonna** 30. If you suspect slap face and there are joint pains, call your homoeopath for help.

Impetigo

Impetigo is an outbreak of itchy, pus-filled spots on the skin. It is associated with staphylococcus or streptococcus bacteria though the underlying cause lies within the patient's immune system. Though impetigo is regarded as a vicious scourge and highly infectious, it is worth looking at the condition from the homoeopathic viewpoint: it is an opportunity for the immune system to detoxify the body. Those who suffer its symptoms and recover by natural means, rather than through suppression by antibiotics, tend never to have the problem again and afterwards go through a period of positive development. This falls in line with the results of any of the other common childhood complaints. The main problem is that to allow the patient to go through the process can require far longer than parents and school curricula are prepared to give. The usual time needed is anything up to 2 weeks though many cases are cleared up on appropriately chosen remedies within 7 – 10 days. However, there are cases that require expert homoeopathic assistance because the patient's body has more to process than simply the outward manifestation of spots; such cases can go on for 4 or 5 weeks and should not be interfered with by suppressive treatment. It is a condition that 'teaches' the system to recognise when to employ the 'home guard' of lymphocytes. One likely benefit is that the patient will not suffer nearly so much from teenage acne.

Impetigo does not always appear on the skin in the same way. There are different types of spots with different coloured matter that exudes. The differences are what make it possible to choose the appropriate remedy. Usually the spots are on the face, arms or legs but they can appear anywhere. They may come up as blisters or they may be red pimples. The spots usually come with itching that is more or less severe. Scratching always causes the problem to spread and it can do so extremely quickly. The most likely site of origin is a small cut, an insect bite that will not heal, a sore under the nose from runny mucus or a lesion in a patch of eczema. Sometimes the eruptions become septic-looking; this does not necessarily mean that the remedies are not working! What is happening is that the patient has a lot of toxicity to process. Contrary to popular belief, not everyone is susceptible to impetigo though those who produce it are likely to be 'doing' the disease with such energy that it triggers off susceptibility in those who need to go through the same thing. Proximity to someone who is affected can energetically spark off the same susceptibility in another person ready to do the same process. (This is true of all the childhood diseases.)

The main remedies for impetigo are:

Antimonium Crudum covers pimples and spots that erupt on dry skin with burning and itching. The surrounding skin looks scaly or rough and as if the patient is rather unclean. The spots develop by producing either a white head or, more usually, a thick crust of honey-coloured scab with a red surround. If it is on the face sores and cracks are likely to appear at the corners of the mouth. The itching is < from warmth and < night time in bed. The spots bleed from scratching. The patient is likely to be irritable, sullen and fretful. The tongue might be white-coated especially if they have a poor appetite (though **Ant-crud.** can cover the opposite, a ravening appetite). Unless the patient has a particularly strong constitution or is ultra-sensitive to remedies, it is worth using high potencies early on. Use the 200 twice daily and tell the homoeopath what you are doing. If this doesn't hold then use 1M at the same dosage. Sometimes it is a good idea to discuss the use of **Staphylococcus** 200 with your practitioner. This is a remedy made from the bug itself and it is invaluable if given once daily along with **Ant-crud.** in difficult cases.

Graphites is needed by those who have dry, rough skin that has begun to look unhealthy and that has scabby eruptions which ooze matter that looks like semi-runny honey. On the edges of the crusts the exudate dries to leave a little deposit of what looks like granulated brown sugar. It is commonly seen around the mouth. The eruptions are very slow to heal and they are worse in folds of skin. It is likely that the glands of the neck or under the jaw will be swollen. The patient is chilly, miserable and weeps at any little thing. Start off with the 30 3 times a day but consult the homoeopath if it does nothing despite indications.

Merc-sol. covers moist eruptions especially on the scalp which have a yellowish look and that tend to bleed on scratching. The pus might smell rank and the patient is likely to produce unpleasant sweat with alternation of chills and heat especially at night. The breath will smell and there will be a strong thirst for cold water. Glands around the head may be swollen. Use the 30 3 times a day.

Mezereum is not a usual first-aid remedy but is mentioned here as it is sometimes needed in impetigo. Around the eruptions there is deep redness of the skin. The spots leak fluid that burns the surrounding flesh making it sore. Itching is intolerable especially at night or after contact with water. Thick crusts form and the gluey moisture beneath can be white or pale before oozing out onto the skin. Can easily be mistaken for an **Ant-crud**. case. Use the 30 3 times a day.

Viola Tricolor (the common pansy) covers eruptions on the face that itch furiously and burn and have thick, sticky yellow pus. The skin on the face feels less elastic, more tense. The face might feel hot. The patient is likely to want to pass more water than usual and the urine will smell unpleasant. Use the 30 3 times a day.

There are other remedies so ask your practitioner's guidance if remedies that seem indicated do not work. It is not at all uncommon for a homoeopath to have to prescribe **Sulphur, Psorinum, Syphilinum** or **Medorrhinum** (depending on symptoms) in order for indicated remedies to finish their work. This reflects the depth of the condition and its vital importance in the scheme of the body's defence mechanisms.

Hand, Foot and Mouth

This is another skin condition that is unpleasant. It is a bacterial condition which is similar to impetigo though less fearsomely speedy. It manifests as eruptions on the extremities and sometimes around the mouth as well. The most commonly needed remedy for it is **Merc-sol.** though **Graphites** runs it a close second. See the description of these remedies above under 'Impetigo'. It is important to let the homoeopath know about this condition as it is not always susceptible to first-aid treatment and it is a condition that might have implications on the general constitution. Use the chosen remedy in the 30th potency 3 times a day. If no better within 48 hours then call the homoeopath.

Molluscum Contagiosum

Molluscum are small, lentil-sized, pink warts that erupt in clusters in favoured areas such as the groin, the buttocks and under the arms and down the sides of the chest. Some doctors want to lance the warts though, fortunately, most will not feel it necessary to interfere with them. It is officially an infection of the skin caused by a pox virus; under the microscope the virus looks very similar to smallpox. This is important because it means, in homoeopathic terms, that the body is attempting to recognise what to do about pox infections in general. If it has dealt satisfactorily with one form of the pox, the body is likely to be able to deal with others by dint of its biological memory. (It is significant that smallpox also has a predilection for similar sites for eruption; even if smallpox has been officially eradicated, the body's inherited memory has not forgotten this terrible disease.) So this is another condition that parents should be grateful for though it is one that it is really important to report to the homoeopath. This is because the hereditary implications call for constitutional treatment. The main remedies for molluscum include **Thuja, Medorrhinum** and **Carcinosin** all of which should be prescribed in the context of the homoeopath's long-term treatment. However, there are occasions when molluscum can become complicated by impetigo. It is likely that the patient would need remedies such as **Antimonium Crudum, Lachesis, Staphylococcus** and even **Syphilinum** because such a situation would mean that the patient is going through a lot of negative energy clearing.

Head Lice

Lice and their nits are a universal nuisance yet only those who are susceptible will support them. Though many children appear to be susceptible at the same time, this is because they have constitutions that need to go through similar development patterns and these include being prone to parasites; an affected child, just by being in close proximity, can awaken another child's latent psoric susceptibility. For this reason it is necessary to have constitutional treatment as well as using well-tried domestic means of solving the lice problem. Once a child has been treated appropriately with internal medicines that reflect the developing energy state, it is unlikely that they will suffer lice again. It is not enough to use aromatherapy oils, nit combs and hair conditioners. These will kill off the parasites in situ but do nothing about the constitution that supports them. While there are several remedies that have a reputation for dealing with the problem (**Staphysagria, Lycopodium, Sulphur**), it is sensible to consult the homoeopath as the indicated remedy might be one that has constitutional effects that should fit into the context of long-term treatment. Practical treatment is relatively easy: cut the hair as short as is reasonable, massage olive oil mixed with a drop of lavender oil into the scalp and wrap the head in a hot towel for three quarters of an hour; wash the oil out thoroughly and then apply plenty of conditioner before nit combing; rinse out the conditioner and dry the hair. Repeat the process each day for 3 days. Many object to cutting the hair but bear in mind that lice can only live in a narrow band of temperature and cutting will make their habitat a chilly place. The homoeopath may recommend the use of other oils but beware of tea tree as this, when massaged into the scalp, can undermine the efficacy of remedies and will often antidote them outright. It is likely that the homoeopath would need to give **Psorinum** at some point in the treatment as this is a cornerstone remedy for those who support parasites. For some people the problem will occur only once but for others the lice will pay a return visit. Do not despair; the child is learning to cope with the psoric miasm and will eventually grow out of it. See the whole event as an opportunity for constitutional treatment which will contribute to the patient's full growth and development.

Thread Worms

Worms are potentially another universal nuisance. They are in the food chain all the time though most of us are able to kill them off chemically within the gut before they reach maturity. Worms like an acid system. They flourish best in a body which is fed with dairy products, sweets and excessive carbohydrates. These foods cause the body to secrete mucus, ideal for worms and candida (a yeast infection) to breed. In terms of homoeopathy worms are, paradoxically, beneficial unless they create an infestation. Worms feed on the excessive mucus and make the environment less conducive for candida to thrive. However, the host is more than likely struggling with an addiction to the very foods that are at the root of the problem. The first practical thing to do for anyone with worms is to cut out those foods which allow the worms to proliferate: cut out milk, cheese, cakes, buns, biscuits, all but the minimum of bread and pasta and all sweets. Meals should be made up of plenty of vegetables, either raw or cooked, protein such as light meats and fish, and carbohydrates such as rice or corn that will not encourage acidity. Hot water with a squeeze of lemon juice twice a day is very cleansing; lemon and lime juice turn to alkali when they reach the stomach. Put the patient on a course of **Nat-phos** tissue salts as this redresses the acid-alkali imbalance.

The life cycle of worms is short; they have a 4 – 6 week cycle and they are often influenced in their behaviour by the cycles of the moon though this cannot be relied on for prescribing. The first sign is usually anal itching; this happens more at night when the patient is likely to scratch in sleep. This is ideal for the worms as it causes a sequence of events to occur: the female lays her eggs on the anus and in the process causes the prickly itching; then the nose is caused to itch which brings on scratching of the nose. The eggs, which attach to the fingers because of their sticky coat, are thus transferred to the nasal passage and thence into the body, starting a new life cycle. Some people advocate the rather drastic measure of inserting a spliced clove of garlic into the rectum as garlic is known to kill worms. The rectal membrane is quite tough but not especially designed to take raw garlic juice – though there are those who have noted the efficacy of this odd suppository. What can be effective is to take a leaf out of a reflexologist's book and rub a sliced clove over the soles of the feet. This will work well enough to cause the patient to have garlic on their breath, evidence that the chemical effects of garlic have been drawn into the system. Other people will apply copious amounts of vaseline to the anus before bed thus giving the female worm a hard time with laying her eggs. What is certain is that frequent washing of the area and frequent changing of linen and towels are sensible. If these suggestions do not work then consult the homoeopath. Prescribing will often follow a non-specific line; there are many remedies for worms but few of them have such clear worm-inspired pictures that they can be prescribed therapeutically. The exception is **Cina** which is for infestations which cause itching of the anus and then picking the nose, grinding teeth, twitching, bed-wetting and a foul temper. The face is pale and there are dark rings round the eyes. Sometimes, however, despite every effort, even remedies are ineffective except in the short term and it is then a good idea to consult a kinesiologist to carry out muscle testing to determine whether there might be a **hidden** chemical imbalance in the body or if there is a need for particular herbs. Ultimately, it is the restoration of a natural balance of chemicals in the system that will clear the body of parasites. Worms cannot live in a body that is in chemical balance.

4   FEVER AND ASSOCIATED CONDITIONS

Fever is the body's natural reaction to a number of stimuli: infection, allergic reaction, excessive exercise, excessive exposure to the sun, brain damage from injury, autoimmune disease and hormonal imbalance. In all cases the hypothalamus, the thermostat of the body, causes blood flow to concentrate more in the core of the body thus preserving more heat and slowing the cooling of blood at the surface. Raised body temperature initiates the body's defence mechanism. In the orthodox view infection by virus or bacteria can come from outside the body or inside; they are seen as predatory. From outside there are pathogens such as cold and 'flu viruses (which are legion) and viral or bacterial pneumonia. From within there are bacterial infections from harboured bugs that make their home in organs where they produce local symptoms as well as triggering more general fever when the acute phase works to a climax. (Bacterial infection of the bladder, kidneys or heart are examples.)

The alternative view is that, in the case of infection (the most usual cause of fever), the whole process is a natural method of triggering self-healing and therefore not to be suppressed without negative consequences. It is a condition that should be promoted so it can come to a natural resolution. This is because the bacteria or virus are not the *cause* of the problem. They are the *result* of a negative susceptibility in the patient; a susceptibility that means that the body has become a viable environment for the pathogens to proliferate. It is the condition of susceptibility that needs to be eliminated by the body itself. In a well-balanced whole body the ecosystem is not a viable environment for pathogens to proliferate. When the body falls out of balance it can express this in an acute way by becoming susceptible to infection and fever. What is remarkable is that it will do this in different and specific ways.

For example, there are fevers that are brought on by getting chilled in an east wind, by getting one's feet wet, through the suppression of another illness such as inflammation of the middle ear, by getting furiously angry, through suffering acute grief, from fear after a traumatic incident or from many other causes. In children there are often less obvious reasons for becoming susceptible. It is remarkably common for the very young to throw a fever because the constitution needs to teach itself how and when to use its immune system. The need to do this lies in heredity. Such diseases as otitis media, tonsillitis, bronchiolitis and bronchitis – all of which are usually accompanied by fever – are typical examples of what homoeopaths consider to be 'tubercular' fever conditions in which the system is attempting to *imitate* the chronic disease pattern of the tubercular miasm (which is virtually universal) so that it can learn how to cope with the long-term implications of inheriting this chronic disease pattern. By activating the immune system before puberty, the body is preparing itself to deal with any later pathology. Children who have had the childhood ailments and fevers are stronger, healthier individuals.

Remember, it makes little difference in the treatment of children if the fever is associated with a bacterium or a virus. We are not treating a bug or a fever; we are treating a body. *The intention behind giving a remedy chosen for its similarity to the particular fever in a potency that is superior in force to the disease, is to trigger the body's immune response to match this remedy energy and thus eliminate the underlying susceptibility.*

Always inform your homoeopath if:

- a fever persists for longer than 24 hours
- a fever continues to rise despite you giving an indicated remedy
- a fever rises above 103°F.
- a fever comes on after a wound (especially if red streaks advance towards the body). This could suggest septic fever.
- a rash appears on the body at the same time. This is a possible sign of meningitis.
- the patient complains of a severe headache (especially in the back of the head). This too is a possible sign of meningitis.
- the patient complains of headache, abdominal pains and nausea. This might suggest appendicitis.

The following is a repertory of common remedies in fevers associated with common symptoms:

1. Fever in childhood: **Acon., Bell., Cham., Coff., Ferr-phos., Gels., Puls.**
2. Fever with inflammation of the middle ear: **Bell., Calc-c., Calc-sulph., Cham., Hepar-sulph., Lyc, Merc-sol., Puls., Sil.**
3. Fever with sore throat: **Acon., Arsen-alb., Bell., Ferr-phos., Gels., Hepar-sulph., Lac-can., Lach., Lyc., Merc-sol., Merc-iod-flav., Merc-iod-rub., Phyto., Puls., Rhus-tox., Sabad.**
4. Fever with vomiting: **Arsen-alb., Bapt., Eup-perf., Ipecac., Verat-alb.**
5. Fever with teething: **Acon., Bell., Cham., Ferr-phos., Gels., Phyto., Sil.**
6. Fever with swollen glands: **Acon., Bell., Calc-c., Hepar-sulph., Lach., Lyc., Merc-iod-flav., Merc-iod-rub., Merc-sol., Phyto., Rhus-tox., Sil.**
7. Fever after head injury: **This condition must be treated in hospital!**
8. Fever with headache: **Apis, Arn., Arsen-alb., Bell., Bry., Chin., Eup-per., Lach., Nux-vom., Puls., Sabad., Sil.**
9. Fever with allergic reaction: **Apis, Bell., Puls.**
10. Fever after getting soaked: **Calc-c., Puls., Rhus-tox.**
11. Fever from overexertion: **Chin., Rhus-tox.**
12. Fever from exposure to the sun : **Acon., Arn., Bell., Glon., Puls., Verat-alb.** This condition should be treated professionally though remedies are listed in case you are on holiday and cannot get the advice.
13. Septic fever (blood poisoning): **This condition must be treated in hospital!**

Aconite: the keynotes are sudden onset, high temperature, dryness, restlessness, thirst for cold water and waves of chills that run through the body. Waves of chill and heat alternate. Patient wants to throw off the covers for relief. Eyes, nose and throat feel dry and burning. Fever is brought on by exposure to icy winds (north or east). In very high fevers there is a marked degree of fearfulness or an anguished expression. < or starts at around midnight. The patient may wake with a fever and a nightmare. Sweating can relieve the symptoms; sweat appears on uncovered parts or parts lain on. **Aconite** fever comes on with viral and bacterial infections such as 'flu, cystitis, childhood diseases, teething and otitis media. Use the 200 for high fever. If for the start of a cold use a 30 but be careful: using an **Aconite** can suppress a cold for a few days unless the match of symptoms is good. It is tempting to use **Aconite** to stop an incipient cold in its tracks. This is bad prescribing. If you are not sure whether to use **Aconite** or **Belladonna** then wait until the picture is clearer or give **Ferr-phos.** 6.

Apis: burning heat with chills on moving < in the early afternoon. Very restless; sleepy and very irritable when disturbed. The face can look puffy. Fever can be the result of anger, allergy and jealousy. Use the 30 or the 200. **If the temperature is very high and there is a severe headache with high-pitched crying or screaming you must take the patient to hospital and inform your practitioner! Give the higher potency on your way there.**

Arnica: fever felt mostly in the head; face is red. Body might be cold but the patient wants to be uncovered. Fever < after injury. Use a 200. **If there is fever with sleepiness after a head injury you must seek professional advice and take the patient to hospital!**

Arsen-alb.: fever with icy coldness and shivering. Patient is restless and anxious and has a pinched expression. Wants fresh air around the head but to be wrapped up and to have warm drinks (unless there is nausea and vomiting). See 'Gastric 'Flu'.

Baptisia: chills with soreness all over the body; muscles feel bruised and achy. Foul-smelling breath; thick, sticky mucus/saliva. Gums and tongue are sore and ulcerated. Heavy, dull and stupid expression on the face as if drunk with a dark reddish hue. Patient can appear to be deathly ill; can't sit up in bed and can't answer questions clearly. May have a gastric bug, 'flu, tonsillitis or septic fever. Use 30 but contact your practitioner as well if there is no response in 24 hours.

Belladonna: the key words are red, hot and throbbing. Red face and/or ears, throbbing carotid arteries (in the neck), hot head, glazed eyes, cool or cold extremities are the common picture (though sometimes the patient may have a pale face; nevertheless, the heat will be there). The heat can be intense enough to feel it radiating off the body. The patient is likely to be thirsty for a cold drink. If the fever is high enough

(103–104°F.) delirium may follow. There are visions of monsters or animals or bizarre scenes; shapes may appear on the walls. In some **Belladonna** fevers there is nausea and vomiting. The tonsils, neck and mesenteric glands (in the abdomen) may be swollen and painful. **Belladonna** is often called for in viral and bacterial infections, teething and fevers that have no known cause. The usual recommendation of the 30th potency is often insufficient. Depending on the intensity of the fever, use the 200 (102–103°F.) or the 1M (103–104°F.). It is not uncommon to need to use the 10M though it is always vital to contact your homoeopath for a condition that would need this potency. Give one dose of the chosen potency and wait for 2 hours. Only go up in potency if nothing has happened and you are sure that the picture is **Belladonna**. If **Belladonna** is indicated and does nothing or the patient relapses, despite several doses, then contact your practitioner. He may have to prescribe **Calc-c.** or **Tuberculinum**. If there is a delay in his responding to your call and you are worried then give a dose of **Calc-c.** 30.

Bryonia: fever with a cold. Heat in the head with reddened face and dryness with extreme thirst. Wants to be left alone and doesn't want to move at all. Wants to be at home to be ill. May have a bursting headache or migraine. Can't have the room too warm. Common in spring and autumn. Use 30.

Calc-c.: is not usually regarded as a first-aid fever remedy but it should be. Chills with sweating especially of the head or night sweats. The patient is very thirsty and shivery. The fever might come on at around 2 p.m. Use 30. This remedy is sometimes needed after **Bell.** fails; see above.

Calc-sulph.: this is not a usual first-aid remedy but is worth knowing as it is often needed in fevers associated with conjunctivitis or otitis media. **Puls.** is often mistaken for this remedy as both cover the characteristic whinging and clinginess with dirty yellow mucous and/or pus discharges. **Puls.** patients tend to elicit more sympathy from the carer than **Calc-sulph.** as the latter can be sullen.

Chamomilla: heat and chills alternate or one part feels very hot and another very cold. Does not want to be uncovered. The mood is very characteristic: nothing satisfies; they ask for this or that and then reject the request with irritation or fury. Wants to be carried around. Very ugly mood. Often accompanied by pain depending on the condition. Crops up mostly in teething and earache but can occasionally be useful in mastitis and milk fever. Use the 30 or the 200.

China: chills are followed by thirst and then fever. This is followed at night by drenching sweats. Sweats on least exertion. The patient is weak and the fluid intake needs to be closely monitored. **China** patients suffer severely from dehydration; it is worth having Dioralite, to help restore the body's salt and fluid balance, in the house for this one. Use the 30 or, in prolonged and intermittent cases, the 200.

Coffea: fever from getting overexcited or from a combination of loss of sleep and fatigue (perhaps after a long journey) or after a painful injury. Feverish when there are severe pains; weeps with the pain. It is as if the pain overexcites the nervous system causing restlessness, fever and emotional overload. Use the 30.

Eupatorium Perfoliatum: onset of the fever is marked by tremendous aching in the bones (as one gets in some types of 'flu). There may be a strong thirst and chilliness with shivering. The fever is often accompanied by headache (back of the head), nausea and sometimes vomiting. The patient is extremely weak and feels beaten and bruised especially in the back. Common in autumn. Use the 30 or 200.

Ferr-phos.: is most useful for the early stages of a fever. The patient is debilitated, sensitive and chilly. There is flushing and pallor of the face by turns. There will often be catarrh in the nose, sinuses and throat. The temperature is not as high as **Belladonna** and there is less redness. The fever may be out of the blue with no known cause or there may be a sore throat, painful ears, teething or tonsillitis. The eyes can be bloodshot. Use the 30. There is often a need to follow on with another remedy in viral and bacterial infections.

Gelsemium: first symptoms are chills up and down the back with weakness and drowsiness. This is followed with muscular soreness, headache and light-headedness. There is an absence of thirst despite the temperature. Patient might ask to be held because of the trembling;

might say that they can't see or focus well. The eyelids droop and they look almost in a stupor. The complexion is flushed but duskier than **Belladonna**. **Gels**. is needed in sore throat, 'flu, otitis media, colds, sunstroke, teething and childhood diseases. Common in spring. Use the 30.

Glonoin: fever after too long exposure to the sun. Always accompanied by a bursting, explosive headache. Heat comes with sweat and a full pulse. Nausea and vomiting may follow. The heat often feels as if it sweeps up the body from the low abdomen to the head. The **Glonoin** fever and headache is fierce and may need a 200 to resolve it though for those who are quite sensitive to remedies the 30 should be enough.

Hepar-sulph.: the fever is characterised by alternation of heat and chills with sweating. The most characteristic symptoms are that the patient is very intolerant of being disturbed, very irritable and sensitive to noise and draught. They will tell you not to bother or fuss. The slightest draught will set off shivering. The skin feels highly sensitive and even painful to touch. The fever comes on with a sore throat, tonsillitis, earache, 'flu or even in the early stages of bronchitis.

Ipecacuanha: is usually needed in conditions that have fever as part of a wider picture: whooping cough, bronchitis, gastric conditions or from becoming overheated. There is the characteristic persistent nausea which is not > from vomiting. There is a lot of salivation with the nausea and the patient is irritable and very hard to please: they want something but don't know what. The patient becomes impatient with suggestions. Children cry and even scream with these feelings. Use the 30 or 200 if symptoms are particularly severe.

Lac Caninum: the patient feels chilly inside but hot to touch. They seem to brew the fever over a few days with the temperature going up and down. Other symptoms are unsettled: soreness of the throat or swelling of glands may alternate sides, first one side and then the other, back and forth. They may wake in the night drenched in cold sweat or may wake from sleep in the morning with a high fever and sweat. A marked symptom is that they, if old enough to express it, feel that the condition is incurable and that they will not get better; wake in a state of doom and gloom or fearful. They feel weak and depressed. Of service in tonsillitis and sore throat, often severe enough to be labelled quinsy. Use the 30 or 200 depending on the severity.

Lachesis: very marked symptoms make this remedy easy to spot. Useful fever with sore throat, earaches, headache, laryngitis and tonsillitis. Pains and swelling start on the left side and move over to the right. Discoloration of the mucus membrane is purplish or dark red. The breath is foul. The patient finds it difficult to open the mouth to show the throat or tongue (and may refuse to try). There are flushes of heat up into the head and the patient can't stand pressure of clothing or bedclothes. There is hot sweat especially about the neck and head. Swallowing is painful and difficult so fluids become a problem. Use the 30. (See **'Sabadilla'**)

Lycopodium: becomes chilled and shivery at 3 – 4 p.m. The patient feels chilly with the fever which is not much over 101°F. They are drowsy and dull; unwilling to move and want to be left alone though they have an unexpressed need to know that someone is there to look after them. One foot might be cold and the other hot, an odd but telling symptom. They feel better for warm drinks and sound snuffly. Use the 30.

Merc-sol.: fever is characterised by strong sweating that makes the patient feel very uncomfortable; it is most noticeable at night. In addition there is strong thirst for cold water which is unquenchable and salivation even to the point of dribbling onto the pillow. The breath is foul and there is a metallic taste in the mouth. They complain that one moment they feel chilled to the marrow and the next, too hot for any covers; the temperature is very unstable. Useful in sore throat, tonsillitis, ear infection, colds, 'flu and childhood diseases. Use the 30 or 200.

Merc-iod-flav.: has some characteristics similar to **Merc-sol.** in the temperature variation, thirst and odour but is marked by fever with right-sided swollen glands, yellow base to the tongue, light-headedness on getting up and flatulence. Most common in tonsillitis; use the 30.

Merc-iod-rub.: similar to **Merc-sol.** but has swollen glands on the left side of the neck, stiffness so that it is painful to turn the head, rheumatic pains in the muscles and dark red mucus membranes in the throat. Most common in tonsillitis; use the 30.

Nat-mur.: temperature with chilly body especially of the chest, feet and hands; loss of appetite but strong thirst for cold water; constipation with fever. If there is susceptibility to cold sores, fever brings herpes out onto the lips. Patient is withdrawn and weak. Use 30.

Nux Vomica: burning hot to touch but can't bear not to be covered up – even moving under the covers causes chills with excessive shivering. The patient is thirsty when chilly but doesn't want drink when hot. Irritable and extremely sensitive to noise and draught. Easily confused with **Hepar-sulph.** which is more intolerant of assistance and more likely to be needed in ear and throat problems. Useful in colds and 'flu and especially useful in those who are overstressed and irritable. Use the 30.

Pulsatilla works on lower grade fevers. It won't be useful for fevers above 101°F. The patient is generally warm, weak and wimpish. They might complain of feeling too hot or chilly by turns; they want cool air circulating and feels < for stuffiness. The face is hot but pale and the hands are warm. They might complain of a tummy ache with the feeling of a lump in the stomach. There is a marked absence of thirst and this can threaten dehydration. They might appear to be thirsty for drinks other than water but this is because they are hungry and cannot be bothered to eat. The preference is often for milk which can cause a problem with excessive mucus formation. **Pulsatilla** fevers sometimes resolve when the patient vomits quantities of mucus that has been swallowed. Do try and get the patient to drink water otherwise there will be a need for Dioralite to restore the electrolyte balance. It is not unusual for a patient to alternate between a **Belladonna** and **Pulsatilla** state. This is confusing and may require you to give first one and then the other several times. When the fever goes up beyond 101°F. give **Belladonna**; when the fever comes down and the patient feels weepy and clingy then give the **Pulsatilla**. If this see-saw persists for more than 24 hours call your practitioner; a dose of **Calc-c.** or the use of higher potencies may be needed. If the fever is clearly **Pulsatilla** then start with a 30 but expect to go up in potency. If you have to alternate with **Belladonna** then use 200. Useful in sore throat, otitis media, 'flu, colds and childhood illnesses.

Pyrogen: high fever with aching, soreness in all the limbs. Chill starts between the shoulder blades and spreads all over; patient can't get warm. Heat and sweats follow while the temperature keeps rising. The face is dusky red and the expression is like a drunk person. The fever can be high enough to bring on delirium. The breath smells foul. **Pyrogen** might be needed in tonsillitis or 'flu. **It is also one of the most important remedies for septic fever which is very serious and must be treated in hospital and by a professional.** In ordinary circumstances use the 30 or 200.

Rhus-tox. covers fever with alternating heat and chills. The keynote symptoms are sore muscles, aching limbs and restlessness. The throat glands might be up. The patient can't bear to be uncovered as this brings on chilly shivers that make the stiffness and aching much worse. They want to stretch and yawn but this brings on the chills again. Often needed in sore throat, tonsillitis and 'flu. Common in autumn and winter. Use the 30 unless the symptoms are severe (200). (Can be confused with **Merc-sol.** but it does not have the foul odour, unpleasant sweats or thirst symptoms.)

Sabadilla: this remedy is useful in sore throat and tonsillitis and is easily confused with **Lachesis** (see above). The marked difference with **Lachesis** is that **Sabadilla** wants warm drinks. It also is > warmth generally. Feels wretched and that the disease is really dangerous. Use the 30.

Silica: the fever is not usually especially high though there is burning heat of the body. The patient is very sensitive to cold air and easily becomes shivery which makes them irritable and feel like crying. Sweat breaks out as soon as they fall asleep. Silica can be confused with **Belladonna** (both have red faces) and **Hepar-sulph.** which is even more irritable. **Silica** gives the impression of being less robust constitutionally.

Verat-alb.: marked external coldness with internal heat. The patient is prostrated with exhaustion, extremely thirsty for cold water and prone to sweating on the face; it stands out in beads on the forehead. It is often called for in gastric fevers when there is diarrhoea, nausea and vomiting. Every drop of water drunk is purged or vomited. This condition can leave the patient seriously depleted of fluids; it is important to call the practitioner for the best advice about follow-up treatment. A few days-worth of Dioralite is likely to be needed. (**Phos-ac.** 30 is often a useful follow-on remedy.)

The Common Cold

Most people prefer to treat a cold with decongestants and over-the-counter preparations. This is usually to avoid missing school or work; just to keep going. Even those who are alternatively minded will reach for **Aconite** to stave off the dripping nose, blocked up ears and the feverishness. A cold is the body's way of clearing out rubbish from the lymphatic system; it is good housekeeping. Sooner or later a suppressed cold will catch up with the patient. If it has been suppressed for long enough the result will be that much more severe, even to the point of causing bronchitis or pneumonia in those with a chesty susceptibility. It is not wise to dose up with **Aconite** unless the symptom picture is appropriate (see **Acon.** in the fever section on pages 90–91). Some people, especially those associated with teaching, are naturally able to stave off developing a cold until the first days of the holiday. This is great for the institution they work for but miserable for the patient. Things are always made worse if the symptoms are then suppressed at a time when they do have the space to 'do' the cold properly. A healthy body will always want to express a cold in terms of nose, sinuses and throat. If the ears and chest are involved then there is greater need for the condition in the first place as a clearing-out process. If a cough follows then it is advisable to be in touch with the practitioner who will guide you through what is necessarily a series of remedy pictures. After the process is cleared, the patient should feel better energy than before it began.

There are quite a few remedies for colds. Cross-reference them with the fever section above if there is an obvious rise in temperature.

Aconite: (see above) colds caused by being out in a cold, dry wind. Sudden onset.

Allium Cepa: lots of sneezing (< walking into a hot room) with copious amounts of hot, watery mucus which makes the nose and top lip sore. The eyes are light sensitive and watery. The patient is hot and thirsty and wants fresh air. The throat is likely to be tickly and sore. And there is a cough which tears the throat. Headaches come on with the catarrh and feel worse in a hot room (like **Puls.**). There is sometimes a severe aching pain in the nape of the neck. Colds brought on in cold, damp weather. Use the 30.

Arg-nit.: flowing white nasal mucus with violent itching (has to keep rubbing the nose) and watery eyes which look red and swollen. Headache over the eyes with inability to think or function at work (patient presses into the forehead with hands). Very weary; has to lie down. Sense of smell is gone. Use 30; may have to repeat it several times for a couple of days.

Arsen-alb.: (see above) nose drips with fluent, watery mucus which tends to burn the inside of the nose and top lip which gets red and sore. Raw burning in the naso-pharyngeal area, where the back of the nose joins the throat. Paroxysms of sneezing with a feeling of blocked up sinuses. Sneezing < from going into a cooler temperature. The throat is often sore and dry and there is a need to moisten the mouth with frequent sips of cold water. Use 30.

Arsen-iod.: this is not a usual first-aid remedy except in hay fever. It is worth mentioning that it is very similar indeed to **Arsen-alb.** except that the person tends to be generally warm rather than chilly. Use 30.

Arum Triph.: Very stuffed up nose with so much blockage that it is impossible to breathe through the nostrils which are raw and might bleed from the patient trying to clear them manually or by blowing too hard. The mucus from the nose is often blood-streaked. Lips are dry, swollen and cracked and tend to bleed. The voice often becomes hoarse and there is a lot of mucus to clear from the throat.

Belladonna: (see above in 'Fever')

Bryonia: very dry nose, mouth and throat with sneezing that brings on mucus with shooting and aching pains in the forehead. There is a strong thirst for water. The lips are dry, parched and cracked. Eyelids are sore, red and swollen. Symptoms travel downwards; colds that threaten to go onto the chest. (See 'Cough' section.) This is the patient who is often described as 'a bear with a sore head' – very grumpy and intolerant of being disturbed; might well be anxious about work while feeling ill. Use 30.

Calc-c.: lots of sneezing and watery mucus with heat in the head, stiff neck, post-nasal drip that runs down the back of the throat and a pain at the root of the nose from obstruction of sinuses. Lies awake and worries that things might not get done: a usual condition that is exaggerated during the cold. The patient may not want to give in to the cold. Use 30.

Calc-sulph.: thick yellow mucus that is lumpy and that blocks up the sinuses; wiping the nose makes it sore. The right nostril discharges mucus in the day with dryness in the left; vice versa at night. The patient is likely to complain and whinge, feeling very put out by the condition. They have little energy and tend to lie around moaning and feeling negative. Use 30.

Camphor: this is not a usual first-aid remedy but is included here as it is a very useful remedy for old people who, caught by a sudden change of weather, start symptoms of a cold that might threaten worse symptoms. The patient feels the cold acutely and has cold skin and yet does not want to be wrapped up warmly. There is frequent sneezing and watery mucus and the face looks pinched and tired. Use 30.

Dulcamara: summer colds when the nose gets stuffed up with no flow of mucus. The voice goes hoarse and the cold may be accompanied by diarrhoea. Use 30.

Eupatorium-perf.: see above in 'Fever'.

Euphrasia: profuse watery mucus by day, stops at night and leaves the patient blocked up. The eyes feel sore from the acrid tears that flow during the cold. There is a bursting headache, light sensitivity and there is frequent yawning. Use 30.

Ferr-phos.: for the initial stages of a cold when the patient is chilly and pale with easy flushing of the face and a frontal headache. There is sometimes a nosebleed as well. Use 30.

Hepar-sulph.: see above in 'Fever'.

Kali-bich.: useful in the second stage of a cold when the mucus thickens up and is yellow or greenish, sticky and very difficult to shift. There are sinus pains in the forehead, hoarseness of the voice and pressure and tightness at the root of the nose. Use 30.

Kali-iod.: this is not a first-aid remedy but it is worth knowing that if you have cold bland mucus with a swollen, red nose and sometimes a mouth ulcer with a white base then your practitioner is likely to supply this in the 30.

Kali-mur.: this is a remedy for the later stages of a cold. Thick, white or grey mucus with blocked ears and hoarseness of voice. Use 30.

Kali-sulph.: last stages of a cold when thick, yellow mucus blocks the nose and spoils the sense of smell; spouses are likely to complain of the snoring. The ears are blocked and the eyes may discharge bland yellow matter. The mucous membranes of the nose feel swollen. The patient's general energy is likely to be feeble. Use 30.

Lycopodium: very snuffly breathing with sneezing and thick, yellow or green mucus though the pharynx is dry. There is a frontal headache. Has to breathe through the mouth; snoring at night. The patient is likely to be flatulent and bloated and, though hungry, inclined to leave meals unfinished. Use 30.

Merc-sol.: (See above in 'Fever'.) The remedy to consider for 'rising colds': symptoms that start in the larynx or chest and that travel up to the nose and sinuses.

Nat-mur.: thick mucus like white of egg with aching in the cheekbones. The eyes feel dry and puffy, can be sore and red; sometimes watery. Tickling and wriggling sensation in the nostril (< R) with profuse sneezing. There is loss of sense of smell and taste. Very thirsty for cold water and inclined to snack on salty things. If the patient is prone to cold sores then they are likely to have them during a cold (see 'Cold Sores'). They also feel emotionally withdrawn and might be tearful. Use 30.

Nux-vom.: starts with dry and blocked up nose with irritability and a heavy head. Progresses to sneezing early in the morning and fluent watery mucus, little thirst, raw pharynx and more irritability. By the evening, there is heat in the face with more runny mucus unless they go outside when the nose goes dry. Goes to bed feeling morose and frustrated and then has a restless night. Cold may have come on from being caught in a cold dry wind (or in cold air conditioning). This remedy is very useful if you have got into a muddle with over-prescribing; if you can no longer see what to do and you have given lots of other remedies then give a single dose of **Nux-vom.** and wait – usually it will sort out the confusion and complete the cure or it will bring out the symptoms of another remedy. Use 30.

Phosphorus: feels weak, sleepy and stuffed up in the head. Can't make any effort. Runny mucus which can be clear or coloured causes much blowing of the nose which results in bloody streaks on the handkerchief. Face can be flushed and pale by turns. Thirsty for cold drinks; may want ice. Not hungry: don't try and feed this patient; it will take them much longer to get better. Likes to be petted and needs company. Use 30.

Pulsatilla: one of the most common and useful remedies for colds. Can have all sorts of symptoms that keep changing. The mucus might be fluid or thick; might be clear, yellow or green. Mucus is always < in the morning and evening. Feels << for being in a hot and stuffy atmosphere. Frontal headache with feeling muddled and unable to think clearly. There is a strong tendency to be tearful in children and women; a man might be described as 'feeling sorry for himself'. Has a dry mouth but is not thirsty. Use 30 or 200 if 30 does not complete the cure.

Rhus-tox.: this is the cold with aching and stiffness in muscles and joints that are > from moving about. The patient is restless and can't get comfortable. There is a lot of sneezing and mucus and the throat glands might be swollen and tender. The origin of the cold might be from getting wet or from sitting on damp ground. Use 30.

Sepia: this remedy might come up after initial doses of **Nux-vom., Nat-mur.** or **Puls. Sepia** follows well after any of these. There is thick yellow or green mucus from nose and throat with dry blockage of the sinuses. Patient feels fed up, dragged down and is likely to be unguarded about comments on the family. It is not uncommon for this remedy to be needed if a cold is on at the same time as a period. If so, there is every chance that there will be a back ache in the sacrum. Use 30 or 200 depending on the severity of the symptoms.

Silica: alternating of dryness and fluent clear mucus. Soreness in the nose with blockage and sneezing especially in cold air. The ears feel blocked up and itchy and they may 'pop'. May be chilly but go out without much clothing and then get worse or feverish. Is often useful at the end of a cold to help clear up catarrh especially if the ears are blocked. Use the 30 or 200. There is a very good combined remedy: **Kali-mur. + Silica** which is specifically noted for clearing the eustachian tubes. (Use this in 12x up to 4 times a day or 30 twice a day.)

Sulphur: lots of mucus which feels hot and burns the nostrils so that they are sore. Blows out blood-streaked mucus. Is generally warm and > for fresh air. Wants lots of water to drink though might be thirsty and forget to drink. Might have a very unkempt appearance and blotchy complexion. The room is likely to smell stale and rather unpleasant. Sometimes the cold is accompanied by frequent loose motions. Can't be bothered mentality; slumps on a sofa and watches television and seems to expect to be waited on. Very useful if other remedies have done nothing because the patient's energy cannot respond. Use 30.

Otitis Media or Inflammation of the Middle Ear

This is a common problem for young children and one that worries parents because of the degree of pain that it often causes and because of the threat of a burst eardrum. Unfortunately, antibiotics have a very good record in the prevention of pain and damage to the drum which means that there is little incentive in treating this condition with homoeopathic remedies. This is a pity as remedies are far superior to antibiotics, do not suppress anything and resolve the problem so that it does not recur. Furthermore, good practice can ensure that there is a minimum of pain and that the eardrum, even if it does burst, heals with no damage to the tissue or loss of hearing. Herein lies a caveat. It is a good idea to treat this condition with the advice of your practitioner unless you are very familiar with the remedies and with the possible problems that can arise. There are not that many remedies to know about in an acute attack but they are often best given in 200. Bear in mind that otitis media might not be the only problem going on; it is not uncommon for it to be associated with fever, teething, a cold or as a long-term chronic result of the DPT (diphtheria, pertussis and tetanus) vaccine though this certainly needs professional experience to treat. When checking for signs, do not poke anything down the ears; handle the head gently because there might be tender swollen glands around the neck. It is a small thing, but warm your hands first; if the patient needs **Hepar-sulph.** they are likely to react angrily to cold fingers. Always ascertain whether it is the right or the left ear that is suffering as this may help in the selection of the appropriate remedy. Unless the ear is actually exuding matter, it can be soothing to drop warm oil into the ear; use verbascum oil from the pharmacy if you have it, or olive oil. If in any doubt then ask for professional advice on this. **If the mastoid process, the bony area behind the ear, is inflamed, red and hot and painful to touch then you must consult your practitioner at once!** (This is likely to be mastoiditis and needs swift and expert treatment; the main remedy is **Capsicum** but it, or any other remedy, should be administered and monitored by the homoeopath who may well want to keep your doctor informed or send the patient to hospital.)

Aconite: sudden onset usually at night with the worst symptoms around midnight. External ear is red and hot and the opening may look inflamed. Anxious, sensitive and restless. Give a 200.

Belladonna: otitis usually with fever. The outer ear is red and hot; the inner opening is inflamed and the pain is both in and around the ear. There can be shooting or tearing pains. The right ear is usually the one affected. Wants to avoid eating as chewing < pains. Otitis with teething. (See 'Fever' above.) Give a 200 and call the practitioner for support.

Calc-c.: might be needed if **Belladonna** fails when there is a fever and loss of hearing and teething. See 'Fever' above.

Chamomilla: this remedy is for intolerable, unendurable sharp pains in the ear. The patient holds the ear and screams. Often associated with toothache or teething. This remedy might encourage the eardrum to split painlessly and release pus held in the Eustachian tube. It is common for the patient to fall asleep on being given the first dose and to wake up with no pain and the matter on the pillow. This is perfectly natural and normal. When the inflammation is gone, follow on with **Silica** 30 to ensure the expulsion of any further pus from the ear and then give **Calendula** 30 (twice per day for 2 days) in order to repair the drum. This will happen in complete safety.

Ferr-phos.: For the first stage of inflammation. The patient feels below par, tends to be a bit pale and flushed by turns and complains intermittently of ear pain. The pains are not as strong as with **Belladonna** or **Chamomilla**. This remedy, if given soon enough, can abort a full-blown otitis attack. If you miss it you will possibly have to deal with one or other of these other remedies. Sometimes **Silica** will need to follow on if there is deafness and popping in the ear. Use 30. (**Ferr-phos.** tissue salt can be given at the first hint of ear symptoms if the problem is recurrent; this sometimes is sufficient.)

Hepar-sulph.: can almost rival **Chamomilla** for pain but **Hepar-sulph.:** is not likely to ask for help. The patient is chilly, sensitive to noise and draught, extremely irritable and doesn't want to be touched or fussed. Check for swollen glands in the neck. This is usually a right-sided remedy. Use 30 or 100.

Merc-sol.: a right-sided remedy that is sometimes accompanied by its characteristic symptoms of foul breath, alternating extremes of temperature, strong thirst for cold water and excessive salivation. If there is any muck from the ear it might be yellow/green and will smell foul. The pains are < at night. Glands are very likely to be swollen around the ear; check in the mouth to see if the tonsils are swollen. Use 30 unless you know that 200 of this remedy works better on your family.

Pulsatilla: is chiefly left-sided though it can fool you. There is a sensation of a blocked ear with aching and sharp pains though not as excruciating as **Chamomilla**. There is heat and redness and sometimes a sensation of crawling. The patient may say that there is pressure on the ear. They will be tearful and pathetic and wanting help. Give the 200 and follow it with **Silica** 30. Sometimes a dose of **Pulsatilla** will speed up the whole process and bring on a **Chamomilla** picture; be ready to give this when you see it but don't give it unless the child has changed from being tearful and clingy to demanding and impatient; **Chamomilla** tends to antidote **Pulsatilla!**

Silica: itching and soreness of the inner ear so that they want to bore finger into ear or press into it. Ear feels plugged up and might pop with yawning. Generally lacking in energy, subdued and veering towards a **Pulsatilla** picture though can be uncharacteristically uncooperative. Usually a left-sided ear remedy. **Silica** often has problems that develop slowly; the patient is one who needs lots of tolerant handling. Check for heat behind the ear and for matter inside. Can be used to encourage the discharge of slow-flowing pus. Use 30.

Tonsillitis

Tonsillitis is often diagnosed as 'a throat infection', 'Strep throat' or 'viral sore throat' and treated with antibiotics. In the case of the first two, the antibiotics are more or less successful and in the third they are prescribed not for the virus but for opportunistic bacteria that thumb a lift on the situation. The presence of streptococcus is, from the homoeopathic viewpoint, irrelevant to treatment unless indicated remedies all fail to work (in which case your practitioner might choose to prescribe **Streptococcus** in potency to break the lack of reaction or because the symptoms fit the picture of this rare remedy). The tonsils are the first line of internal defence. They are an integral part of the lymphatic waste-disposal system. If tonsils swell then there is some eliminative process for which they are being used by the body. Antibiotics stop this process happening and, despite apparent success when the fever abates and the tonsils reduce in size, it is ill-advised suppressive treatment to stop them from completing their acute purpose. Repeated suppression is extremely unwise as it leads to a number of results: susceptibility to otitis media, frequent colds with swelling of other glands, asthmatic breathing, kidney infections, cystitis and glandular fever and a generally weakened immune response. Chronically swollen tonsils are now a commonplace among the younger generations and are, in the alternative view, one of many direct results of artificial immunisation against whooping cough. Acute tonsillitis, diagnosed by looking into the back of the mouth and seeing the characteristic globular swellings at the sides of the entrance to the throat, is usually quickly responsive to homoeopathic remedies unless there is a long family history of chronic glandular and chest conditions. Chronically swollen tonsils should be treated by a professional homoeopath because prescribing in such cases takes experience in knowing how hereditary disease patterns (miasms) are expressed in a variety of different ways by individuals. Children of any age can develop the symptoms. You may not realise that the tonsils are swollen in the very young; the first sign can be a refusal to eat and a tendency to rub the ears which might lead to you diagnosing teething. There may or may not be fever though it is common; fevers might be either high, medium or low grade. Vomiting will occur if in the throat there is a lot of mucus which is then swallowed. Sometimes there is a headache as well, a lot of saliva and bad breath; in some there is just inflammation of the membranes of the throat. It is advisable to stop feeding any dairy products during the condition as milk and cheese cause the body to produce more mucus which raises the level of acidity in the system. Sometimes tonsillitis can be extremely severe with thickened membranes in the throat and difficulty breathing past grossly enlarged tonsils. This might well be a streptococcal infection that is known as quinsy. If you suspect this then call for professional help even if you think that you have the remedies in your kit. Quinsy requires close attention not just because of its severity but also because it is often a major opportunity to treat the patient through an underlying chronic state that has hereditary implications. (Chronic inflammation of the mucous membranes of the throat can indicate that a forebear had diphtheria badly.)

The following list is a mini-repertory of throat remedies:
- Right side: **Apis; Bell.; Hepar-sulph.; Lac-c.; Lyc.; Merc-sol.; Merc-iod-flav.; Phytolacca**
- Left side: **Lac-c.; Lach.; Merc-iod-rub.; Sabad**.
- Stinging pain: **Acon.; Apis; Bell.; Merc-sol.** (on swallowing).
- Pains like a splinter: **Apis; Hepar-sulph.; Lac-c.; Lach.; Merc-sol.; Sil.**
- Pains extending to the ear: **Calc-c.; Hepar-sulph.; Merc-sol.; Phyto.; Sulph.**
- Burning pains: **Acon.; Apis; Bell.; Calc-c.; Hepar-sulph.; Lac-c.; Lach.; Lyc.; Merc-sol.; Merc-iod-flav.; Merc-iod-rub.; Phyto.; Sulph.**
- Painless: **Bapt.**
- Feeling of suffocation: **Apis; Lach.; Phyto.**

- Sensation of constriction around throat: **Acon.; Apis** (throat pit); **Lach.; Puls.**
- Has to keep swallowing: **Bell.; Calc-c.; Hepar-sulph.; Lac-c.; Lach.; Lyc.; Merc-sol.; Sabad.**
- Impossible to swallow: **Apis; Bapt.; Lac-c.; Lach.; Lyc.; Sabad.; Sulph.**
- Hard of hearing: **Hepar-sulph.**
- On attempting to swallow fluid, drink is forced through nose: **Lac-c.; Lach.; Lyc.; Phyto.**
- Worse for thick, sticky mucus: **Apis; Bell.; Calc-c.; Merc-sol.; Merc-iod-flav.; Merc-iod-rub.; Phyto.; Sil.**
- Sensation of a hair in the throat: **Lach.; Sabad.; Sil.; Sulph.**

The following remedies are the main acute remedies that are worth keeping in the kit. Cross-reference them with those in 'Fever'.

Aconite: sudden onset especially < at midnight or midday. Fever with red throat and burning and pricking sensations which can go into the ears; has to keep swallowing at first but when throat starts to close up swallowing becomes difficult. Use 30.

Apis: inflamed, dry throat with dreadful stinging and burning pains. The membranes of the throat look swollen and puffed up as if with water. The right side of the throat is likely to be <. The patient is generally hot, dopey, restless but enervated and extremely irritable especially when disturbed. They want only cold water to soothe the throat. Compare with **Belladonna**. Use 30.

Baptisia: dark red tonsils with no pain but the patient appears to be very ill indeed and the foetid smell in the room is obvious. Use 30.

Belladonna: < the right tonsil which is bright red and hot. Other glands may also be affected. They find it hard to swallow past the obstructing tonsils. Use 200 or higher.

Calc-c.: may be needed to complete the cure begun by **Belladonna** or **Apis**. The uvula and palate also appear swollen; there is pain going into the ears on swallowing. Yellow/white ulceration appears on the tonsils. Use 30.

Ferr-phos.: swollen, raw tonsils with a climbing fever. Useful in the early stages and can abort the condition. Alternating pallor and flushing with general weakness and sensitivity. Swallowing is extremely painful. Use 30.

Hepar-sulph.: mostly a right-sided remedy though both sides can be affected. Pains are like a splinter or fishbone and the pain goes up into the ear on swallowing. Symptoms can take a while to brew; you may miss the start of this remedy but it will be evident as soon as you see irritability, less acute hearing, a desire to be left quiet and alone and a reduced appetite. Use 30, 100 or 200 depending on the severity.

Lac Caninum: though this is not a typical first-aid remedy it is worth knowing about as it is quite common in this condition. Very swollen tonsils which almost close the throat with sharp pains felt first in one side and then the other in alternation. The external throat is very sensitive to touch. The chief characteristic mental symptoms are despondency, tearfulness and a conviction that the condition is very threatening and dangerous. There can sometimes be delirium in the fever. Use 30.

Lachesis: the patient will not be able to open the mouth wide enough for you to see much though the breath is likely to be foul and the tonsils purplish or dark red. This is a left-sided remedy though pains and swelling will characteristically move from the left side to the right. Swallowing is unbearable causing much grimacing. They cannot drink anything for the pain. There is a feeling of suffocation and constriction of the throat. They will not tolerate anything near the throat such as clothes or blankets. They are very nervous and full of poisonous emotion; they may say spiteful things. Poor sleep because every time they fall asleep they wake with a lurch in a panic. Use 30 but see **Sabadilla** below.

Lycopodium: right-sided but symptoms go from right to left. Tonsils have ulcers which may exude yellowish matter. Wants to be well wrapped up and given warm drinks even though these cause pain on swallowing. Use 30.

Merc-iod-flav.: mostly right-sided though the left might follow. The base of the tongue is yellow, the glands are swollen like a string of beads down the side of the neck and the patient is light-headed on standing up from sitting or lying. They are also flatulent. Use the 30 unless you know the patient does well on 200.

Merc-iod-Rub.: the left-sided **Mercury**. Submaxillary glands are swollen, the neck is generally stiff preventing turning the head to the left and there is general muscular aching like rheumatism. The tonsil is dark red and the tongue is furred. Use the 30 unless the patient does well with 200.

Merc-sol.: foul breath, dribbling saliva and alternation of heat and chills with sweating on becoming hot which makes him feel uncomfortable. Tonsils are horribly swollen with white pus exuding from them. They can look a little like golf balls. They are very thirsty for cold water which is not quenching. Use 30 or 200 depending on severity.

Phytolacca: this is known as the 'vegetable mercury' because of its similarity to **Mercury** (see above). Pain in the right tonsil with a sensation of a hot lump in the throat. The tonsil might be rather blue-looking. They feel thoroughly weak and prostrated. There also may be muscular soreness. The breath is less smelly and the thirst is less marked than **Merc-sol.** Use 30.

Rhus-tox.: swollen tonsils with yellow matter exuding from both sides. They are very restless and anxious. After any resting they are likely to feel stiff and achy and irritable. Getting wet and chilly might have triggered the symptoms. Use 30.

Sulphur: is sometimes called for when indicated remedies do nothing. This is especially true of the mercury remedies and **Lycopodium**. Give a single dose of **Sulphur** 30 or 200 and wait. If still no change then call your practitioner.

Chest Infections

The diagnosis 'chest infection' is not precise. It is generally applied to a cough with more or less mucus in the lungs and is usually the result of not looking after a cold. However, a chest infection can lead to various other more serious conditions: bronchitis, bronchiolitis, pleurisy or even pneumonia. Bronchitis (which often affects older people) is inflammation of the main tube into the airways; bronchiolitis (which is increasingly common amongst weak-chested children) is inflammation of the smaller tubes leading into the lungs; pleurisy is inflammation of the lining sac of the lungs; pneumonia is a viral or bacterial infection of the air sacs and surrounding tissues in the lungs. Fever is associated with all of them at some point in their process. Antibiotics are the usual preferred orthodox treatment even when the associated 'causative agent' is viral because doctors are anxious to prevent opportunistic bacteria from colonising an already indisposed area. The alternative view is that the viral or bacterial element is always the result of a prior susceptibility and indisposition. What is most significant is how the body signals its distress with its individual symptom picture. Read the picture for minor chest infections by cross-referencing the 'Cough' (pages 166–73) and 'Fever' (pages 88–97) sections and the remedy pictures in part III. The main remedies that will come up are **Acon., Ant-tart., Arsen-alb., Arsen-iod., Bell., Bry., Caust., Carbo-veg., Kali-bich., Lyc., Merc-sol., Nat-mur., Nux-vom.** and **Phos.**

It is really important to recognise the symptoms indicating a serious turn in chest complaints. You should not attempt to treat anything more serious than an uncomplicated cough; for everything else you should be in touch with your practitioner. Chest infections can quickly spin off into a serious condition in those who are hereditarily susceptible, old, weak, highly stressed, depressed and poorly motivated, using recreational drugs (including nicotine) or on long-term medication. The old and the very young are particularly vulnerable. (Having said which, it is very common for those who suffer a serious chest complaint to be expressing a condition that is the outcome of long ignoring their need to stop what they are doing, slow down or change. It usually has the positive outcome of obliging them to rest and recuperate.) To tell when a minor complaint is becoming something more threatening here are some indicative signs:

- Pains in the chest become persistent especially if they are there even when not coughing.
- Sharp pains shoot through the chest area on moving about.
- The patient coughs up thicker and more purulent catarrh.

- Coughing produces blood streaked mucus.
- A fever develops especially with alternating chills and heat with intermittent sweats.
- Wheezing and rattling develop and cause difficulty with breathing (asthmatic).
- Hyperventilation (rapid breathing) and sleep apnoea (breathing stops for long periods during sleep) occur.
- The face goes blue with the effort of coughing or breathing.
- Nausea and vomiting accompany gagging with the cough.
- There is loss of appetite over a period of several days.

The most important remedies to have in the kit for those who are susceptible to chest conditions are **Aconite** 200, **Arsenicum Album** 30 and 200, **Antimonium Tartaricum** 200, **Bryonia** 30 or 200, **Carbo Vegetabilis** 30, **Cuprum** 30 or 200, **Phosphorus** 30 or 200 and **Natrum Sulphuricum** 30 or 200,. (**Nat-sulph.** is not included in the list of first-aid remedies in this book but it is very useful for thick green or green/yellow mucus that is fetched up from the lungs with pain in the lower left chest; this is like **Phos.** though **Phos.** is much thirstier and weaker while **Nat-sulph.** is heavy, sad and sluggish.) Where there is a choice regarding potency be guided by whether those in your care respond quickly enough to 30 or if they usually work well with 200. If in doubt consult your practitioner or start with 30 anyway and only go to 200 if no progress is made quickly enough and you are sure of your remedy. When dealing with threatening coughs stay in touch with your practitioner as you are their eyes and ears; teamwork can avoid the need for antibiotics and suppression.

Swollen Glands

Adenitis is the term given to swollen lymph glands. Glands occur everywhere in the body and they swell when the system needs to eliminate toxicity but cannot do it as quickly as it usually does through the bowels, bladder and skin. The swelling often accompanies a fever. The most commonly affected glands, apart from those in the throat and neck, are those in the abdomen and the groin. They can be painful to touch. The most common remedy for adenitis in fever is **Belladonna** though **Calc-c.** may well be needed before they resolve. The other remedies associated are **Aconite, Apis, Hepar-sulph.**, **Merc-sol.** and **Silica.** Check these remedies in 'Fever' (pages 88–97) to see if the rest of the picture fits. Children often have swollen glands around the neck; this indicates a chronically afflicted immune system mostly as a result of vaccine damage. This must be reported to your practitioner as it will form an integral part of constitutional treatment. **Any swollen glands appearing without fever should be reported to the homoeopath at once. Swollen glands that persist with a recurrent 'flu or 'viral' infection and a cough must also be reported.**

Bladder and Kidney Infection

Bladder and kidney infections are associated with one or other of the legion of different bacteria that seem to bedevil us. They can be associated with fever symptoms. If the patient has a fever and obvious urinary tract symptoms then you must be in touch with your practitioner. Even if the picture is straightforward and you can see exactly what remedy is needed, it is important that a professional offers advice. The reason for this is because bladder infections with fever symptoms can quickly become kidney problems with severe pains and bleeding. Remember that the kidneys lie higher up the back than most people think; they are either side and just below the bottom ribs. Any persistent aching there should be reported. If in doubt, give **Berberis Vulgaris** 30 twice daily and call the clinic for advice as soon as possible. See 'Cystitis' (pages 232–5).

Emergency Fever Conditions

There are two conditions that involve fever for which you absolutely must seek hospital treatment: meningitis and Kawasaki syndrome.

Meningitis: is associated with both bacteria and viruses. Susceptibility to meningitis is due to a number of causative factors: head injury, a lowered immune system due to stress, alcohol, vaccine damage or frequent use of suppressive or recreational drugs and as a result of unresolved childhood diseases such as measles or mumps. There has been a suspiciously swift increase in the number of cases of meningitis since the MMR inoculation was introduced in

1990; this is less than surprising given that the body is intentionally prevented from expressing any of these diseases in the way that it should and meningitis is a known complication. The signs to look for include:

- High fever
- Headache with pain at the back of the head
- Stiffness of the neck
- Rolling the head from side to side or arching the neck and back
- Delirium and stupor
- Vomiting and diarrhoea
- High-pitched, piercing screaming
- Red rash which is blotchy and can sometimes be purplish in hue

If you become aware of any three or more of these symptoms then **take the patient to hospital and call your homoeopath!** Give **Belladonna** or **Apis** in the highest potency you have (10M is usually the most effective) as you get on your way. (To differentiate between these two remedies remember that **Apis** is more restless and irritable but drowsy while **Belladonna** is mostly hot in the head and upper body and more likely to be delirious with strange delusions.) If the cause of the dangerous symptoms is definitely a head injury then give **Nat-sulph.** 200 but still **take the person to hospital!** The reason for this is that the speed of meningitis can be extremely alarming.

Kawasaki syndrome: is a different condition altogether and one that has only been known about since the 1960s. It mostly affects children of five and under though there have been cases amongst teenagers. Kawasaki is harder to diagnose than meningitis as it often starts off as some other condition such as scarletina (which is like a weaker relative of scarlet fever), measles or another condition of apparently viral origin. It is characterised by fever, rashes and swollen lymph glands; sometimes there are swollen and painful joints and heart symptoms that are not easily detectable by untrained eyes. Sometimes it can be mistaken for the early signs of meningitis. It is so important for the patient to receive expert professional care because there are severe complications to Kawasaki: inflammation of tissues of the heart and the pericardium (the sac around the heart), heart failure and infarction (death of the heart muscle). There are other threatening complications: inflammation of the inside tissues of the eye, meningitis, rheumatic inflammation of the joints and cholecystitis (inflammation of the gall bladder). In addition there may be exhausting diarrhoea and anaemia. Though most children recover, some go on to suffer problems from weakened or damaged heart tissue. One of the major problems of this condition is that often the indicated homoeopathic remedies seem to be ineffective. For this reason, if **Belladonna** or **Apis** seem to be indicated but do nothing in high potency, it is essential to call your practitioner and get the opinion of your doctor as well. **If in doubt take the patient to A & E anyway!**

5   INFLUENZA

There are two types of influenza: stomach and systemic (the bone-achy kind). Gastroenteritis is associated with certain types of bacteria creating toxicity in the alimentary canal. It results in purging by diarrhoea and vomiting. The main remedy is **Arsen-alb.**. Cross-check between fever (pagres 88–97), gastroenteritis (pages 181–2), tonsillitis (pages 106–110) and colds (pages 98–103). Systemic 'flu can also be complicated by diarrhoea and vomiting in some. With gastric bugs there is not always the same degree of fever or body pains – though **Baptisia** and **Eupat-perf.** are exceptions. The main remedies for systemic 'flu are: **Aconite** (only as a first prescription when the symptoms are of sudden onset); **Arsen-alb.; Baptisia; Bell.; Bry.; Eupat-perf.; Ferr-phos.; Gels.; Hepar-sulph.; Merc-sol.; Nux-vom.; Puls.; Phos.; Rhus-tox.; Sabad.**

Gastric influenza is self-limiting in that once the body has purged itself of the offending bacteria it will restore itself as long as there is no dehydration from loss of fluids (this is really important to monitor in the very young and the elderly). Systemic 'flu, on the other hand, can become a chronic problem if it is neglected or suppressively treated especially if the lymphatic system has been strongly represented by swollen glands. Influenza is treated by antibiotics when mucus production is heavy enough to threaten a bacterial chest infection. The mucus does clear up but the whole ecosystem is weakened. Unfortunately this is compounded by the patient going back to school or work too soon which compromises the recovery; this results distressingly often in glandular fever especially in stressed teenagers.

6   GLANDULAR FEVER

If glandular fever (mononucleosis in the US) is suspected, a blood test is taken. A negative test is absolutely no guarantee of not having glandular fever. Though glandular fever is associated with the Epstein-Barr virus we should diagnose the condition by dint of the symptoms which can be similar to tonsillitis though more glands are involved: those in the armpits, abdomen and groin may be swollen and painful. This is a condition that can affect any age group though it is commonly a complication with teenagers who become considerably stressed by peer pressure and scholastic expectations. In the US it is reckoned that up to 50% of children have had Epstein-Barr related symptoms by the age of five. The statistic in Britain is less likely to be so alarmingly high though poor nutrition and the appalling pressures to perform well, imposed on school children by the rigid demands of uncreative academic curricula, contribute significantly. It is imperative that anyone suffering from glandular fever should allow considerable time for recuperation. While many parents feel that it is important to get their children back into school as quickly as possible, it is essential that recovery from the condition should be complete first. This means that the patient is restored in energy as well as having normal glands. Those old-fashioned necessities of rest, fresh air and good nutrition are prerequisites to this recovery. This is important because those who do not recover fully before going back to their previous routine could easily succumb either to another bout or to myalgic encephalomyelitis (ME or chronic fatigue syndrome) – a long name for a serious condition in which the immune system is severely compromised and the person is struck with lethargy, lack of will power and motivation and, frequently, a hidden agenda of not wanting to get thoroughly well.

Glandular fever is not a condition for first-aid treatment; it requires experienced professional advice. It can sometimes seem that even this expert help is insufficient; it can take time to prescribe adequately as the body's energy is often so depleted by the illness and its underlying causes that dealing with what homoeopaths call 'lack of reaction' is a priority. Patience, sharp observation and perseverance are needed on the carer's part. Having said which, most of the remedies that you find listed for tonsillitis are called for by acute glandular fever. **Aconite** (unlikely to bring about cure on its own), **Apis, Belladonna, Hepar-sulph., Merc-sol.; Merc-iod-flav.; Merc-iod-rub.; Phyto.; Sil.** In addition there are other remedies that might be called for though some may not qualify for the first-aid kit: **Ailanthus, Arsen-iod., Baryta-carb., Baryta-iod.; Calc-c. Ailanthus** and the two barium remedies are characterised by extreme mental fatigue and are indicated in cases where the patient has vastly overworked their adrenal glands. Sometimes glandular fever does not resolve until a dose of **Carcinosin** is administered showing what miasmatic influence is involved. It is well known as a remedy to unlock difficult cases that do not respond either in the acute, as in glandular fever, or in chronic ill health as in ME. **Please do not underestimate the depths of the roots of this condition!** A lot of recuperation is needed and children should never be encouraged to go back into the school system too soon especially if they would face pressure and stress! As a rough guide, it can take as long as 6 to 8 weeks to recover fully from glandular fever.

7 THE HEAD AND HEADACHES

Headaches are among the most difficult things to treat in homoeopathy. One of the reasons for this is that there are so many different causative factors. Acute headaches are often only one part of a more generalised condition and frequently they are the tip of a more chronic iceberg. Apparently uncomplicated headaches result from such things as physical trauma, drinking too much, overuse of the eyes or mind, overindulgence in eating, lack of sleep, an emotional upset or outburst of rage, or sitting in the sun too long. Headaches as an expression of a deeper problem can arise from postural problems, menstrual complaints, high blood pressure, liver and gall bladder complaints, addiction to nicotine or other recreational drugs, having to take long-term medication, eating a diet that is unsuitable or working or living in a place that is suffused with bad energy that causes sick building syndrome.

Migraine headaches are not to be confused with ordinary headaches. Migraines are an expression of a deep and underlying chronic state that takes expert professional help to unravel. There is almost always a relation between the state of the liver and the onset of the typical visual disturbances, pains and gastric derangement. While remedies found in the first-aid kit might relieve the acute symptoms, the long-term fundamental reasons for migraines should be treated by a professional.

To help you to deal with relatively uncomplicated headaches, the following repertory should be a guide to selecting a remedy for the causation as well as the symptomatic results. For chronic headaches consult the homoeopath.

- < alcohol: **Arsen-alb.; Bell.; Bry.; Chel.; Chin.; Gels.; Ign.; Lach.; Lyc.; Nat-mur.; Nux-vom.; Puls.: Sulph.**
- < anger: **Bry.; Cham.; Ign.; Lyc.; Nat-mur.; Staph.**
- < beer: **Bell.; Nux-vom.; Rhus-tox.**

- Bilious (liverish) headache: **Bry.; Chel.; Ipecac.; Nux-vom.; Puls.**
- < coffee: **Bell.; Bry.; Cham.; Ign.; Lyc.; Nux-vom.; Puls.**
- < with a cold: **Acon.; Bell.; Bry.; Nux-vom.; Phos.; Puls.; Sil.; Sulph.**
- < constipated: **Bry.; Nat-mur.; Nux-vom.; Puls.**
- < coughing: **Bell.; Bry.; Calc-c.; Chin.; Ipecac.; Lach.; Lyc.; Merc-sol.; Nat-mur.; Nux-vom.; Phos.; Puls.; Sepia; Spongia; Sulph.**
- < dehydration: **Chin.; Nat-mur.; Nux-vom.; Puls.; Sepia; Sil.; Sulph.**
- < drinking ice-cold drinks (especially when overheated): **Acon.; Bry.; Lyc.**
- Drowsiness with headache: **Chel.; Gels.**
- < drug abuse: **Nux-vom.**
- < eating too much (especially rich food): **Nux-vom.; Puls.**
- < emotional upset or grief: **Cham.; Gels.; Ign.; Puls.; Staph.**
- < exhaustion from overwork: **Arsen-alb.; Chin.; Gels.; Sepia.**
- < eyestrain: **Calc-c.; Lyc.; Nat-mur.; Phos-ac.; Phos.; Ruta; Sil.**
- Flushed face with headache: **Acon.; Bell.; Gels. (dark); Glon.; Nat-mur.: Nux-vom.**
- Faint feeling or light-headedness with headache: **Calc-c.; Gels.; Glon.; Lyc.; Nat-mur.; Nux-vom.; Puls.; Sil.; Sulph.**
- < fasting or missing a meal: **Lyc.; Phos.; Sil.; Sulph.**
- < fatty food: **Carbo-veg.; Puls.; Sepia.**
- Fever with headache: **Acon.; Apis.; Arn.; Arsen-alb.; Bell.; Bry.; Chin.; Eupa-perf.; Hepar-sulph.; Lach.; Nat-mur.; Nux-vom.; Puls.; Rhus-tox.; Sil.**
- Gastric headache: **Arsen-alb.; Bry.; Carbo-veg.; Chin.; Eupa-perf.; Lyc.; Nux-vom.; Puls.; Sulph.**
- < hangover: **Bell.; Bry.; Carbo-veg; Nux-vom.; Puls.**
- < excitement: **Coff.; Phos.**
- < reading too much: **Nat-mur.; Ruta.**
- < shopping: **Sepia.**
- < smell of tobacco smoke: **Ign.**
- < strong scent (i.e. of flowers): **Phos.**
- < stuffy atmosphere: **Lyc.; Puls.**
- < sun: **Acon.; Bell.; Bry.; Glon.; Lach.; Puls.; Sulph.**
- < eating sweets: **Arg-nit.**
- < after swimming in the sea: **Arsen-alb.; Rhus-tox.**

- < travelling by car: **Cocc.; Petroleum; Sepia.**
- < weather changes: **Bry.; Calc-c.; Puls.; Rhus-tox.**
- < wind: **Acon.; Hepar-sulph.; Nux-vom.; Puls.; Rhus-tox.; Sil.**

NB For most headaches the 30th potency should be adequate. The exceptions might be those which are part of a fever picture or during menstruation in which case the 200 might be necessary. The more severe the headache the more frequently you can give the remedy: i.e. **Bryonia** 30 can be given every hour for several hours and **Rhus-tox.** can be given every half hour (as it expends so much energy being restless). **Arsen-alb.** is best given once and then wait; sometimes the patient will be sick which >. On occasion **Glon.** needs to be given every 15 or 20 minutes as the symptoms can be so violent.

Aconite: hot, pulsating and heavy in the head; hair feels as if being pulled. Burning sensation. May be dizzy.

Arg-nit.: head feels squeezed in a vice; wants to press head with hands; head feels as if expanding; chilly and trembly with brain fatigue. Likely to be light-headed or dizzy.

Arsen-alb.: burning pain > from a cold flannel or cool hands; if generally chilly, wants to wrap up but keep head cool; scalp is sensitive < combing hair. Restless and frowning.

Belladonna: pounding, throbbing pain < temples or forehead; red face and/or radiating heat from head; << bending down or lying flat; waves of pain; comes on with fever. Might be dizzy. Can be < after washing or cutting hair or with earache or teething. Thirsty for cold drinks.

Bryonia: bursting, splitting pains which are << any movement; wants to remain absolutely still. Very irritable. Very thirsty for cold water. < business worries.

Calc-c.; hot head with pale face, can be confused with **Bell**. Also: icy-cold head with light-headedness (especially on sudden movement) and muddle-headedness. < stooping; < mental exertion; > lying down and closing eyes. Hammering pain through the forehead to the back of the neck. Light-headed or even dizzy.

Carbo-veg.; heavy, dull pain < in the back of the head; pain is present on waking and goes through to the eyes; head feels hot but the body is cold though the headache is < for being in a warm room. Wants to sit quietly, leaning back. < gastric discomfort.

Chamomilla: throbbing on right side of head; wants to lean backwards; < earache or teething; pain extends into ear or jaw; pains are unendurable = fury, screaming and crying.

Chelidonium: drilling pain over the left side of right eye on the orbital bone which extends back over head to the right side of the neck; can extend further over the back of the right ear and to the bottom of the right shoulder blade. Back of the head feels heavy. Might be light-headed. > and + very hot drinks. Origin of headache is in the liver which may have pain as well. (But see **Lyc.**)

China: throbbing, bursting pains that make the brain feel bruised; blood vessels pulsate; generally > for being in a warm room and for pressure. Useful after dehydration after acute diarrhoea and vomiting; disordered digestion with flatulence, rumbling and tummy cramps; thirsty for water. No hunger but will eat snacks of delicatessen-type food.

Coffea: as if a nail is being driven into the head or throbbing and tension all over. < from getting overexcited or from excessive enthusiasm over anything.

Eupatorium Perfoliatum: pains at the back of the head that spread all over especially during 'flu; throbbing < movement; nausea and > after vomiting. Pains << from cold air = feels as if scalp contracts. Bones might be deeply aching as well.

Gelsemium: sensation as of a band especially around the back of the head; dull, heavy pains that make the brain feel bruised; pain can start in the nape and go over the head to the forehead and settle over the eyes; patient is dopey and weak; apathetic and dizzy. Scalp is sore to touch and there is soreness and stiffness in the neck muscles. If the headache precedes a cold then there are chills that go down the back.

Glonoin: waves of throbbing and exploding pain; head feels ready to burst; flushes of heat rush up to the head; light-headed; head feels very heavy and congested but is << from lying down. < from the sun or during the menopause.

Hepar-sulph.: short, sharp stabs of pain in the right side as if a nail were being driven in; < with onset of a cold, earache or 'flu. Very sensitive scalp: < least touch.

Ignatia: intense pressing pains often in a small area (< temple which can feel as if a knitting needle is being forced out or behind the eye); wants to lean forward as this > pressure. < from coffee, smoking (passive or active) and alcohol.

Lachesis: pains settle over the left eye with tremendous pressure and heaviness in whole head; feels bursting and hot with < from every change of position; generally feels < on the left side, though if the pains move over to the right as well then this indicates the remedy strongly. Patient is likely to be extremely snappy and not very coherent. Commonly needed during periods and the menopause – consult your practitioner.

Lycopodium: pain in the temples as if they are being gradually pressed together; pain is < right side though pain in the forehead behind the right eye might move over to the left. Often the result of stress and pressure at work with < from missing a meal or dehydration from forgetting to drink. Most **Lycopodium** patients are windy. (Can easily be confused with **Chel.** which is not a first-aid remedy except for those who respond to it better than **Lyc.** Check with your practitioner.)

Nat-mur.: throbbing, hammering headache with sensation of numbness at times; visual disturbance. < sun, bright lights, reading, studying, inflamed or blocked sinuses; > sleep. Pain < over the eyes or in a band around the head. Light-headed. Patient is usually thirsty and dry mouthed. Sometimes it is better to give **Bryonia** (especially around the middle of the day) as this remedy is very close to **Nat-mur.** and less likely to cause an aggravation. If neither **Nat-mur.** nor **Bryonia** do anything positive then consider **Nat-carb.** which is a very sensitive state and << for sun.

Nux Vomica: headache from overindulging or drinking too much: hangover. Feels very liverish and may feel nauseous and dizzy. Also spasms of pain with pressing and heaviness in the forehead after working too hard or too long to meet deadlines. Head can feel bruised. Often has biliousness with head pains. Is to be seen pressing forehead with hands or leaning against something.

Pulsatilla: any pain and location might be dealt with by **Puls**. Often one-sided (usually left) with throbbing or bursting sensations; pains may wander from place to place. Any dizziness is < from looking up. Symptoms are accompanied by dryness with thirstlessness and watery eyes. Almost always has the typical mental picture.

Rhus-tox.: pain in the back of the head which is tender to touch; pains also < in forehead and extending backwards. Brain feels loose; feels as if it falls to the side lain on. Patient is restless and achy generally.

Ruta: the most useful remedy for headache from reading, sewing or close work which causes eyestrain. Eyes feel hot and look reddened.

Sepia: pains shoot into the left eye and heaviness especially on the top of the head, pressing down; pain can also shift from one side of the back of the head to the other. Headache with exhaustion, nausea and tearfulness; patients would feel much > for exercise though all they want to do is to lie down in a dark room. Easily confused with **Nux-vom**.

Sulphur: hot head especially on the top; throbs and feels sore and heavy; pressure in the temples; all < for standing; > sitting or even > lying down. Weekend headaches of intellectuals: they 'live in their heads' and look exhausted and droopy; want to flop on a sofa; very thirsty though may forget to drink which will make their breath smell rank.

Warning Symptoms to be Aware of

- Persistent headaches with visual impairment and dizziness in someone not prone to headaches or migraine. **This suggests the need for specialist investigation.**
- Headache in the temple region with swollen blood vessels, tender scalp

and either double vision or blind spots; chewing food may aggravate the pain and there may already be some muscle pains. **This suggests temporal arteritis and requires immediate professional attention from a specialist and the homoeopath.**

· Headache with flushed face, easy exhaustion, shortness of breath, light-headedness, frequent indigestion (sometimes with nausea) and possibly nosebleeds suggest seriously high blood pressure. **Seek immediate professional advice.**

· Any combination of the following should be referred for professional treatment: dizziness with mental confusion, slurred speech or inability to choose the appropriate words and say them, staggering gait or a tendency to fall, feeling faint, double vision, jerking movements, numbness or weakness of a limb or one side of the body. This suggests a transient ischaemic attack when the normal blood supply to the brain has been interrupted. **Immediate professional advice is essential as this condition can lead quickly to a stroke!**

8 VERTIGO AND DIZZINESS

'Vertigo' is usually associated with the fear of heights; this is a general symptom of underlying psychic stress. Dizziness and loss of balance and spatial coordination are symptoms of various different illnesses. Some remedies cover vertigo or dizziness felt in acute conditions: **Pulsatilla**, **Cocculus** and **Nux Vomica**, for example. Once the remedy has been given, the dizziness should be one of the first symptoms to be relieved as the normal blood supply to the head is restored (see 'Fainting' on page 54). Persistent dizziness is a condition that should be treated by a professional as it can be a warning symptom of a deep-seated chronic problem.

Dizziness can be associated with alcoholism, transient ischaemic attack, labyrinthitis, Ménière's disease and calcification in the inner parts of the ears which all need long-term treatment and careful monitoring. Dizziness can also be the result of chronic musculo-skeletal displacement and should be treated by a cranial osteopath. Accidents, birth patterns and orthodontic braces are examples of what can cause changes in body structure that can cause balance problems and dizziness. However, there are other, acute conditions in which dizziness is a central symptom that can be treated with first-aid remedies.

- Sea and car sickness: **Cocc.**
- Results of overwork or loss of sleep with stress: **Cocc.**
- Being too long in a hot environment: **Lyc.; Phos.; Puls.**
- From dehydration: **Nux-vom.; Lyc.; Puls.**
- Getting drunk: (see 'Hangover' on page 120)
- After smelling strong scents or chemicals: **Nux-vom.; Phos.**
- From smoking or passive smoking: **Gels.; Nat-mur.; Nux-vom.**

- After exhausting bout of diarrhoea, sweat and vomiting: **Chin.; Phos-ac.; Phos.; Sep**.
- After strain from lifting heavy weight: **Puls**.

Cross-refer these remedies with their descriptions in part III. Use the 30th potency for these conditions unless you know that the patient responds best to either higher or lower potencies.

EYE CONDITIONS

The eye is a highly complex structure and any chronic or worrying acute pathology should be treated by a professional to ensure that the vision is safe. However, lumped together under the general term 'eye conditions' are problems with associated structures: the tear ducts, the eyelids, the sclera (the white of the eye) and the blood vessels that run through it, the conjunctiva (the protective covering of the surface of the eye) and the muscles of the eye. The following headings will help you decide whether you should call your practitioner or treat the problem yourself. Apart from the remedies in the first-aid kit you might think of keeping a bottle of **Euphrasia Ø** (mother tincture). This herbal preparation is universally acknowledged as one of the best medicines for the relief of eye conditions. Use one drop in a quarter of a cup of tepid water either to swab the eye or for use in an eyebath. An alternative would be a cold (moist) tea bag placed over the eye; this can afford relief for tired or painful eyes. For eye conditions in babies still breastfeeding bathe the affected eyes in breast milk; an ancient and well-tried treatment.

Blepharitis or Inflammation of the Eyelid

With this condition, which can affect either one or both of the eyes, the eyelid becomes sore, red, itchy and/or burning. The eye might be dry or watery and the patient may want to rub the eye. Sometimes there is crustiness and flaking of the skin. In the morning there is usually yellow matter in the inner corner, or the eye might be stuck together and difficult to open without being bathed. The condition is usually associated with staphylococcus though it can occur when acne rosacea (see pages 249–50) is present which is often a menopausal problem. The main remedies include: **Arg-nit.**; **Apis**; **Lyc.**; **Merc-sol.**; **Nat-mur.**; **Puls.**; **Rhus-tox.**; **Staphysagria**.

Styes

A stye is a small abscess, usually containing pus, in a gland on an eyelid though sometimes it can be more like a blind boil. It is usually associated with staphylococcus and can appear along with blepharitis. It can be very painful or not so and orthodox treatment (antibiotics) is often ineffective. The old wives tale about rubbing a stye with a gold wedding ring is not so fanciful: **Aurum** (gold), though not a first-aid remedy, is sometimes called for with a stye and the ring has sometimes proved effective if it is used early on. A condition that is similar to a stye is a chalazion, a swollen oil gland at the edge of the eyelid. The swelling is red and irritated for a while before settling down to being an indolent lump. The main remedy is **Silica** (see below) though **Pulsatilla** and **Staphysagria** are common too. Styes are often the result of suppressed anger (see **Staphysagria**).

Blocked Tear Ducts

The cause of a blocked tear duct might be an infection, an injury to the face or, in babies, an underdeveloped duct. This latter situation is best left to professional treatment and, in some cases, may require surgical assistance. Straightforward infection may respond to an indicated first-aid remedy but if nothing has been effective within 48 hours call your practitioner. Symptoms that can be treated at home include swelling and pain with redness at the inner corner of the eye; oozing pus (usually yellow). Gentle massage of the tissues around the affected area can also help. Sometimes there is a general state of malaise occasionally with a low-grade fever. In addition to remedies you can think of applying a warm compress to the area. If there is a chronic repeated pattern of forming such a problem then the patient must see the homoeopath, not least as there may be an underlying chronic miasmatic pattern emerging (usually sycosis). The main remedies are **Apis**; **Arg-nit.**; **Calc-c.**; **Borax**; **Merc-sol.**; **Puls.**; **Sil. Graphites** should also be considered (even though it is not in the first-aid list) as it covers the typical symptom picture: swelling, redness, itching, soreness, oozing pus with crusty deposits. Another very useful remedy is **Calc-sulph.** which has yellow pus, redness and soreness with lack of reaction to well-chosen remedies (it is often mistaken for **Puls.** but is more morose than weepy and clingy) and it is excellent at dealing with infections that are associated with staphylococcus.

Conjunctivitis

Inflammation of the conjunctiva can be the result of infection, injury or allergic reaction. Susceptibility to infection might be acute or chronic; to allergy, it is always a chronic condition. Any chronic tendency must be treated professionally. In very young babies this condition can be the result of acquired gonorrhoea. Even if the mother had no apparent symptoms of gonorrhoea at the time of the birth it is essential that the homoeopath should treat the child as there will be a strong hereditary (miasmatic) influence at work on the patient's constitution which will need deeply acting remedies to lift it. The main features of the problem, whether acute or chronic, are the same. The eye is irritated and the white appears bloodshot. If there is a bacterial element then there is white, creamy or yellow pus. There is often intense itching. The most usual remedies are **Apis; Arg-nit.; Arsen-alb.; Bell.; Calc-c.; Merc-sol.; Puls.; Rhus-tox.; Sil**.

Photophobia (Light Sensitivity)

Sensitivity to light can be the result of allergy, infection or hereditary susceptibility of some form. It can occur acutely (as in a cold or conjunctivitis) or be a chronic state (as part of hay fever or as a permanent condition). There are over 140 remedies that cover this symptom. If it is the main focus of a chronic condition then take the case to the homoeopath, otherwise regard it as a temporary symptom of an acute that will resolve with the chosen remedy.

Lachrymation (Watering Eyes)

Watering eyes is a common symptom of many complaints. If it is a chronic symptom that is irritating enough to be a main complaint then ask the homoeopath. It is very likely that the underlying problem lies in 'the heart' and the watering is a physical 'metaphor' for not having resolved a historical emotional issue. Watery eyes during a cough is covered by **Euphrasia,**

Nat-mur. and **Puls.**; during a cold it is covered by **Allium Cepa**, **Euphrasia**, **Nux-vom.** and **Puls**. If a headache is accompanied by watery eyes then think of **Puls**.

Dry Eye Syndrome

Chronically dry eyes is a condition common to a variety of diseases: rheumatoid arthritis, Sjögren's syndrome (in which eyes, mouth and mucous membranes dry out) and systemic lupus erythematosus (which is associated with rheumatic pains, skin rashes and fevers). The other state that has dry eyes is the menopause; the lack of hormones causes this irritating problem which is usually treated with artificial tears. It is a useful symptom but it is a part of a larger picture that needs professional treatment.

Corneal Ulceration

Ulcers can develop either because of susceptibility to bacterial, fungal or viral infection or because of injury. Occasionally dry eye syndrome (see above) might be part of the picture. This is potentially a very unpleasant condition and must be treated as an emergency, professionally and very speedily. Homoeopathic remedies are perfectly capable of resolving the symptoms but be ready to see an ophthalmologist if your practitioner advises it or wants a second opinion. The typical symptoms include sore or burning pains, photophobia, watery eyes and white or yellow pus on the surface of the eye. The ulcer may be so small as to make it hard to see it or it may be quite apparent. (DIY accidents need A & E attention to remove debris that would possibly cause permanent damage. See **Silica**.)

Herpes Simplex on the Cornea

Herpes needs expert prescribing (see 'Herpes Simplex' pages 250–2). The cornea can sometimes be affected and causes acute soreness, redness, photophobia and watering. It does not respond to antibiotic creams which are often prescribed as initially it can be hard to tell herpes from a staphylococcal infection. Avoid the follow-on suggestion of antiviral drugs as these suppress the symptoms without weakening the herpes virus. Even if this condition is one that the patient usually leaves to resolve itself (in mild cases), it is worth consulting the homoeopath as treatment would be to address the underlying chronic susceptibility to harbouring the virus. These comments are even more relevant to herpes zoster (shingles) which can be very persistent and extremely painful and distressing.

Remedies in Acute Eye Conditions

Aconite: sudden onset; red, inflamed, sore and hot. Photophobic. Conjunctivitis and blepharitis. Use the 200 especially after exposure to a cold wind.

Apis: blepharitis, stye, conjunctivitis, ulceration. Always puffy around the eye, swollen, red and watery conjunctiva with stinging and burning pains that are maddening; can feel as if there is sand under the lid. Whites are inflamed and reddened with blood vessels. Use the 30; 200 when symptoms are severe.

Arg-nit.: blepharitis, blocked tear ducts, conjunctivitis, ulceration. Swelling of the conjunctiva with redness in the inner corner and copious amounts of pus < on waking. Thick crusts on the margins of the eyelids; hard to open eyes on waking. Eyes feel strained. Wants to keep the eyes cool. Use 30.

Arsen-alb.: conjunctivitis, ulceration. Burning pains with hot tears, light sensitivity and scaly skin on the lids. > if warm flannel is applied. Sand under the lid sensation. Eyes appear sunken and with a dark ring around. Use 30.

Belladonna: conjunctivitis: red, hot and swollen sometimes with pulsation felt in the eyes. Eyes appear staring and glassy and the pupils are dilated. Photophobia. Use 30 or 200.

Calc-c.: conjunctivitis; yellow matter from eyes in the morning with watering eyes later especially in the open air. Babies affected may appear to have a slight squint. Photophobia; pupils dilated. Use 30.

Euphrasia: conjunctivitis; profuse, hot, burning tears with redness of the lids and sensation of sand under them. Thick yellow pus from inner corner and has to blink to clear mucus from the surface of the eye. Remedy can be used in both 30 and in tincture.

Graphites: blepharitis; red, swollen lids with sore even cracked edges to the lids and flaky skin. Honey-coloured deposits which dry and are painful to clear away. Recurrent stye especially of the lower lid. Use 30.

Hepar-sulph.: conjunctivitis with extreme sensitivity to touch and cold; yellow matter in the eyes and red, inflamed lids. Even cool air < the sensations. Use 30 or 100 which will have to be ordered from your pharmacy.

Hypericum: stye on the lower left eyelid but which is only part of a more generalised picture of low spirits, even depressiveness. Use 30.

Ipecac.: conjunctivitis – an unusual remedy for this but accompanied by the odd symptom of nausea on looking at moving objects; < watching television. Also shooting pain through the eyeball with inflammation and watering. Use 30.

Lycopodium: stye near inner corner of eye (< on the right side); redness and soreness of area. Often accompanied by flatulence and bloating. Use 30.

Merc-sol.: conjunctivitis especially with cold symptoms; lids are swollen, sore, red and scurfy. This is a remedy that can go on to more serious conditions so if there is no response to it when you feel it is well indicated then do not hesitate in calling your practitioner. Use 30 (sometimes needs to be repeated quite frequently: up to 4 times per day).

Nat-mur.: blocked tear duct; blepharitis, ulceration; inflammation with itching, burning and profuse watering. Lids are red and sore and feel as if sand is underneath. Wants to rub eyes all the time which <. Symptoms are usually < during a cold. Photophobic< sunlight. Use 30.

Pulsatilla: one of the most common remedies for eye conditions in children; conjunctivitis; blepharitis; styes. Yellow matter from the eyes especially on waking with watering in the rest of the day; itching and burning of the lids and feeling of sand beneath. Stye (recurrent) on the upper lid, often with no head. Use 30 or 200.

Rhus-tox.: conjunctivitis, blepharitis, stye. Inflammation, swelling, photophobia and lots of yellow pus; profuse watering < cool air. General restlessness and great anxiety about the condition. If the symptoms do not begin to clear within 12 hours then you must call your practitioner as **Rhus-tox.** symptoms can be very serious indeed. Use 30.

Sepia: blepharitis, styes; usually accompanied by exhaustion and being fed up and 'down'.

Silica: blocked tear duct; styes; blepharitis. Slow developing swelling of the inner corner of the eye with blocked tear duct or (recurrent) stye on the upper lid toward the inner corner. Gritty feeling in eyes. Sharp pain sometimes strikes through the eye but mostly painless. It is the general state of the patient that suggests this remedy. Useful if tiny particles of debris are lodged in the tissues of the eye. Use 30.

Staphysagria: blepharitis; conjunctivitis; styes (recurrent); chalazion. Itching on the edge of the lids. Upper lid and inner corner affected most. Eyes can feel hot; less mucus or pus than with other remedies. The emotional picture can help determine whether this remedy is indicated (see **Staphysagria** in part III). Use 30.

Sulphur: most conditions of the eye come under this remedy. Eyes are inflamed, dry, hot, sore and gritty. Eyes look tired and droopy. Recurrent styes especially of the upper lid. Use 30.

Other Eye Conditions which Need Professional Help

Pterygium: is a jelly-like growth that advances across the conjunctiva; it is usually off-white or pink and harmless except that it can interfere with the field of vision. It is usually peeled away by the ophthalmologist though it may grow back again. The homoeopath will regard this as only a part of a more general picture that requires treatment.

Iritis and scleritis: are extremely unpleasant and potentially dangerous conditions which can result in the loss of sight. Symptoms of both include severe pains, usually boring or burning, and dark discoloration of the eye, sometimes angry red or purplish. There is often a relation with rheumatoid arthritis and the usual orthodox treatment is with corticosteroids and immuno-suppressive drugs. Even if the patient has had to resort to this drastic treatment because of the need for speedy removal of the symptoms, it is important to use homoeopathy as well in order to limit the likelihood and strength of a return of the symptoms.

Squint: is most commonly a problem in very early childhood and, though it concerns muscles, is treatable with homoeopathic remedies especially if started early on. To complement the remedies it is extremely advisable to consult a cranial osteopath. This is important because the osteopath should be able to determine to what degree the bones of the head are out of alignment so as to cause the problem and how to encourage them to set back in their correct position.

Cataract: is the formation of a cloudy mass within the lens of the eye and can be the result of several circumstances: injury, surgery, exposure to sunlight or X-ray, as a complication of diabetes or some other chronic disease and as part of the ageing process. Occasionally babies are born with congenital cataract. Cataracts are usually removed surgically once they are 'ripe'. Homoeopathic treatment needs to be begun early on. (See 'Eye Injuries' pages 23–4)

Floaters: are the result of dead cells floating in the vitreous fluid within the eye itself. The body has been unable to break down these cells and they have clumped together and form 'clouds' that float back and forth across one's vision. Nothing can be done about them in orthodox medicine. In homoeopathy, however, they are seen as originating in sluggish liver function and the slow and gradual development of gallstones. It is likely that the patient would be given liver drainage and support remedies; treatment can continue for some while before the condition is alleviated.

Seeing zigzags or colours: is usually a sign of migraine. The symptoms may appear with dizziness, feeling faint, nausea, vomiting and/or headache but can be there with no other symptom.

Signs to report immediately include: the appearance of black spots, 'bubbles', blurred vision in the centre of the visual field, diplopia (double vision) and hemiopia (half vision which can appear as lost vision of the top or bottom half or the left or right side of the visual field). Frequently bloodshot eyes and persistent sensations of pressure in the eyes should also be reported without delay.

Sudden partial loss of sight after blurring and seeing floating shapes can indicate a detaching retina. Tired eyes, seeing halos of light around objects, and pressure and throbbing sensations in the eyeball all suggest glaucoma. **Seek appointments with both the doctor and the homoeopath immediately for both these conditions!**

10   EAR, NOSE AND THROAT

Ear Conditions

Apart from acute earache (see 'Otitis Media' page 137) the other conditions of the ears need professional advice: chronic earwax, pus discharges (especially with blood), catarrhal deafness, labyrinthitis (inflammation of the inner parts of the ear), Ménière's disease and tinnitus (noises in the ear) are all problems that have chronic implications and are likely to need several consultations to resolve. Popping and cracking in the ear along with aural distortion and pressure within occurs when there is trapped wax or fluid deep inside the ear or in the Eustachian tube, behind the eardrum extending down into the throat. The most common remedy for popping is **Silica**. It is especially indicated for pressure build-up and popping when descending in a plane or driving down a steep hill. Use 30 for this unless there is sharp pain which calls for 200. One other acute is when water gets into the ear after swimming or scuba diving. If **Silica** is not indicated then **Sulphur** is often curative; it covers the symptom of a swashing in the ear after submersion in water. Use the 200.

Catarrhal deafness: is often the result of long suppression of frequent bouts of otitis media. If not then it is likely to be due to poor liver function and an underlying miasm. **Kali-sulph.** (yellow and slimy muck in the ear) and **Kali-mur.** (thick and paler matter) are useful tissue salts for ears: one 3 times a day; either might be indicated in a higher potency if the symptoms are persistent.

Labyrinthitis: is usually associated with a virus and causes transitory dizzy spells. If it persists then consult your homoeopath.

Ménière's disease: has officially no known cause but often results from a great deal of stress (even of short duration). As it engenders a lot of anxiety patients tend to seek suppression of the symptoms. This is a pity because suppression covers up the underlying emotional cause. It is not uncommon for antidepressants to be among the drugs considered for treatment while those chosen for the distressing symptom of vertigo are not without unpleasant side effects. The very fact that the **China** remedies (**China Officinalis, China-sulph., China-arsen.**) are so often indicated in Ménière's tells us that the patient is likely to be sensitive, weak, over-stretched in the nervous system and in need of a great deal of rest irrespective of the distressing symptoms.

Tinnitus: is one of the most difficult conditions to treat; it can take years of frustrating work or it may resolve after one visit. There are many causes for tinnitus and they are rarely acute but of long standing. One cause is long-term taking of aspirin. Deafness and damage to the ear can also be caused by other drugs: antibiotics (especially neomycin) are particularly at fault while streptomycin causes balance problems. Quinine can cause permanent hearing loss which should be borne in mind by frequent travellers to hot countries. There may also be a hereditary aspect and there is often a stress factor to deal with.

Hay Fever and Allergic Rhinitis

'Hay fever' suggests a seasonal condition that is triggered or exacerbated by particular allergens; allergic rhinitis is more chronic and covers symptoms that can be permanent or intermittent but not dependent on season. The symptoms may include headache, inflammation of the eyes, nose and throat and difficulty breathing with either dryness of the mucous membranes or profuse manufacture of mucus which might be of any shade from clear to green. It might be a condition that springs up in children as a complication of suppression of childhood acute states and immunisation; young people often 'grow out of it'. It may be a problem that suddenly starts in middle age and lasts for many years. Whatever the symptoms and triggers, hay fever is miasmatic in origin. While it is often possible to find a first-aid remedy to deal with symptoms when they appear, it is extremely unlikely that such a remedy would deal with the genetic causative factor; this needs long-term constitutional treatment from an experienced practitioner. Even if the patient is well in every other way apart from annual attacks of the symptoms, it is sensible to go for pre-seasonal consultations aimed at lessening the susceptibility to the allergens. The process can take up to 3 or 4 years. It is extremely worthwhile to go through long-term constitutional treatment especially to avoid passing on the same genetic inheritance to children.

It is not unusual these days for a patient to show signs of needing a particular hay fever remedy this year and a different one next year. Occasionally, a patient will do well on a remedy for a few weeks only for the symptoms to change subtly which will mean switching to the next indicated remedy. Very severe cases will need to be monitored by the practitioner as intercurrent doses of one of the nosodes may become necessary to deal with underlying blocks to cure. This is particularly true of those who develop nasal polyps, not an unusual tendency in those with allergic rhinitis.

Patients should try and resist the temptation to use decongestant medicines or antihistamines as they tend to add a layer of negative energy onto the already difficult picture and they may antidote the beneficial effects of remedies. Worse, they tend to cause the body to involve the lungs with symptoms because the nasal passages have been interfered with. There are well over 70 remedies listed for hay fever, each one with its own individual picture. Below are only the most common ones. Use the 30th potency up to 3 or 4 times per day. Only go up to the 200 if there is an initial response that is not holding. Do not go back down in potency once symptoms have started to abate! You will antidote the beneficial effects of what you have done so far.

Allium Cepa: the symptoms are very similar to those one feels when cutting up onions; smarting in the eyes and nose, with watering and itchy soreness; wants to rub the lids which <. Sneezing with watery mucus which makes the inside of the nose sore and the upper lip becomes red and sore. Very sensitive to the smell of flowers: symptoms are << in the height of the summer when flowers are out. Pressure felt in the middle of the chest especially with a cough. Breathing begins to sound asthmatic.

Arsenicum Album: airways all feel congested forcing mouth-breathing. Nose drips clear watery mucus which makes the top lip sore; cannot lie down from nasal obstruction at night; must sit propped up to breathe.

Eyes burn and smart from watering hot tears. Around the eyes feels swollen and waterlogged. Breathing can become asthmatic; < on the in-breath.

Arsenicum Iodatum: this is not a common first-aid remedy but should be considered here as it is very useful in hay fever. The symptoms are very similar to those of **Arsen-alb.** though **Arsen-iod.** is more likely to have a warmer body temperature and the mucus from the chest or throat will be thicker and more coloured; it might even be greenish. From the nose the water is hot and burning; the posterior part of the nose and the pharynx can feel particularly sore. The nose appears and feels swollen and may well be red. There may be night sweats as well. Asthmatic breathing.

Arum Triphyllum: only considered as a first-aid remedy in hay fever. Easily differentiated from others by the raw palate, cracked corners of the mouth, acrid discharge from the nose and constant desire to pick the nose.

Arundo Mauritanica: only considered as a first-aid remedy in hay fever. The itching of the palate with burning, prickling and itching of the eyes are characteristic. With sneezing there is itching in the nostrils.

Dulcamara: only considered as a first-aid remedy in hay fever. < from mown grass; < from being outside and > being indoors. Constant sneezing and nose blowing but nostrils feel obstructed. Generally > by the seaside.

Euphrasia: hot, watery tears which burn and irritate the eyes; profuse watery mucus that is bland from the nose (opposite of **All-c.**). Nose runs in the daytime but blocks up at night. Light sensitivity and sneezing. Coughing in the morning brings up mucus from the lungs. There may also be a loose cough and loose stools.

Iodum: not a usual first-aid remedy but useful in hay fever. Violent sneezing with swollen red nose; skin feels hot and the patient is restless and feels > for being outside and moving around being active. There may be rawness and tickling in the larynx and the lungs. Becomes ravenously hungry; mentally restless. Appears to be a bit 'speedy'. If **Iod.** seems indicated but does little then consider **Kali-iod.** as this has similar symptoms but the patient is weaker, less active and more irritable; violent sneezing with watery eyes < on getting up. Breathing is wheezy and asthmatic < on the in-breath.

Natrum-mur.: < for sunshine. Eyes stream and feel sore and burning. Coughing brings on watering from the eyes. Profuse white-of-egg mucus with feeling of obstruction in nose. Copious sneezing with loss of smell and taste. Hay fever with cold sores on the lips. Blisters tingle and itch and scab over.

Natrum-sulph.: the remedy for thick, yellow or yellow/green mucus from nose and/or throat with yellowish eyes and light sensitivity. Eyes feel achy, hot and itchy. Throat is also sore.

Nux Vomica: rough throat with rawness and/or tickling; throat and ears feel connected with swallowing. Frequent and profuse sneezing with snuffly breathing and much blowing which does nothing to shift the obstruction. Sneezing or coughing can < headache. Eyes can be bloodshot and exertion, sneezing and coughing = a red face. Very irritable indeed.

Sabadilla: frequent sneezing with prickling itching in the nostrils. Patient constantly rubs the nose to relieve the itching. Very sensitive to smells and << from the scent of flowers. Soft palate tends to feel itchy and hot food feels too hot. Eyelids burn and water with sneezing and coughing and in the fresh air. Eyes feel pressed in and there might be a severe frontal headache. Breathing becomes wheezy. Can be confused with **Sanguinaria** which covers similar symptoms but is dryer with soreness in the upper chest and a cough at night and a constant need to take a deep in-breath.

Sinapis Nigra: distinguished by the nasal blockage that alternates between right and left nostrils. The blockage can be < in the left side with little mucus to show for it but the eyes will have hot tears. There is thicker and more coloured mucus from the back of the nose that has to be hawked out. Feels better if they can get on and do something.

Wyethia: indicated by its dry, hacking cough with tickling and swollen feeling in the throat with difficulty swallowing. The palate is itchy and there is a constant and irritating need to clear the throat.

Sinusitis

Sinusitis can be misleading. There are several areas of sinuses in the head, all susceptible to producing mucus from membranes that line them: frontal, above the brow; maxillary, beneath the eyes and beside the nose; ethmoid, above and behind the bridge of the nose. There are two other sinuses deeper in the head called the sphenoid sinuses. Sinusitis may be acute as the result of an infection or chronic as the result of repeatedly suppressed infections or it can be due to allergic reaction, or a combination of these. The symptoms of the two kinds are similar and can be treated with the same remedies though chronic sinusitis needs long-term constitutional treatment as indicated remedies rarely hold on their own. Frontal sinusitis causes pain over the eyes and across the forehead; the brow feels heavy and it can cause photosensitivity. You may see the patient putting pressure on the area to alleviate the pain. Maxillary sinusitis causes pain and pressure in the cheekbones, neuralgic pains in the teeth and obstruction of the nasal passages. Ethmoid sinusitis tends to cause pressure and pain at the bridge of the nose and behind the eyes as well as a splitting headache and a post-nasal drip. Mucus can be anything from clear water to thick green plugs; the more colour in the catarrh, the more bacterial proliferation there is. In homoeopathic terms, the more disgusting the catarrh, the more the body has been in need of a detoxification. The bacteria is not the *cause* of the illness; it is the patient who is expressing a symptom picture while the bacteria are proliferating opportunists which in their turn oblige the body to find a solution to the infection that results in the 'spring clean'. So much is the sick body in charge of the illness that it will even dictate the type of pain felt and the colour and consistency of the mucus: the individual symptom picture that can be read. It is important to differentiate by quality of pain and mucus; by location of pain and mucus; by concomitant symptoms such as behaviour of symptoms. (Do the pains alternate sides? Does the colour of mucus vary at different times of day? Is the patient thirsty? etc.). There are not many remedies that are uncomplicated in this condition hence the small number in the list below. If there is a state which is not described among the remedies below it needs to be relayed to the homoeopath. Chronic sinusitis is characterised not just by sinus pains and mucus but also by a post-nasal drip, a constant flow of catarrh that runs down the throat and is often swallowed. It is a condition that should be treated as it can lead to persistent susceptibility to sore throat and chest infection; constitutional treatment will almost inevitably involve the nosodes.

Use the 30th potency unless specified otherwise. You may need to repeat 2 or 3 times per day for several days. If you get no result within 2 days then reassess; you may need a higher potency after all or you may not have been wrong in your first choice but the patient might have moved on to a related remedy. Occasionally, it is necessary to alternate two indicated but related remedies to achieve lasting benefit (i.e. **Puls./Kali-sulph.; Lyc./Arsen-alb.; Kali-bich./Puls.**)

Arsen-alb.: thin watery mucus constantly drips from the nose but the sinuses (especially the frontal and maxillary) feel obstructed. Sometimes the right nostril feels blocked. Raw, sore or burning sensations in the sinuses and nose. Colds that will not resolve and feel as if they are going down on the chest. Stuffy head that can become a headache. Sometimes **Arsen-alb**. is well followed by **Kali-mur.** when what remains is stuffiness in the nose and white/grey mucus; confirmed by the whitish grey coating on the tongue.

Calc-c.: root of nose feels swollen; yellow catarrh blocks sinuses and patient is aware of a rotten smell (rotting vegetation). Edge of the nostrils feels dry and sore; may have ulcerated patch inside. Nose is dry and blocked at night and runs in the day. Nosebleed on blowing. (See **Sticta** in **Nux-vom.** below.)

Kali-bich.: thick, sticky, yellow mucus that clogs up the nose and sinuses with a sensation of obstruction or pinching at the root of the nose. Pains in the frontal sinuses with headache; patient wants pressure on the forehead and maxillary area. Sneezing can bring out strings of foul catarrh that are difficult to detach. If severe, the inside of the nostrils will be full of crusty plugs of mucus that are hard to pick off without causing bleeding. Mouth breathing with nasal sounding voice. Sometimes **Kali-sulph.** or **Hydrastis** do better: **Kali-sulph**. is often used to finish off a simple cold when yellow catarrh is all that needs to be cleared away;

Hydrastis covers thick yellow (even fluorescent coloured) mucus especially from the back of the nose.

Lycopodium: blockage of the nose forces mouth breathing with constant sniffing; hard to blow anything out. At night the nose is dry and blocked causing snoring and a frontal headache. The right nostril may have blocked up first, followed by the left. Mucus rattles in the throat and chest. Feels > for warm drinks which slightly alleviate the blockage temporarily.

Merc-sol.: yellow-green mucus is too thick to run but causes rawness and soreness. Bones around the sinuses feel swollen and painful. Breath smells foul; metallic taste in the mouth. Viscid clear saliva with dribbling in sleep. Very thirsty for cold water. Temperature goes up and down. If the condition keeps relapsing and there is obviously a build-up of phlegm in the chest then you may need to ask your practitioner for **Merc-sulph.** This is especially true if the patient is consistently warm or overheating.

Nat-mur.: cheekbones feel achy and sinuses feel dried up and yet stuffed up. Inside of nose feels sore and swollen; painful to blow hard. Sudden flow of white-of-egg mucus with loss of smell and taste which is brought on by a bout of violent sneezing. Very thirsty and not hungry for anything but savoury snacks. This remedy can be mistaken for **Nat-carb.** which is similar but covers soreness and redness of the nose with great sensitivity to draughts, the sun and dairy products; very cross mood too. **Nat-sulph.** is also similar but less affected by cold; thick yellow mucus with salty tasting catarrh and the tongue is greenish or brown.

Nux-vom.: stuffed up and snuffly breathing with blockage alternating between left and right. Blocked up at night and outside in the cold; running mucus in the day. May complain of ache in gums or teeth as well. Prickly tickles felt in the nose. Especially suited to those who are driven and irritable. **Sticta Pulmonaria** might be considered for a blockage at the root of the nose, dryness of the mucous membranes and a constant need to blow without any discharge.

Pulsatilla: thick, yellow catarrh with dry mouth and throat and no thirst. Loss of smell and taste. Blocked nose > when out in the fresh air, < for being stuffed up indoors. Tongue might be yellowish. Use the 200. Sometimes a **Pulsatilla** is greatly supported by a daily dose of **Silica** 6 or 30.

Sepia: thick, green or yellow ropy mucus which has to be hawked up from the back of the throat. Crusts in the nose. Useful when patient is exhausted and fed up or has just had a period. Nostrils feel sore as cold air is drawn through.

Silica: nose crusts up and bleeds when these are picked out; edges of nostril can crack and be sore. Mucus is whitish and frothy but nose feels dry. Patient complains of sensations in the ears: cracking and popping.

Nosebleeds

The causes of nosebleeds include: trauma, vigorous nose blowing, congestion of the sinuses, rupture of a capillary from removal of crusts, a staphylococcal infection, high blood pressure, liver disease (including alcoholism), anaemia and narrowing of the arteries. Some women with menstrual disorders may have vicarious nosebleeds which are those that take the place of menses. There are also some hereditary diseases which will cause nosebleeds as will certain chronic diseases such as leukaemia. There are some additional reasons why an otherwise healthy person might have a nosebleed; one is consistent use of or living in close proximity to mobile phone technology and another is taking excessive amounts of vitamin B. Bleeding may come from just inside the nostrils or further back towards the bridge. Profuse nosebleeds tend to be of bright red blood; slow ones tend to be of darker blood. Nosebleeds in adults that persist for more than 24 hours may be a sign of hypertension. **Take the patient to hospital.**

It is always sensible to allow a nosebleed to flow for a short while. It is often nature's way of releasing tension, lowering pressure in the system. Common sense should dictate how long is needed, though with some sensitive people loss of even a little blood can cause them to feel faint so advise them to sit forward or to lie down. Pinching the sides of the nose firmly for a minute or two is the first thing to try. If this does not work then run the cold tap and ask the patient to snuff up the cold water; the cold will cause the blood vessels to constrict. If the patient is too young or unwilling to do this then get cotton wool and soak it in the cold water and apply it to the nose. If the patient has been lying down or has the head thrown back then there is a likelihood that a lot of the blood will flow back into the throat and be swallowed which can lead to vomiting. Do not be alarmed if hawked up blood appears dark and clotted. **If the nosebleed is consistently of dark blood then it must be reported to your practitioner.**

There are dozens of remedies for nosebleed. It is easier in first-aid prescribing to go by causation than diagnosis:

- < anger: give **Arsen-alb.** if the patient is bad-tempered from frustration or **Ferr-phos.** if the patient is weak and delicate and coming down with a bug.
- < blows or blowing: from a blow or too vigorous blowing give **Arnica** 30 or 200; for nose blowing in sensitive people who are brewing a cold give **Ferr-phos.** 30.
- < coffee: from getting 'hyped up' and irritable with the need to drink coffee give **Nux-vom.** 30.
- < coughing: **Drosera** 30 (when there is a tickle in the throat) or **Puls.** 30 (when there is dryness and no thirst).
- < emotions: for those who get overemotional and overexcited then feel weak give **Phos.** 30.
- < exertion: give **Arnica** 30. If the bleed comes on after lifting a heavy weight then give **Rhus-tox.** 30.
- < fever: for bleeds during a fever give **Ferr-phos.** 30 or, if very morose and disinclined to move at all, give **Bryonia** 30.
- < headache: for sudden onset during a headache give **Acon.** 30; for a pale feeble person brewing a cold give **Ferr-phos.** 30. If the nosebleed comes on *after* the headache lifts then give **Sepia** 30.
- < menopause: nosebleeds during the menopause are best treated by the professional; if there is a sense of great pressure in the forehead behind the nose which feels < for bending over or sitting down and the bleed comes on from blowing then give **Lach.** 30. (The blood may be thick and dark, bright red or clotted.)
- < overheating: if the patient is hot, light-headed, flustered and air-hungry then give **Puls.** 200. If the patient is too warm, fed up and cross then give **Sepia** 30 or 200. **Belladonna** is needed when the face is flushed

red and the head feels too hot.

- < period: if a bleed comes on during the period give **Sepia** 30 if she is fed up, tearful and lacking in energy or **Bry**. 30 if very thirsty, irritable and fretting about work commitments. If weepy, pale and wanting company give **Puls**. 200. **Sulphur** 30 if tired, floppy, thirsty, hot and 'can't be bothered'.
- < perspiration: if the patient bleeds and sweats at the same time give **Phos**. 30 or 200.
- < straining to pass a stool: give **Phos**. 30.
- < washing the face: **Arnica** 30. If there is a cough as well then give **Drosera** 30.

Children who have frequent nosebleeds are often found to need either **Ferrum Metallicum**, **Phosphorus** or, even more likely, a dose of **Tuberculinum**, any of which should be administered by a homoeopath who will judge the potency and sequence of remedies. Anyone who has a nose that is sensitive and that readily bleeds on slight touch or blowing – a 'bleeder' – is likely to need **Phosphorus** at some point, but in order to select the appropriate potency and timing consult the homoeopath. If a patient feels thoroughly weak after a nosebleed give one dose of **China** 30.

The Thyroid Gland

The thyroid is a butterfly-shaped ductless gland that spans the lower throat just below the Adam's apple. It is integral to maintaining balance in the metabolism. It is notoriously difficult to regulate once its functioning is upset. It is possible to have a malfunctioning thyroid with no sign of it in the blood test; even if a test does show pathological changes, it is not always a good basis for treatment as the organ can be so changeable.

- An overactive thyroid can cause congested sensations in the throat with fast heart rate, trembling, insomnia and a feeling of being rushed. There also might be weight loss and overactive bowels.
- An underactive thyroid is characterised by tiredness, sluggishness, weight gain and constipation; there is chilliness and a low heart rate, dry skin and cold clammy sweating.

However, individuals do not always fall neatly into one or the other of these two categories and may show a mixture of symptoms. As the thyroid is a vital part of the endocrine system, it is necessary to seek advice and treatment from the homoeopath as soon as possible. Though the advice is very likely to include going to the doctor for blood tests remember that homoeopaths are always principally guided by the general and particular symptoms of the individual.

11. CONDITIONS OF THE MOUTH, TEETH, TONGUE AND GUMS

Buccal thrush

Thrush is a version of candida, a fungal infection. It is common in babies, in the old and in those who have an impaired immune system possibly as the result of taking antibiotics or steroids. The symptom picture includes white or off-white patches inside the cheeks which can be scraped away, leaving sore, red areas. For babies who are breastfeeding it is best for the mother to look at her diet: it may be that she is eating things that encourage candida such as too much sugar, dairy products or gluten based food such as bread and pasta. Sometimes mothers have cracked or sore nipples at the same time. For older people with false teeth it is worth considering the state of the dentures which can cause abrasion in the delicate membranes of the mouth. A mouthwash of **Calendula Ø** + **Salvia Officinalis Ø** (in equal parts) is very useful in soothing soreness and maintaining oral hygiene: 5 drops of the tincture in half a glass of water used as a gargle and rinse twice a day. (This is also useful for those who have a tendency to frequent sore throats.) Alternatively, aloe vera from health food shops has anti-candida properties. The most commonly recommended remedy for buccal thrush in children is **Borax** but it only resolves the condition if the rest of the picture is present: sore mouth makes the baby cry when attempting to suckle or eat; there are little ulcers on the inner cheeks and the tongue which might bleed easily; the mouth feels hot and the palate feels burnt; in addition the baby has a dread of being put down into the cot or of being carried downstairs. Without this whole picture **Borax** 6 or 30 may slow or stop the thrush for a while but the condition is likely to need a more thorough approach. In older people the most common remedy is **Nat-mur.** which is indicated when there are small white ulcers with red tops in the mouth which are sore and burning; a 'mapped' tongue (irregular smooth patches on it which make it look like a map); cracked lips and even cold sores. Use 30. The following are other remedies which will help differentiate:

Lac-can.: increased mucus and saliva with swollen glands around the neck and jaw which < and > first on one side and then on the other. Gets cross very quickly but gives the impression of being worried about something.

Merc-sol.: foul breath, dribbling of excessive saliva and strong thirst; the edge of the tongue is indented with teeth marks and the tongue looks enlarged; little, painful ulcers which might bleed.

Kreosotum: this is the remedy to consider for thrush during pregnancy. There is usually a picture of weakness and exhaustion with foul breath and strong thirst.

Nux-vom.: back of the tongue is white and coated; gums also affected and tend to bleed easily; bitter or sour taste. < from getting run down and overstretched at work.

Sulphuric Acid: not a usual first-aid remedy but useful when someone is weakened after a long illness and has gums that bleed easily.

Bryonia: chiefly useful in babies who are thirsty and irritable every time they are disturbed.

Bleeding Gums

Persistent bleeding of gums is a reason to consult your practitioner; though the symptom may not appear threatening it is sometimes a herald of other problems that need professional attention. It might be symptomatic of poor nutritional balance, vitamin deficiency, mercury poisoning from amalgam fillings, anaemia, menopausal changes and unresolved emotional issues. Poor liver function can also contribute to bleeding gums; alcoholics and those on long-term chemotherapy are both susceptible. If the symptom is accompanied by halitosis (bad breath) then it is likely that there is either bacterial infestation of the mouth or that the digestion is disordered. In either case, the problem is not simply local but general and constitutional. For bleeding gums after a tooth extraction (and a dose of **Arnica**) the main remedy is **Phosphorus**: helpful in those who tend to bleed easily and feel weakened by the blood loss. **Calendula** is very helpful when surgery has left a wound that needs to heal quickly. For all three conditions use 30 unless otherwise directed by your practitioner. Apply **Calendula Ø** to the wound.

Mouth Ulcers

Ulcers can appear on the gums, lips, palate or tongue. They may be small, red or white and sore like tiny blisters (aphthae) or large, open sores which exude matter or bleed. Pains range from sharp and pricking to burning. They usually indicate that the patient is run down and in need of rest or a better diet or both; ulcers are a very common reaction to stress. Certain things aggravate ulcers: spicy hot food, acid fruits like tomatoes and citrus fruit, smoking and sometimes sweets. Persistent large ulcers can be the result of mercury poisoning from amalgam fillings, which would be ample reason to have the fillings removed, or because of the syphilitic miasm becoming prevalent. Ulcers on the lips can be the result of the herpes virus; this suggests that long-term constitutional treatment is needed. When looking for identifying symptoms check the colour, shape and quality of the surface of the tongue. To assist the indicated remedy a mouthwash of **Calendula Ø + Salvia Officinalis Ø** (5 drops in a quarter of a glass of water) is soothing; if unavailable then a solution of salt and warm water can do well.

Remedies for small ulcers (aphthae):

Arsen-alb.: white or bluish ulcers on inner cheek or tongue which burn and feel sore; < to touch. Dry mouth with need for sips of water. Tongue is likely to be coated white.

Borax: white ulcers on the tongue or on the inner cheek which tend to bleed; much < from salty or sour food. Mouth feels hot and breath may be hot too. Particularly indicated in children's cases.

Merc-sol.: very sore little ulcers which might be white or yellowish; foul taste with excessive salivation and strong thirst for cold water. Tongue is coated and flabby; can be yellowish or white; teeth indentations along the edges. (Confusingly, sometimes the salivation and thirst symptoms are missing.)

Nat-mur.: small, white ulcers on the tongue, gums and inner cheek which are sore, burning and tend to smart. Breath feels hot and mouth feels dry; very thirsty for cold water. Loss of taste. Dry lips which might be cracked.

Sulphuric Acid: white ulcers on the gums and palate which are sore and tend to bleed; tend to be more common in those who are going through a long illness or are chronically ill, especially children who do not put on weight, have poor nutrition and weak digestion.

Remedies for large ulcers (note that persistent large ulcers should be a reason to consult your practitioner):

Kali-iod.: ulcers on the inner cheeks or gums which have a milky-white surface; the edges are irregular. Pains are burning. (Not a first-aid remedy but if needed for persistent ulcers it is worth keeping a supply. It is a very deep-acting remedy so discuss its use with your practitioner.)

Merc-sol.: ulcers which spread and have irregular jagged edges; grey surface. Foul metallic taste, salivation and strong thirst. (If this form of ulcer persists then strongly suspect mercury poisoning from amalgam fillings and/or the syphilitic miasm; consult your practitioner.)

Nitric Acid: ulcers from biting the inside of the cheek; pains are sharp and needle-like. Tongue is fissured with lots of tiny cracks; might be flabby or swollen. Gums can feel spongy. Usually the patient feels very sensitive, negative and pessimistic.

There are many other remedies for mouth ulcers but they are indicated in conditions that should be handled by your practitioner. On occasion, ulcers might not be healed until deep, constitutional and miasmatic work has been done. This is why ulcers can be a way into deeper healing.

Halitosis – Bad Breath

Bad breath can be caused by poor dental hygiene when bacteria build up in between the teeth and around the gums, or by poor digestion with any attendant problems such as poor nutrition, liver congestion, microbial parasites or food allergy among the causes. Breath might also smell rank after an acute illness or a hangover; it can be unpleasant when there is copious infected mucus. Smokers are also susceptible to foul breath not just from the cigarettes but because inhaled smoke affects the lungs and causes them to be congested. Sometimes certain odours are associated with specific diseases: the smell of urine on the breath is a sign of advanced kidney disease; the smell of acetone (like nail varnish remover) is a sign of severe diabetes. **Both require immediate professional treatment!**. If the cause is in the mouth then the answer lies in better oral hygiene. Use dental floss and interdental brushes to remove all particles of food and follow up with gentle brushing. A mouth wash of aloe vera or a combination tincture of **Calendula Ø** and **Salvia Officinalis Ø** can also be helpful: 5 drops in a quarter cup of water. If there are microbial parasites in the liver, a course of black walnut and wormwood capsules is recommended in addition to milk thistle supplement from the health food shop. **Nux Vomica** 6 or 30 is indicated for bad breath with hangover.

Tooth Abscesses

Abscesses in the gums and around the teeth are never simply local affairs. They are a local manifestation of a deeper condition that involves both the immune system and the liver, the organ that generates heat in the body. It is important to see abscesses in this light because the usual treatment is to take antibiotics which suppress not only the local infection but also the body's chosen manner of elimination. The best treatment is to promote and speed up the process to a quick resolution. Sometimes amalgam fillings contribute to tooth abscesses. It may be that the abscess is developing where there is a root canal filling; this is not uncommon and it is a reason to consider carefully whether this form of treatment is a good idea in the first place. Consult your homoeopath about both of these matters. In other cases it may be that the liver is congested from poor diet or alcohol. Occasionally the abscess represents a safer mode of elimination and a better site for pus formation than previous acute inflammation e.g. if someone with mastitis has been treated with antibiotics several times and now produces an abscess below a molar. If there has been previous suppression then it is best for the homoeopath to be involved. If not then the following remedies are common solutions:

Hepar-sulph.: abscess forms in the gum with sharp, splinter pains; very sensitive to any touch or chewing. Generally does not want to be touched or questioned too much; irritable! See **Myristica** below.

Lachesis: decay below a filled molar (upper left) causes pressure, swelling and heat in a developing abscess. Pains can vary but are always bad: throbbing, drawing and boring. Pains in limbs on the other side of body and < if the period is due are also characteristic. Patient may not be particularly coherent and will be bad-tempered.

Merc-sol.: abscess with increased salivation, foul (metallic or bloody) taste and strong thirst for cold water. Pains are sharp and tend to go up into the ear or jaw. Use 30 or 200.

Myristica: is a blood cleansing remedy and is similar to **Hepar-sulph.** and sometimes works even more swiftly. When used in conjunction with **Silica** (see below) it is often all that is required to deal with uncomplicated abscesses. Give the 200 one per day and **Silica** 30 one twice a day. Continue for up to 10 days. If progress is halted or slow after a week then consult your practitioner in case there is an underlying constitutional reason for lack of complete success.

Pyrogen: is a powerful blood cleansing remedy that is only needed if there is a deep-seated constitutional toxicity. The abscess will be deep, slow to develop and darkish red. The breath is putrid. The patient will feel as if 'flu is coming on with aching all over and a dark flushed complexion. Use 30 or 200 but bear in mind that your practitioner should be advising you.

Silica: is a remedy for slow-developing abscesses with intermittent sharpish pains. It can encourage an indolent abscess to come to the surface or to be dispersed by the body by absorption. It can also be used in tandem with **Myristica** (see above).

Teething

Teething pains without complications are often quite simple to treat. The remedy is indicated by its keynote symptoms:

Aconite: sudden onset with heat in the face, redness and need to chew on something. Fretful and whiny with disturbed sleep. The child is thirsty for cold water. Pains may be accompanied by a persistent cough. Use 30.

Belladonna: pains come on with a fever; radiant heat from the face with glassy eyes and red cheek. Restlessness and whining mood with foul nappies. Use 30 or 200.

Chamomilla: pains with a very disagreeable mood. Child cannot tolerate the pain and becomes inconsolable and very angry; demands things that they reject when they are given; wants to be carried everywhere. Use 30 or 200.

Unfortunately, teething can be complicated. The following is a common list of teething complications:

- < constipation: **Kreosotum** (pains < at night with hard, dry stools; child is weak and delicate; new teeth may come through with signs of decay); **Silica** (sweaty feet and hands with straining to pass stools which start to protrude but then recede). Use 30.
- < diarrhoea: **Borax** (watery, yellow stools); **Calc-c.** (usually slow dentition in general); **Calc-phos.** (with restlessness, irritability, flatulence, greenish stools, weakness and a desire for salty or savoury things); **Cham.** (stools smell like rotten eggs); **Podophyllum** (stools are yellow, frothy and accompanied by loud and foul wind); **Rheum** (sour smelling diarrhoea; whole child smells sour and is very irritable and restless). Use 30.
- < high fever (and even convulsions): **Belladonna** 200.
- < eye symptoms: **Belladonna** (dilated pupils, glassy look, red conjunctiva and photophobia); **Calc-c.** (red, swollen, itchy and watery in the open air; sometimes has a squint while teething); **Puls.** (pus exudes from the eyes, < left). Use 30.

- < insomnia: **Coffea** (too wide awake with restlessness); **Cypripedium** (wakes with a cry then wide awake with agitation or playfulness); **Scutellaria** (wakes from a nightmare and feels restless and irritable). Use 6 or 30.
- < intolerance of milk: it is advisable to consult your practitioner for this though either **Aethusa** (vomiting of thick curds of milk with thick congestion of the airways, general weakness and sweat, crying and marked dopiness), **Calc-c.** (baby smells sour and has a sweaty head) or **Mag-mur.** (regurgitates white frothy mucus, passes milk undigested and has a bloated, hard abdomen) might be needed. Use 30.
- < sores on the gums: **Arsen-alb.** (blisters on gum above tooth that is coming through; pale, shrivelled, anxious look; restlessness and easy vomiting of food; < night time); **Borax** (little sores on the gums that are very sensitive to least touch; salivation; child screams in pain and distress when lowered into the cot). Use 30.
- < swollen gums: **Bryonia** 30 (dry, red lips with hot, dry swollen gums; child averse to being moved; very thirsty).

For children whose teeth take an unconscionable time to come through it is sometimes helpful to give them **Calc-phos.** tissue salt twice daily. (If they are undergoing constitutional treatment discuss this with the homoeopath.) Chamomilla teething granules are available from the pharmacy; these are tiny grains that are easy to administer and baby-friendly. They will alleviate symptoms when **Chamomilla** is homoeopathic to the condition.

Toothache

Mild toothache might be caused by little more than inadequate oral hygiene: food stuck between teeth can cause irritation, swelling and sensitivity in the gums. Interdental brushes, floss and gentle brushing are all that is necessary unless the symptoms have gone too far and infection has set in. Otherwise toothache is usually the first subjective symptom of dental decay. It often begins with mild sensitivity to hot and cold and to chewing on hard food. If this is ignored it can lead to excruciating pain which can seem to extend beyond the affected tooth. Toothache might also be caused by an infection in the sinuses closest to the tooth that seems to hurt most, though the nerve affected, the trigeminal, can cause confusion by referring pain sensations to another site such as the teeth and gum directly opposite in the lower jaw. Pain may also start up in teeth below where an abscess is forming; when this happens it is characteristic that pain comes and goes intermittently which encourages delay in consulting the dentist. Sometimes, congestion and infection in the maxillary sinus (under the eyes and beside the nose) can aggravate a chronic, slow-developing abscess around the incisors which only seems to be a problem when the immune system is lowered enough to allow the sinusitis. Taking decongestants might alleviate the immediate pressure on the abscess but it does nothing for the chronic condition. Most people take analgesics for toothache and hope it will just go away. This is not a good idea as delay can cause deeper trouble. Even if you ask your homoeopath or find the indicated remedy for the pain, make an appointment with your dentist! It is not advisable to use oil of cloves as it is likely to antidote remedies! In most cases use the 30th potency: one every 2 to 3 hours.

Aconite: pain is excruciating, throbbing and < at night; < after catching cold. Redness of the cheek on side affected. Sudden onset especially < after being in a north or east wind. Often needed by children. Pain can appear in healthy teeth. Use 30 or 200.

Arnica: the best remedy for pain after dentistry. Give a 30 every 4 hours for the first day. If severe then use a 200 twice per day for several days. Can be alternated with **Hypericum** which will help with nerve pain.

Belladonna: gum feels swollen and hot with sharp or digging, boring pains; face might be hot and red on affected side or toothache comes on with fever. Pain comes on a little while after eating and gradually increases to a high point and then wears off. Teeth on the right side are particularly affected. Cheek can appear swollen.

Bryonia: pains are all < for warm food and drink and > for cold water. Pains < any movement but > from pressure. Tooth characteristically feels too long. Cheek swells on affected side < right. Molars are especially affected. Pain can be confusing as it often seems to be in a healthy tooth referred from one with decay.

Chamomilla: unendurable pain in one side of jaw without being able to pinpoint the offending tooth. Area is swollen and red and has sharp, digging pain < eating or drinking anything warm or cold or becoming too warm in bed. Pains always stoke a very bad temper; peevish and no one can do anything right for the patient. Babies want to be picked up and carried about. Pain in healthy teeth. (Use the 200 when pain is severe.)

China: pains << from touch; < left side; < during breastfeeding; < upper teeth. Often accompanied by digestive disturbance: flatulence, bloating and belching with a strong thirst and desire for easily digested but piquant food. < from eating fruit. Pains come on intermittently and are throbbing as if blood were filling up the tooth. Pains > for pressing teeth together. Very irritable with the pain.

Coffea: unendurable pains that cause weeping and throwing oneself about in agony. Wants to hold ice in the mouth or to drink fridge-cold water to relieve the pain. Pains are < night-time; < after eating a meal with warm food. Especially useful in excitable people. Pain in healthy teeth. Wants to bite teeth together.

Gunpowder: useful for toothache with abscess; can be given while waiting for the dentist when there is pain in a gathering abscess with or without suppuration; useful when other indicated remedies do not help. Can be alternated with **Hecla Lava**.

Hecla Lava: toothache with abscess especially where there is infection deep into the bone.

Hepar-sulph.: during the pain teeth feel hollow or too long. Very sensitive in every respect: irritable and < from touch or pressure. Can't bear to bite teeth together. Gums may bleed easily.

Kreosotum: patient is likely to have advanced tooth decay. Pains usually < in the upper left-side molars and extend into the ear and jaw. Likely to have foul breath; soft, bleeding gums which look unhealthy. Sometimes indicated in pain during pregnancy.

Lachesis: pains are usually < left side and < into the left ear. Sensation of pressure in gums that appear slightly bluish. Bad breath and dry lips.

Waking from pains at night. (See 'Tooth Abscesses' above.)

Mag-carb.: perhaps the main remedy to use for cutting the wisdom teeth: pains are boring, sore or throbbing and there is swelling of the cheek. Pains > cold drink. Generally < being still too long; > for moving about doing something. Also consider for toothache during pregnancy. (The 200 is useful when dealing with wisdom teeth.)

Merc-sol. pains from decay in the teeth usually < right side. Excessive salivation, metallic taste and bad taste usual concomitant symptoms. < at night; very thirsty for cold water. Pain feels burning and aching; wants to rub the gum below.

Nitric Acid: pains with swollen, bleeding gums or soft, spongy gums; are pale. Teeth feel loose. Pains are sharp and stabbing and < just before bedtime and through the night. Patient is excessively peevish and difficult to live with; inclined to be quarrelsome with the pains.

Nux Vomica: pains are < cold drinks and food but > warm drinks. Cheek becomes swollen and pain can shoot along the jaw from bad tooth and even up into the temple. Glands nearby might swell. A remedy for gumboils: swollen and ready to burst.

Plantago: often useful when other remedies are not indicated clearly; pains in tooth which is decaying rapidly. Usually there is a lot of salivation while the pain is there. This remedy can be used both in the 6th or 30th potency and in mother tincture form (Ø) and applied directly.

Puls.: typical is that pain is > for holding cold water in the mouth around the affected tooth (which feels loose). Pains are always < in the evening and through the night. Pains are > when outside in the fresh air. Sometimes indicated in toothache during pregnancy. It is often best to use the 200 here.

Sepia: usually indicated in those with period symptoms (see general picture in part III). Decay in molars causes dull, stupefying pains that drag the patient down; > when out for a walk or doing exercise.

Silica: teeth feel too long and loose. Useful in children who are losing their baby teeth. Pains can be boring or sharp and might go into jaw, the cheekbones or up into the ear. Gum looks sore and red; gumboil with sticking pain. (See 'Tooth Abscesses' above.)

Staphysagria: pains from teeth blackened by decay; gnawing, drilling pains that feel to be in the roots deep below the gums (which bleed easily). Teeth have a history of being crumbly and in need of filling. Glands below the jaw may be swollen.

Tooth Decay

The remedies for the pains of tooth decay are listed above. Decay occurs in various ways:
  • on the smooth surface especially between the teeth when care is not taken to remove particles of food with floss or interdental brushes;
  • on the slightly ridged surface of the back teeth and the grooves of the chewing surface of the molars when brushing is insufficient to remove the build-up of bacteria between teeth and cheek where they can eat away at the enamel;
  • on enamel that has been chipped and left unattended;
  • in the root when gum has receded and left bone exposed that is not carefully cleaned.

Things which can contribute to tooth decay include sweets, saccharine-rich drinks, junk food, alcohol, tobacco, poor dental hygiene, a lowered immune system, chronic ill health (especially when aggravated by pain) and heredity. As I mentioned above the best way to avoid decay is careful brushing with a relatively soft-bristled brush, cleaning between the teeth with dental floss and, where possible, with an interdental brush. Fluoride in any form is NOT a good idea as it is a poison! Despite its use by the dental profession and by toothpaste manufacturers, it has toxic effects which compromise the immune system; the tonsils are particularly affected.

It is always best to be in consultation with your practitioner about early tooth decay as it is indicative of chronic conditions even if these do not have any other serious manifestation. Despite the list of contributory factors, teeth only start to decay if there is any problem with nutrition, excessive acidity or poor elimination of waste and toxicity, or if there is a hereditary disposition to easy decay (which very often involves the other problems). Decay can begin very early indeed; milk teeth are increasingly susceptible and sometimes come through grey or even black in very young children. Although nothing can be done to save such teeth, this must be treated by a dentist *and* the homoeopath because a lot can be done to boost the constitution and limit the indicated miasmatic influence that would otherwise affect not only the adult teeth but other aspects of general health as well. Teeth with white staining suggest a constitution that has been medicated with multiple antibiotics.

Orthodontic Work

Many children see the orthodontist in order to have braces fitted to change the position of teeth and to create a more satisfactory 'bite'. Sometimes teeth are removed to achieve this though it is always best to consult an orthodontist who is not too ready to create space by taking teeth out; removing teeth can change the shape of one's jaw and features. (There are other methods which encourage the jaw to grow to fit the teeth.) If braces or 'railtracks' are fitted it is worth knowing about **Calc-fluor.**, a remedy that is unrivalled for that aching, gnawing discomfort stemming from tension in teeth and jaw from tightening the apparatus. Use the 6 (or 30 if the pains are bad) up to one 3 times per day while the discomfort persists. The remedy made from **Sycamore Seed** is also excellent in this situation and complements **Calc-fluor.** The 30 can be given 2 or 3 times per week while the process of change is continuing. It is very important to have cranial osteopathic treatment during orthodontic work because the changes wrought on the shape of the jaw alter the balance of the head and the way it 'sits' on the spine. Without making sure that the spine is also prepared for the changes it is likely that back problems would ensue in the future. There are many who develop chronic back pains partly as a result of not having been aware of the significance of the influence of altered balance from braces round the teeth!

Mercury Fillings: Amalgam

Mercury fillings are NOT safe whatever you may hear to the contrary; the British Dental Association still sees little wrong with amalgam fillings despite the gradual shift in worldwide opinion. Though some people are more susceptible to the effects of the metal than others, it is vital to understand that mercury is a poison and has a wide range of side effects that are well documented. Mercury is an unstable liquid metal which is mixed with four other metals to create a flexible but hard amalgam filling for cavities. When mixed with other metals or heated, mercury becomes 'active' and starts to 'leach' its toxicity into the system. (Gold fillings in the same mouth as amalgams exaggerate this.) Not only are tiny particles given off into the system but also the amalgam acts like a battery and gives off electrical current which interferes with the central nervous system. Particles leached out into the saliva whenever one chews or has a hot drink eventually find their way into the bloodstream and thence to the soft organs such as brain, liver and kidneys where they are most readily stored. The side effects of these two events can range from the insignificant to the catastrophic.

The following is what can be ascribed directly to mercury poisoning: excessive salivation, foul taste, halitosis, swollen glands, susceptibility to oral infection, swollen tonsils, mouth ulcers, tooth abscesses, acidosis and heartburn, excessive thirst, gastric disturbance, alternation of diarrhoea and constipation, sudden incontinence of stool, imbalance of bowel flora, susceptibility to candidiasis and yeast infestation, anaemia, severe pruritis (itching), depression, poor memory, clumsiness, slow reactions and senility. Such side effects can appear as part of the description of diagnosable conditions and thus not as symptoms of toxicity; many cases of candida, thrush, heartburn, irritable bowel syndrome, chronic fatigue, diabetes and high blood pressure (among others) may be derived from mercury poisoning.

Removal of fillings has to be done with great care and by a practitioner well-versed in the protocol necessary. It is always advised to go to a dentist who is sympathetic to alternative methods and can work alongside your homoeopath. Where possible they should use rubber dams that prevent tiny particles of mercury becoming embedded in the tongue and soft palate as the amalgams are drilled out.

You should be given the choice of 'white' fillings, which are made of acrylic, and porcelain ones which are derived from clay. The white fillings are better because porcelain fillings tend to absorb X-ray radiation quite readily. White fillings are more difficult to work with because they have to be put in in stages, each level being allowed to dry.

The replacement of amalgams is not available on the NHS so it is expensive. Nevertheless, it is extremely important to do it if mercury is at the root of any health problem.

Remedies to be taken during the removal process may include **Merc-sol.** and **Amalgam** in potency. **Sarsaparilla** 3, 3 times daily is advisable as it encourages the system to remove mercury from the soft organs, the so-called chelation process. Remedy, potency and frequency should be decided by your practitioner. A dose of **Emerald** 30 before each extraction can help with the removal. A dose or two of **Arnica** 30 or 200 afterwards is often a good idea to relieve strain from the jaw. After the removal of all the amalgam fillings it is well worthwhile consulting a nutritionist who can suggest supplements for chelation: using chemicals such as chlorella to bind with the mercury and carry them out of the body.

12   THE CHEST AND UPPER RESPIRATORY TRACT

Croup

Croup is a condition associated with the activity of any of various different viruses – too many to be of any significance in making a diagnosis. It is usually a climax of the development of a cold or influenza in very young children and sometimes it can be part of a process that leads into whooping cough (see pages 79–80). It is characterised by narrowing of the airways from swollen mucous membranes which brings on difficulty in breathing and a harsh, 'barking' cough. It is often hard for the child to breathe in. There can be rapid, short breathing, or deep and laboured breathing in and short breathing out. In some there is rattling of mucus in the chest and in others it sounds as if the lungs must be dry. The cough is spasmodic and often wakes the child. It is usually much worse at night and easier again in the day. Croup may or may not be accompanied by fever. It is a condition that does require careful watching as it occurs in the very young and the symptoms can change rapidly. It is often necessary to ensure that the airways are kept open by propping the patient up and also that fluid intake is maintained. **If vomiting is a symptom then involve your practitioner at once as choking on vomit is dangerous.**

'Steaming' can be very helpful if the throat and cough sound very dry though do not use any eucalyptus or other oils for inhalation. A child who has croup several times often does not lose the cough in between bouts and they are then suspected of having asthma. Beware of this diagnosis as it leads to permanent use of inhalers which will keep the airways open but generally weaken the whole economy of the body and create a chronic state out of a series of acute attacks. For this reason croup **must** be reported to your practitioner; it requires constitutional treatment not least because croup is often a chronic effect of the DPT vaccination complicating the inherited effects of the tubercular miasm. If the patient has been coughing and retching for more than 24 hours, despite initial treatment, call your homoeopath. Occasionally a child will not respond to indicated remedies and the symptoms of croup become so alarming that hospital becomes the only course to take. This situation usually occurs when there is a hereditary disposition to lung conditions and the child, unwittingly, is responding to an ongoing emotional crisis within the family. If a child has been taken to hospital for croup and has had to have suppressive treatment, report this to your homoeopath at once so that remedial steps can be taken to relieve the system of chemical toxicity.

Croup often starts suddenly at around midnight. This alone indicates **Aconite** as an initial remedy though it covers many of the other symptoms: dryness, heat and fearfulness; hoarse, hacking cough; difficult, short breathing. A dose of the 200 will often ease the symptoms immediately. However, it is often not the only remedy needed; it is followed well by **Spongia** and **Hepar-sulph.** The main remedies for croup are **Aconite, Arsen-alb., Bell., Hepar-sulph., Lach., Phos., Rumex** and **Spon.** (see 'Cough' below). **Ant-Tart.** 200 is a valuable remedy to keep in stock in a family prone to croup or other chest conditions; it is the remedy to give for desperate breathing difficulties while waiting for professional advice.

Listening to the Lungs

Sometimes it is instructive to put your ear to the patient's chest to see if you can hear which part of the lungs is affected. This is because certain remedies have an affinity for specific parts of the chest. The two lungs are made up of three lobes on the right side (top, middle and lower) and two on the left (upper and lower). You need to listen to both front and back for a full picture. In someone who is well you should be able to hear very little apart from the heartbeat which is strongest centrally. In someone with a chest infection you might hear anything from rasping to wheezing, crackling to bubbling. Though it takes a practised ear to tell the difference between remedies from the quality of sound, it is possible to detect whether one or other lobe is most affected. The following list may help to determine the choice of remedy and to describe the situation to your homoeopath over the phone:

- Right upper lobe: **Ant-tart., Arsen-alb., Calc-c., Bell., Bry.** (especially to the side and in the back)
- Right middle lobe: **Ant-tart., Bell., Bry., Chel., Ferr-phos., Lyc., Merc-sol., Sulph.**
- Right lower lobe: **Ant-tart., Bry., Chel.** (extends from right side into bottom of lungs in the back), **Ferr-phos., Kali-c., Lyc.** (over some hours condition spreads from right lung to left), **Merc-sol.,** (extends front to back), **Sulph.**
- Left upper lobe: **Acon., Ant-tart., Phos., Puls., Sil., Sulph.**
- Left lower lobe: **Ant-tart., Kali-c., Lyc.** (after spreading from right side), **Nat-sulph., Phos., Rumex, Sil.**

Ant-tart. is indicated anywhere in the lungs because it covers profuse quantities of bubbling, rattling mucus throughout the lungs with racking cough.

Coughs

Coughs can be hard nuts to crack because of the enormous variety of symptoms and the many different aspects to take into consideration. If the cough is the result of a cold or 'flu it is likely to need one of the common remedies (marked with * in the following list). The symptoms of the cough might be in the pharynx (as you turn the corner from the mouth into the throat), the larynx (the throat down to the throat pit), the trachea (the main windpipe before the lungs), the bronchus (the main tube into the lungs) or the bronchioles (the smaller tubes that carry the air in and out of the lungs) – either on the left or the right side. It might be 'dry' or 'wet'; it might be worse or better for a host of reasons: day or night; hot or cold drinks; inside or outside, etc. The sound of the cough can be deep, explosive, hacking, hoarse, hollow, racking, rattling or ringing and it might seem wheezy, suffocative or teasing. Some cough remedies are identified more readily by the general symptoms (**Bell.**: high fever, redness and pulsation) rather than the specific symptoms of the cough itself. Others are recognisable by the sound alone (**Spon.**: sounds like a saw cutting through a plank of wood). As coughs are difficult to identify, the list of remedies is divided into two sections. If you do not have success then you should consult your practitioner within 3 days; a neglected persistent cough can lead to or indicate other problems. Other reasons which might underlie a chronic cough include: an allergy, liver dysfunction, heartburn with hiatus hernia, chronically held poor posture (ever since an accident, for example), passive or active smoking or a long-unexpressed emotional reason. (Chronic coughs that do not originate from a cold or 'flu should be professionally investigated!)

Emergency Coughs

Aconite: sudden attack of dry, barking cough around midnight with straining to breathe in, great anxiety and fever. < since getting cold in a wind.

Ant-tart.: covers suffocative, rattling cough with much mucus in the lungs though little is brought up. Every cough leaves the patient gasping; they are weak, weary and irritable. There is retching and gagging with the cough and eventual vomiting brings up mucus that has been swallowed. The mucus in the lungs is audible as rattling. The patient wants to sit up but is too weak to do so for long. It is very characteristic for the patient to bend backwards to cough. After coughing and vomiting there is pallor and sleep. Use 200; 1M or even 10M (after discussion with your homoeopath) in those with a history of breathing and lung problems. Very useful in an asthma acute; this is a remedy that can prevent the need to go to hospital.

Belladonna: a short, dry, barking cough which can be violent enough to cause bloodshot eyes. Breathing will be short and shallow and there will be radiant heat. The fever may be general and very high or local to the forehead. The mouth and breath are likely to be hot as well.

Carbo-veg.: catarrhal cough with deep spasms of coughing which leave the patient breathless, sweaty on the forehead and blue round the lips. Must sit up at 45°; sits and pants or gasps between bouts of coughing. Typical in bronchitis of the elderly or in late stage of acute in the young.

Cuprum: dry, suffocative spasms of coughing which prevent any breathing or speaking. Cough comes in bouts of long coughs; often 3 at a time. Cough < 3 a.m. or < hiccoughs. A drink of cold water temporarily eases but may refuse it as they can't bear anything near the mouth.

Lachesis: choking cough with sensation of being throttled and suffocated < lying down. Desperate to take a deep breath of cool air. Coughing exaggerates any pains in the tonsils or throat. Cough < at night and wakes with a start or a paroxysm. Fearful to go to sleep.

Phosphorus: cough with rawness and burning from the throat to the bottom of the ribcage. Tearing sensation at each cough and likely to bring up blood with any mucus. Wants to sit up but is too weak; cannot lie on the left side. Cough is often complicated by a splitting headache.

See also **Hepar-sulph.** and **Kali-carb.** below.

Acute Cough

'Wh/c' indicates a remedy that is useful in whooping cough.

*Aconite: sudden attack of coughing < for being out in a cold north or east wind and getting chilled; short, dry and barking. Breathing becomes strained and cold air <. After taking **Aconite** the symptoms may change to those of a proper cold; if so, leave well alone and allow the symptoms to work themselves out.

*Ant-tart.: one of the main remedies for cough after a cold or 'flu that will not respond to rest and care. Lots of phlegm rattling in the chest which is hard to bring up; weakness and lassitude make it hard to cough. Must sit up to cough; gasps for breath before each bout. Cough is < at night and in early morning. Can usefully be alternated with any other indicated remedy if necessary except **Kali-sulph.** but especially **Arsen-alb., Bry., Carbo-veg., Ipecac., Hepar-sulph., Kali-carb., Phos. Sepia and Sulph.** (Wh/c)

Apis: characteristic ringing sound to the cough which comes on from irritation behind the sternum and from swollen membranes in the larynx. Top of the chest and larynx feel restricted and dry. Child may scream before or between coughing bouts. Panting breathing. Retching with coughing.

Arg-nit.: cough with hoarse voice, thick, tough phlegm and a sensation of either a hair or a splinter in the throat. Back of the throat may be dark red and the trachea is raw and sore. Cough < from laughing, talking, singing, passive smoking and in a hot, crowded atmosphere. Coughing may bring on belching, gagging or retching. (Wh/c)

*Arsen-alb.: short, dry cough with difficulty in raising irritating phlegm; what mucus there is, is frothy and may be flecked with blood. Dry mouth with need to take sips of cold water to lubricate throat. < at night and must sit up to cough. Sensation of vapour in throat pit. < going upstairs or uphill. Words of sympathy during a coughing fit only make it worse. (Wh/c)

*Belladonna: dry, short cough with tickling in the trachea and rapid breathing. Pain in the larynx and stomach on coughing. The tongue has the appearance of a strawberry and the breath may be hot. Child cries before coughing especially if the cough is < night. Stiff neck from coughing. Head is hot even if there is no marked fever. (Wh/c)

*Bryonia: hard, dry cough from a crawling, tickling sensation with very strong thirst for cold water or a warm drink. Very characteristic for the patient to press in on the sternum when they cough. Cough < from eating and drinking which leads to gagging, retching and vomiting. Stitching pains in the chest. If there is a headache as well, each cough feels as if the head will split open. Cough < coming from outside into a warm room; < from any movement. In older people or in menopausal women the cough can cause stress incontinence. This remedy is useful in pleurisy and bronchitis; if you suspect either condition then consult your practitioner! (Wh/c)

Calc-c.: persistent, painless, irritating cough with hoarse voice and sticky mucus that is difficult to shift. Feels as if there is dust in the airways. Cough < for climbing stairs; must sit down after a bout of coughing. Periodically the mucus increases and loosens and comes up yellow and sickly. Useful for those who had a cold which never quite finished.

*Carbo-veg.: effortful coughing with hoarse voice from thick mucus which is yellow/green when brought up. Short of breath; > when fanned. Gagging and retching, even vomiting from coughing. Burning sensations in chest; red nose with bluish tinge round mouth and sweat on brow after coughing. Cough < evening and night; < change of temperature.

Sensation of vapour in throat pit. Long cough comes in threes. (Wh/c)

Causticum: cough with loss of voice < after being in a draught or air conditioning; < overuse of voice. Dry cough with feeling that one can't breathe deep enough; sensation of a streak of rawness down the throat. Cough and rawness > by a swallow of cold water.

Chamomilla: cough with filthy temper. Child is unreasonable and fretful; sensitive to pains and < by coughing. Anger < the cough.

Coccus Cacti: frequent bouts of short, racking coughs from tickling in the trachea which eventually bring up quantities of clear strings of mucus which hang from mouth. Face goes dark red from the effort of coughing. Spasms of coughing in the morning; < from brushing teeth. (Wh/c)

Corallium Rubrum: known as the 'minute gun cough' because of the regularity of the paroxysms of short, barking cough. Gasping for breath before coughing. Cough < for profuse post-nasal drip. Airways feel cold on taking in breath. Palate and throat feel dry and scraped. Patient is often drowsy. (Wh/c)

Cuprum: long, violent, spasmodic coughs which are > from swallows of cold water. Nasty metallic taste in the mouth. Cannot speak from coughing; face looks distorted, pinched and pale or bluish. (Wh/c; see **Ipecac.**)

*Drosera: cough < tickling in the throat which < as soon as one lies down and < after midnight. Spasms of coughing that cause breathlessness. Trachea feels dry and the cough sounds deep, hacking and hollow. Patient has to hold the chest with both hands while coughing. Cough also < laughing, talking, crying and becoming too warm. (Wh/c)

Dulcamara: wet cough < in the winter or early spring from catching cold in cold, wet weather. Despite the copious mucus, must cough a lot to bring it all up. Cough and cold sores on the lips.

*Hepar-sulph.: rattling, very hoarse cough with loose, choking phlegm; child can sound as if they are suffocating while lying in bed at night. Needs to sit up and bend head back in order to cough better. Cough is much < for getting cold or having a cold drink; even for putting an arm out of the covers. Cough with sore throat with stitching pains into the ear (< R). Follows **Aconite** well especially in croup.

Ipecac.: cough with tight chest, rattling mucus and sensation as if something were lodged in the trachea. Cough with gagging, retching and vomiting; cough brings on nausea. Tongue looks shiny and smooth as if covered with glassy saliva. Fit of convulsive coughing makes the whole body go rigid and causes blueness of the face (see **Cuprum**). This is indicated when there is a nose bleed with the cough. (Wh/c)

Kali-bich.: hard, dry metallic cough which is < thick, yellow, stringy mucus that is very hard to shift. Cough with sinusitis and pains in the sinuses above the eyes and tickling in the middle of the chest. Wheezy breathing.

Kali-carb.: cough always < 2 – 5 a.m. or coughs day and night trying to dislodge mucus that only comes up occasionally in small gelatinous gobs or otherwise has to be swallowed. Sometimes small balls of mucus fly out of the mouth with coughing. Whole chest feels sensitive and cold. Stitching pains in chest with the cough (this may be a sign of pleurisy or bronchitis). It is important to be in touch with your homoeopath if you are using this remedy in case symptoms suddenly worsen!

Lachesis: see 'Emergency Coughs' above.

*Lycopodium: cough is deep and hollow from the bottom of the chest with tickling in the airways. Irritation and constant manufacture of catarrh in the trachea with sniffing and snuffly breathing. Right side of chest sounds crackly with phlegm. Catarrh brought up is thick and yellow or greenish. Sensation of vapour in throat pit. Patient is very likely to be windy and bloated. Cough is < between 4 and 8 (a.m. and p.m.).

Merc-sol.: cough with cold and sore throat; hard, racking and violent. < at night. Cough with salivation, enlarged tonsils and foul smelling breath. Cough consists of 2 short coughs in quick succession which is repeated frequently.

Nat-mur.: cough after a cold with dryness of mucous membranes, tickling in the throat; < by being in a draught. Cough can be accompanied by a hammering headache which is < for every fit of coughing (see **Hepar-sulph.**). Stitching pain in the right side below the ribs with every cough. Eyes water with coughing.

*Nux-vom.: cough brings on a bad headache. Dry cough with tight chest which tires the patient; all < for exertion and continuing to work hard. Wants to eat something during the cough. Warm drinks >. Snuffly breathing (see **Lyc.** and **Puls.**). Should avoid coffee and beer.

*Phosphorus: raw, burning chest with the cough; hard, dry, rough and tickling which causes exhaustion. Feels trembly after coughing fit. Wants to hold chest together while coughing. Can't lie down on left side. Sharp stitching pain above one eye with every cough. Brings up coloured sputum which is blood streaked. Sometimes cough is caused by the strong smell of chemicals; feels as if lungs are penetrated by the effects of fumes.

*Pulsatilla: cough keeps changing symptoms; dry cough at night but loose and rattling in the day. Copious expectoration on waking which is thick and yellow. Cough comes in fits of 2 coughs at a time; < from a tickle as from a vapour in the trachea; < as soon as patient lies down (see Dros.). Coughing = watery eyes (see **Nat-mur.**). Gagging and retching with cough. (Patient must avoid milk which they may want.)

Rhus-tox.: dry, teasing cough with tickling in the bronchus, in the upper mid chest. Tearing pains in the chest and sweating on coughing. Taste of blood in the mouth. Comes on with a cold from getting chilled and wet.

*Rumex: suffocative, choking cough which comes on when cold air reaches the throat pit. Patient wants to hold a scarf against nose and mouth to prevent cold air < cough. Chest gets tighter at night and is < at 11 p.m., 2 a.m. and 5 a.m. Cough can be < change of atmosphere and room temperature. Cough is < from talking especially towards evening. Sore feeling in the tops of both lungs below the collar bones. (Wh/c)

Sepia: cough after a cold with thick greenish mucus; tickling in larynx brings on a dry, exhausting cough. Coughs during sleep; on waking brings up foul mucus; leaves a salty taste. At other times of day has to swallow the little mucus brought up as it cannot quite be expectorated. Cough sometimes ends with a sneeze. Feels generally heavy, sagging.

Silica: suffocative cough after a cold with swollen glands (under the chin and sometimes in the nape of the neck). Thick yellow-green mucus with a suffocative cough < at night. Cough < lying down at night; < any effort or drinking, eating or talking. Pale or waxy complexion with sores at the mouth corners.

*Spongia: dry, barking cough that sounds like a saw going through wood. Breathing is difficult with the sensation that the patient is breathing through a dry sponge at the top of the chest. Fearful with suffocative breathing with abdominal muscles working to keep the air going in and out. Wheezing and burning in the chest. Blood floods into the head with coughing. Phlegm accumulates in the chest but cannot be expectorated. Feels as if there is a plug in the larynx; cough > warm drink or eating something (though sweets < the cough) < lying down in a warm room. Often helpful in following **Aconite** and **Hepar-sulph.** in croup. (Wh/c)

Sulphur: short, dry cough (2 at a time) with sharp pains under the left shoulder blade or looser cough with rattling mucus and oppression on the chest as if someone is sitting on it. Very useful when other remedies do not finish the job or at the end of an acute after other remedies have worked well but not brought about complete relief. Lips can sometimes be bright red in acute conditions.

Tissue salts: Kali-mur. is useful for loud, raucous cough with hoarse voice and white sputum at the end of a cold; if there is continued mucus production as well then ask for Combination 'Q' and take one 4 times a day.

Home-made Cough Treatments

Lemon, honey and glycerine is soothing for tickling, teasing coughs. Squeeze half a lemon into half a cup of warm water; add a teaspoon of runny honey and two teaspoons of glycerine from a chemist. Give teaspoon doses as needed. (Do not add boiling water to honey; stir it in warm water till it thins.)

If you grow thyme in the garden you can make use of it medicinally. Though Thymus Serpyllum is traditionally the variety used for coughs and lung problems, the other types have similar properties. Make a 'tea' by pouring half a pint of boiling water over a teaspoonful of leaves and flower tops and leaving to infuse for 10 – 15 minutes. Strain off the leaves and add a little honey to taste. In case of winter coughs, cut enough leaves and flower tops for drying. One old recipe adds a pinch of rosemary to the brew.

Onion syrup makes a useful cough linctus: cut up a pound of onions and boil them in 2 pints of water until they are soft. To this can be added half an ounce (15g) of crushed fennel. Leave the brew to stand for 12 hours in a lidded container. Add 8 ounces (200g) of sugar and bring it up to the boil. Allow the syrup to cool and then give teaspoon doses as needed. (It is not as disgusting as it sounds though it should not be given to hyperactive children.)

Laryngitis and Loss of Voice

Acute laryngitis is inflammation of the voice box and is usually associated with a viral or bacterial infection though the cause is often getting chilled in a draught, getting wet or overstraining the voice (often as the result of expressing or suppressing an emotion). Sometimes an allergy is responsible. The condition is characterised by a change in the quality of the voice or complete loss of it due to dryness of the mucous membranes or an accumulation of thick mucus around the vocal cords. There may or may not be a cough. Chronic changes in the voice may also be due to nodules or polyps on the vocal cords; these should be suspected if indicated remedies do not have any positive effect. Otherwise the usual suspects for chronic symptoms are passive or active smoking, alcoholism, chronic post-nasal drip obliging the patient to breathe through the mouth, and underactive thyroid.

Use the 30th potency of these remedies for loss of voice:

Aconite: sudden loss of voice especially after being caught in a cold wind.

Arg-nit.: lost voice from thick, yellow/green mucus amassing around the vocal cords. Back of the throat appears dark red and is sore.

Arsen-alb.: hoarse with squeaking voice, dry throat and drippy nose. (May be < allergy.)

Carbo-veg.: lost voice with gravelly cough, shallow breathing and mucus expectoration.

Causticum: dry, rasping voice (or lost) in singers or teachers after a cold or getting caught in a draught. Throat feels narrowed and difficult to expectorate. < voice strain; > public speakers with failing voice.

Gelsemium: loss of voice with sore throat at beginning of infection or just before period.

Hepar-sulph.: hoarseness and distorted voice with thick yellow mucus during throat infection that comes on after a chill. Has a sensation of a plug in the throat on swallowing.

Ignatia: voice lost after emotional upset; sensation of a lump in the throat.

Kali-bich.: voice lost or distorted due to very thick, sticky catarrh around the vocal cords; difficult to expectorate but when it does it comes out in sticky strings.

Lachesis: loss of voice with very painful sore throat and sensation of being throttled or acute sensitivity to anything touching the throat (including clothing).

Nat-mur.: loss of voice after a cold; strong thirst with poor appetite. Throat feels dry which makes eating difficult and unappealing. (May be < allergy.)

Nux Vomica: mucus round vocal cords with irritation, soreness and nasty taste; snuffly breathing, tickling in throat and desire for coffee. (May be < allergy.)

Phosphorus: squeaky voice and tickly throat < talking, singing, laughing with tearing pain; dryness of larynx with thirst. (May be < allergy to chemicals or smell of flowers.)

Pulsatilla: thick yellow or green mucus < on waking in a.m. which causes loss of voice. Voice comes and goes < evening and first thing in a.m. (May be < allergy.)

Rhus-tox.: lost voice after straining (teachers, singers) with yellow catarrh and stiffness of neck and limbs.

Spongia: loses voice while attempting to speak or sing; can't control pitch. Constantly hemming to clear throat. Larynx is painful and dry > swallow of water. May be due to thyroid problem.

Asthma and Acute Flare-ups of Asthmatic Breathing

Asthma is a chronic condition of the airways in which there is more or less obstruction in the tubes either from an accumulation of mucus or a narrowing of the airways due to contraction of the tiny muscles that line the tubes – or both. It is usually a condition that has its origins in emotional issues that have never been resolved. Such emotions may have been triggered extremely early, even before speech and may have been a result of an event that occurred during the pregnancy or the patient's birth (such as the cord wrapped round the neck). A miasmatic link is always to be found. Asthma is also often associated with eczema, especially suppressed childhood eczema, the suppression being the trigger for the lungs to suffer the chronic consequences. Asthmatic breathing can also be the end result of suppression of the immune system by artificial vaccination particularly against whooping cough, or from the suppression of otitis media or acute chest conditions by antibiotics and steroids. Allergies can also be a trigger for asthmatic breathing (see 'Hay Fever' on pages 138–42). Asthma is a condition that should not be treated without professional help. However, once started on constitutional treatment with the practitioner it is perfectly reasonable to administer remedies for acute episodes as long as the practitioner is informed. The homoeopath should be able to decide which are the most suitable first-aid remedies in any individual case. If asthma persists despite thorough treatment the likelihood is that the underlying emotional picture is not being addressed. If acute flare-ups of asthmatic breathing persist then it is possible that an allergy causing the problem has not been identified. **'Status asthmaticus', when the patient does not respond to treatment, begins to turn blue and finds it a severe struggle**

to breathe, is a medical emergency; dial 999 or take the patient to hospital! It is always a good idea to complement homoeopathic treatment with cranial osteopathic treatment as the symptoms of asthma include enormous stress and pressure on both the lungs and the solar plexus from tension in the diaphragm. Such pressure inevitably leads to compromised liver and spleen function which in turn affects the eliminative processes and immune system.

The following are the most common acute remedies:

Aconite: sudden attack of dry, hoarse breathing which induces great anxiety and fear. Usually with a hard dry cough. < since being out in a cold north or east wind. Sudden attack of asthmatic breathing around midnight. Chest feels full and constricted as if with a band.

Ant-tart.: asthmatic breathing with copious mucus in lungs that rattles in chest causing wheezing; breathes by using abdominal muscles. Wants small swallows of water. Appears to be suffocating from mucus in lungs. Coughs up balls of jelly-like phlegm. (See 'Coughs'.)

Arg-nit.: attacks of suffocating cough with thick greenish mucus during cold weather in summer. Must get fresh air. Much < in a close or crowded atmosphere.

Arsen-alb.: attack < 1 – 2 a.m. with wheezing and whistling breathing, restlessness, fearfulness and need to stay sitting up. Expectoration: white or yellow with salty taste. Chest feels raw or burning especially under the sternum. Band around chest sensation. (See 'Coughs'.) < allergies (see 'Hay Fever' pages 138–42).

Arsen-iod.: wheezy breathing < between 11 p.m. and 2 a.m. Brings up yellow/green phlegm with difficulty. < allergies (see 'Hay Fever' pages 138–42).

Blatta Orientalis: breathing < from tremendous accumulation of foul mucus in the lungs which threatens to suffocate the patient. Use the 30; is indicated in fleshy or corpulent people. It should be considered when **Arsen-alb.** seems indicated but fails and particularly when the patient is intolerant of heat.

Ipecac.: gasping for breath with wheezing cough, tight chest, nausea and gagging. The face goes pale with blueness round the mouth.

Lycopodium: short, rattling breathing < late afternoon or early hours of the morning with sniffing and snuffling, greenish catarrh and flatulence.

Kali-carb: should be prescribed and monitored by the practitioner. The patient sits leaning forward with elbows on hips or knees or on the table with arms spread wide. < for any activity; wheezing due to sticky mucus in the chest that is difficult to raise.

Nat-sulph.: attack of asthmatic breathing around 4 – 5 a.m. with thick greenish mucus. < in damp weather. Attacks < for frequently catching cold. (See 'Coughs' pages 168–73).

Nux Vomica: asthma brought on by overeating or eating too much rich food. Must loosen clothes for relief. Breathing > for belching. Also asthma from stress, overwork and living too hectic a life.

Phosphorus: attack of asthma provoked by coughing; chest feels hot and tight. Quick, shallow breathing. (See 'Coughs' pages 168–73)

Pulsatilla: asthmatic attacks with oppression of the chest brought on by emotions; often < night. Thick yellow mucus in the airways < on waking up in a.m. Asthma after allopathic medicine. Often needed after antibiotics or steroids to help clear them from the system though this should be overseen by your practitioner.

Sepia: asthma < just before or during a period or through the menopause.

Spongia: wakes up suddenly (after midnight) with feeling as if suffocating with dry throat and gasping for breath. Breathing is > if the head is thrown back.

Sulphur: asthma acute following on from a cold; sits up and must have the windows open. < 11 a.m. or between 4 and 6 p.m. Lips might be red and face pale and wizened.

Mention should be made of **Lobelia Inflata**, a remedy for asthma in smokers who dislike their addiction, feel deathly sick at the smell of tobacco and feel prickling sensations all over due to reduced oxygen level in the blood. This is not a first-aid remedy but can be useful in those who have episodes of asthmatic breathing due to their addiction. (Use 30 unless your practitioner advises otherwise.)

Pleurisy and Pneumothorax

Sharp, stitching pains on coughing, on taking a deep breath or on making any movement accompanied by shallow breathing, and referred pain in the back or shoulders can all indicate pleurisy. If the patient is also very thirsty and irritable, give **Bryonia** 30 and call the homoeopath. Pleurisy is sometimes concomitant with pneumonia. **If there is a fever then inform the homoeopath at once. Pneumonia must be treated professionally or in hospital.**

Shortness of breath, severe digging pains in the back or into the shoulders with a dry spasmodic cough and exhaustion can suggest pneumothorax. **If the symptoms are severe then call the homoeopath and take the patient to hospital at once in case the symptoms progress to a collapsed lung.**

Heart and Circulation

Conditions of the heart and circulation should always be closely monitored by a professional homoeopath, preferably in collaboration with the doctor. This is essential if allopathic drugs are being taken. Homoeopathic remedies do not interfere with heart drugs but the homoeopath does need to know what the patient is taking. The role of the homoeopath in treating patients on allopathic heart medication is that of support rather than cure. However, emergency acutes can be very satisfactorily dealt with by remedies as long as patient (and carer) and practitioner are in close accord about the use of acute remedies. The following descriptions are common acute emergencies:

• Intermittent aching, constrictive or cramping pains in the mid-chest with breathlessness especially < strong, cold winds or going uphill suggest angina. Squeezing pains with a band round the diaphragm or around the chest also indicate this. **Inform the homoeopath at once and, if severe and persistent, go to the hospital.** (Patients who live with this pattern of symptoms chronically would be well advised to keep

Latrodectus Mactans 30 or 200 and **Cactus Grandiflora** 200 in their first-aid kit. **Latrodectus** covers pains into the left arm and **Cactus** covers sharp, sticking pains with a squeezing sensation around the chest. Seek advice from your homoeopath on keeping these remedies. Patients should also avoid any exertion after a meal.)

- Pain that spreads from the mid-chest up into the jaw, left shoulder and arm (occasionally the right) and into the back, especially if tiredness, shortness of breath and debility have preceded the symptoms for a few days, suggests an imminent heart attack. There may be faintness, nausea, anxious restlessness and sweating. **Take the patient to hospital immediately and give an aspirin.** If **Latrodectus Mactans** 30 is to hand give one every 10 minutes until the hospital takes over; if the pain extends into the right shoulder give **Lillium Tigrinum** 30 at the same rate instead. (For those with an existing unstable heart condition it is worth discussing these two remedies with the homoeopath.)

- Any chest pains accompanied by high fever, exhaustion, pains into the left arm and an inability to lie down with any comfort suggest pericarditis, inflammation of the sac surrounding the heart. **Contact the homoeopath immediately or, if unavailable, take the patient to hospital.** (If the patient is acutely frightened give an **Aconite** 200.)

- Swelling and hardness of the calf with pain as if the calf had been in cramp; sometimes with discoloration of the skin which is tender to touch and a puffy ankle all suggests a deep vein thrombosis. If the leg feels tense and part of it is discoloured deep red or purple then give **Lachesis** 30. **Inform the homoeopath immediately; if not available take the patient to hospital at once.**

- Throbbing pain in the abdomen with a severe deep pain into the back in someone with high blood pressure suggests an aneurysm. **Take the patient to hospital at once!** If the patient has wheezing, a cough and pressure in the throat with pain into the left shoulder blade it suggests an aneurysm in the thorax. **Give Lachesis 30 and take the patient to hospital!**

13 THE DIGESTIVE SYSTEM AND ORGANS OF THE DIGESTIVE TRACT

Food Poisoning

The main causes of food poisoning include drinking contaminated water, eating contaminated food or eating insufficiently reheated cooked meat or fish. Various viruses and bacteria are associated with the symptoms of diarrhoea, nausea and vomiting. Whether it is salmonella, E. coli or staphylococcus, it is the symptom picture that will indicate the remedy to use though it is often helpful to know whether the culprit was fish, meat or something else.

Diarrhoea and Vomiting:

- < eating spoiled fish: **Arsen-alb.; Carbo-veg.; China; Puls.**
- < eating bad shellfish: **Arsen-alb.; Bry.; Lyc.; Urtica Urens**
- < eating spoiled meat: **Arsen-alb.; Carbo-veg.; China; Puls.**
- < drinking contaminated water: **Arg-nit.; Arsen-alb.; China; Zingiber.**
  (If giardiasis, caused by a parasite, is suspected then you should call your homoeopath – see below for the symptom picture.)

Gastroenteritis

This is a general term for bacterial, viral or parasitical infection of the digestive system that brings on diarrhoea, nausea, vomiting, loss of appetite and discomfort or pains in the abdomen. Gastric 'flu often arises as a seasonal epidemic; the most common remedy is **Arsen-alb.** which will cover a majority of cases whatever the associated bug: bacteria or virus. However, **Arg-nit.**, **Baptisia, Bryonia, Cuprum, Rhus-tox., Veratrum-alb.** or **Zingiber** might be indicated. It is very common for 'stomach bugs' to be associated with illnesses that are quite capable of changing shape; what begins as a sore throat and a cough becomes a diarrhoea and vomiting attack or vice versa. These episodic bouts of acute illness will often require a sequence of remedies. Take 3 or 4 of the most striking symptoms as your guide at any one time; if the picture shifts then you will need to change remedies. Some viral infections can affect not just the gut but also the lungs, leaving the patient with a persistent cough; this requires very careful professional monitoring in case of dehydration. Make sure the patient drinks frequent sips of water even if they do not want to. (Note that **Arsen-alb.** is the remedy that is most likely to want to drink in sips and that **Pulsatilla** is the most typical remedy to lack thirst.) In patients reluctant to drink water, offer flat Coca-Cola as this helps to restore glucose and fluid. To flatten the fizz add sugar.

Parasites in the Digestive System

Parasitical infection is often difficult to diagnose at first as it can appear similar to gastric 'flu, but it is much harder to clear and patients do not respond so well to remedies; this is the case with giardia and the less common cryptosporidium both of which may require a stool sample to determine whether they are present. **Both must be treated by a professional because they can cause dehydration and malnutrition from malabsorption.** The main remedy, once again, is **Arsen-alb.** but this is often inadequate on its own. As parasites can spread so quickly within families it is important to deal with them as soon as possible; children are particularly affected as their systems are so easily depleted. Both giardia and cryptosporidium are commonly picked up from contaminated water; travellers are particularly susceptible (see **Zingiber**). Sometimes it is difficult for a homoeopath to combat these parasites because of the speed of the condition; to select the appropriate remedies at the appropriate potencies might take more time than the patient and their family have. In this case antibiotics would be used by the doctor. To avoid the scorched earth effect that antibiotics have on the gut it is sensible to consult a herbalist or nutritional kinesiologist who can work on a natural biochemical level alongside the remedies.

Arg-nit.: nausea and vomiting accompanied by belching; brings up thick mucus with the vomit. Burning and constriction in the stomach with fullness and flatulence in the abdomen. Noisy diarrhoea: watery with green stools.

Arsen-alb.: nausea, vomiting and diarrhoea: copious watery, brown, yellow or black slimy stools or very foul smelling stools in small quantities with griping in the abdomen; pains in the gut or at the rectum can be burning. Temporarily > from vomiting or stools. The patient is anxious, restless and apparently exhausted though has energy enough to be demanding. Wants sips of cold water to wet the mouth or might refuse water for fear of vomiting; can't bear the thought of food. Food poisoning from bad meat or fish.

Carbo-veg.: abdomen feels blown out and puts pressure on the stomach; can't bear anything tight around waist. Nausea with sour belching and restricted breathing and faintness. Can't bear the thought of food. Burning in the rectum on passing foul smelling stools. Walks around with a stoop. Wants fresh air though cold to touch. Food poisoning < from eating bad chicken or fish or after drinking ice water.

China: very swollen abdomen with colicky flatulence which gives no relief when passed. Pale stools are acrid and copious, contain undigested food and look frothy and can be involuntary. Patient feels very weak after passing motions. Abdominal rumbling with thirst for cold water. Food poisoning and ill effects of eating bad meat, fish or fruit. Also < from drinking beer or bad water.

Cuprum: diarrhoea and vomiting preceded by hiccoughing. Nausea with colic in abdomen and calves which is so bad that the patient cries out in pain. Liquid, green stools spurt or gush out. All symptoms are temporarily > for drinking cold water.

Lycopodium: main remedy for ill effects from eating oysters. Bloating, churning, fullness, nausea and flatulence. Diarrhoea alternates with ineffectual urging.

Pulsatilla: main remedy for ill effects of eating pork or excessive amounts of rich food, fats and ice cream. Feels as if there is a stone lodged just below the ribs, in the stomach. Can still taste the food which is the cause of the problem. Flatulence and belching. Watery, green stools but doesn't pass as much as would like to.

Rhus-tox.: diarrhoea from drinking cold water or beer after being hot; < eating ice cream after a hot meal. Violent colic in abdomen causes patient to bend forward or to lie on stomach for relief. Very restless and anxious. Passes slimy, foul smelling, watery stools.

Urtica Urens: nausea, vomiting and diarrhoea after eating spoiled shellfish. After passing greenish brown diarrhoea urging persists with little effect. Anus can feel raw or burning.

Veratrum-alb.: terrible colic with extreme symptoms of exhaustion, deathly nausea and desperate unquenchable thirst for cold water which is vomited very soon. With the prostration there are beads of sweat on the forehead.

Zingiber: gastric symptoms from water-borne parasites or after eating melon. Diarrhoea with colicky pains and flatulence and a feeling that the anus is loose; dry mouth and thirst, nausea and a sense of heaviness. (See chapter 26, 'Travelling Abroad'.)

Flatulence

Wind in the digestive tract is only significant if it is persistent, distressing or painful. In homoeopathy we note the difference between belching and passing anal wind because some remedies are better known for the first and others for the second. Causes for wind are various but most usually it is due either to gulping air while eating hastily or fermentation of unsuitable food in the gut which gives off gases. Other, more intractable causes include a faulty diet with regular eating of unsuitable food, enzyme deficiency (which can be a pancreatic problem), an imbalance of natural bowel flora (which can be caused by psychosomatic triggers as well as unwise eating) and the presence of candida, a yeast infection. Certain foods have a particularly bad reputation for causing embarrassing wind: the proverbial baked beans and the cabbage family. Worse still can be farinaceous food, which is any food made from wheat. This can be worse because most modern bread and pasta are made from genetically modified wheat which has been hybridised to create far more gluten than it naturally would; gluten, especially in those sensitive to it, can have the effect of causing poisoning symptoms: wind, constipation or diarrhoea (or both in alternation), mucus on the stool, abdominal pains, breathlessness, constant catarrh of the respiratory tract, weakness, tiredness, lack of motivation, irritability, memory loss, depression, poor sleep and poor skin. Any condition that includes some or all of these symptoms should be treated by a practitioner who might well choose to share the treatment with a kinesiologist-nutritionist.

However, an acute bout of 'wind' can respond to home prescribing. The most usual remedies for belching include **Carbo-veg.** (< after a heavy, rich meal when the patient feels breathless and in need of fresh air and there is > from belching), **China** (when burping does not provide relief and the digestion is delicate), **Lyc.** (when the patient is hungry but then easily full up with a few mouthfuls), **Arg-nit.** (< from eating too many sweets and when there is a bloated abdomen) and **Puls.** (when the burping is accompanied by queasiness and a dry mouth with no thirst).

The most common remedies that will treat flatulence from the bowel include **Arg-nit.**, **Bry.**, **Carbo-veg.**, **China**, **Lyc.**, **Nat-mur.**, **Nat-sulph.**, **Nux-vom.** and **Pulsatilla**. Though the effects may be very similar, the causes which indicate the remedies are different. If the condition is chronic then consult your homoeopath, but if it is the result of unwise eating or an acute problem it will respond to first-aid prescribing. (See the general descriptions in the last section of the book for the main indications.)

• < anger: **Lyc.**, **Nux-vom.**
• < anxiety: **Arsen-alb.**, **Gels.**, **Lyc.**
• < beans: **Bry.**, **Lyc.**, **Nat-mur.**
• < bread: **Bry.**, **Lyc.**, **Nat-mur.**, **Nux-vom.**, **Puls.**
• < breakfast: **Nat-sulph.**
• < butter: **Carbo-veg.**, **Puls**.
• < cabbage: **Bry.**, **China**, **Lyc.**, **Nat-mur.**, **Puls.**
• < carrots: **Lyc.**
• < in children who are anxious but otherwise healthy: **Arg-nit.**, **Lyc.**
• < drinking beer: **Bry.**, **Lyc.**, **Nux-vom.**, **Puls.**

• < fruit: **China, Puls.**
• < heavy food: **Bry., Lyc., Puls.**
• < milk: **Bry., Lyc., Puls.**
• < pastry: **Bry., Puls.**
• < peas: **Bry., Nat-mur., Lyc.**
• < pork: **Carbo-veg., Nat-mur., Puls.**
• < potatoes: **Bry., Nat-sulph., Puls.**
• < raw food: **Lyc., Puls.**
• < starchy foods: **Carbo-veg., Lyc., Nat-mur., Nat-sulph., Puls.**
• < sugar and sugary foods: **Arg-nit., Lyc.**
• < wheat: **Lyc., Nat-mur., Nat-sulph., Puls.**

Colic in Babies

Trapped wind is the most frequent reason for colic in babies. The origin of the wind may be eating too quickly, mother's milk, formula milk, eating solids that are unsuitable, teething, anxiety or anger. Just in case the origin is elsewhere check on the nappies to inspect the urine and stools; colic can be a kidney or bladder problem or a bowel problem such as a twisted gut or worms or it can be an emotional problem with its origins in family dynamics. If colic does not respond to your first choice of remedy then consult your practitioner just to be reassured nothing else is happening.

Mother's milk can be a problem in some circumstances: occasionally the baby has an aversion to it. There are several remedies.indicated in this: **Calc-phos.** (peevish, fretful always restless and dissatisfied, slow teething and poor growth rate) is the most common and the child will refuse the breast, but **Borax** (easily startled, very upset when put down in the cot, crosspatch with a tendency to oral thrush) runs it a close second. Sometimes the baby is intolerant of wheat which can 'come through' in the milk. Occasionally formula milk is unsuitable. Soya milk can be a source of constipation and colic as soya is grown in bauxite (aluminium)-rich soil which can slow the digestion. Cow's milk is hard for humans to digest anyway because it contains four times the amount of salt and grease that we can tolerate; the result is often curd-like stools with abdominal discomfort. (**Aethusa** is an important remedy for intolerance of milk: colic with cold limbs, sunken puffy face, regurgitation after each meal and limpness. If you suspect this remedy is indicated call your homoeopath at once.) Teething commonly causes gut problems especially when the molars are coming through. If the child is rubbing the face or chewing on things, has variable motions and tummy pains these symptoms can be a strong indication of teething (see **Chamomilla**). Anxiety (see **Arg-nit., Bry., China, Lyc., Puls.**) is a prime cause of wind and in babies it often comes with irritability (see **Bry., Cham., Lyc., Nux-vom.**). If the anxiety is related to birth trauma then you should consult your practitioner and a cranial osteopath; if it is to do with family dynamics then call your homoeopath.

The following repertory is a guide to the indicated remedy:
- < from breast milk after mother has drunk coffee: **Cham., Nux-vom.**
- < before diarrhoea: **Arsen-alb., Chin., Coloc., Lyc., Puls., Sulph.**
- > after passing diarrhoea and wind: **Arg-nit., Dios., Lyc.**
- < after eating: **Carbo-veg., Chin., Coloc., Lyc., Puls., Sulph.**
- < after eating fruit: **Calc-phos., Chin., Coloc., Puls.**
- < after eating bread or pasta: **Bry., Cina, Lyc., Nux-vom., Puls., Sulph.**
- < after eating any of the cabbage family: **Bry., Chin., Lyc., Puls.**
- < after eating cheese (especially cheddar): **Arg-nit., Arsen-alb., Coloc., Nux-vom.**
- < from eating too greedily: **Chin., Cina, Lyc., Puls.**
- < after anger: **Cham., Coloc.**
- < with desire to arch back and writhe about: **Dios.**
- < with desire to bend double: **Coloc., Mag-phos.**

The following are the main remedies for colic in babies and infants:

Arg-nit.: colic from anxiety with flatulence and greenish stools. Belching accompanies the pain. Child may have a tendency to conjunctivitis. Causation may be apprehension in the mother or even her eating too many sweets while breastfeeding.

Arsen-alb.: colic after any food; restless and anxious. Only takes a little drink and refuses food. Pains may be accompanied by vomiting and followed by diarrhoea.

Chamomilla: terrible pains that causes writhing and fury. Impossible to pacify the child except by picking up and carrying around.

China: colic after eating fruit; pains accompanied by belching and flatulence which does not relieve. Abdomen looks bloated. Feels > for walking about and for bending double.

Cina: colic from intestinal worms. Bloated, hard abdomen with pains around the navel which feel > for being rubbed. Twitching limbs and filthy temper. Hungry despite the colic. (Consult your homoeopath.)

Colocynth: very severe cutting pain across the abdomen (usually from left to right) that is violent and sudden. Patient must double up with the cramp and put strong pressure on the painful area. Agonised expression on the face. The baby screams when moved; prefers to be lying on tummy. Cause is often anger. (If 30 does not help then use 200.)

Dioscorea: colic from being hungry; > moving about. Writhing in agony with arching of back and stretching out; cannot bend without < of pain.

Lycopodium: colic with flatulence and bloating < after eating and < evening. Warm drink >. Most common remedy for colic in babies who have grown long in the body without filling out much.

Mag-phos.: cramping colic which is > for bending double and being rubbed. Bloated abdomen; possibly < constipation. The baby may also have hiccoughs and be going through teething. Wants warmth and comfort; cries piteously when in pain. (Remedy best given in 30 or 200 in warm water.)

Nux-vom.: colic while breastfeeding especially after mother has had coffee or other stimulants or in children who are very sensitive and irritable unless active and occupied. Pain comes in waves and may be accompanied by hiccoughs and belching especially after overeating.

Pulsatilla: colic in clingy, tearful babies who feel > for being carried about. Rumbling gut with distension < evening. Pains may come on about one hour after feeding.

Sulphur: colic < after eating and drinking (too fast); abdomen is sore and sensitive to pressure. Belches may smell sour or sulphurish like bad eggs. Loose stools follow pains and may cause redness around the anus. Colic in hot babies with big bellies and thin limbs.

Heartburn

Heartburn (acid reflux) is caused by hyperacidity. Acid leaks up into the oesophagus from the stomach and burns the delicate membranes even as high as the pharynx, at the back of the mouth. Overeating may be the obvious cause in which case **Nux Vomica** is the chief remedy especially if the patient is irritable: use 30. Whenever the patient bends or lies down the acid leaks out. This often happens most after main meals or at bedtime. Those who have heartburn should never eat later than 8 p.m. If the problem is persistent it may be due to a hiatus hernia, a chronic condition causing belching and reflux. This condition should be treated by your homoeopath and a cranial osteopath. As a support there is a combination remedy that is very useful: **Arsen-alb.** 6 + **Hydrastis** 6. Ask your practitioner or get the pharmacy to send you 8 grams of pills: take one after every meal. If belching is accompanied by breathlessness then use **Carbo-veg.** 30 (one before each main meal) which works well alongside the combination. **It should also be noted that the symptoms of severe heartburn can be similar to angina.** If in any doubt or if the remedies taken for heartburn do not help within a short time (a few days) then contact your homoeopath. Ask about the advisability of taking **Nat-phos.** tissue salts. (For heartburn in pregnancy see 294–5.)

Bouts of burning pains in the stomach with persistent hunger pangs and a desire for milk may indicate a peptic ulcer. These symptoms should be reported to the homoeopath. **If with the burning pains there is persistent nausea and dark or black vomit (like coffee grounds) this should be reported to the homoeopath immediately as it might suggest that an ulcer is bleeding.** (Patients should avoid antacids and courses of antibiotics as they suppress the condition and offer no lasting cure. Ask your practitioner about supplements such as slippery elm bark. Papaya and an infusion of thyme may also be helpful.)

Loss of Appetite

There are many reasons for loss of appetite: brewing a cold or 'flu, constipation, menstruation, eating between meals, change of season especially from cool weather to hot, excessive eating of sweets or drinking of alcohol, taking allopathic medicine, smoking cigarettes or cannabis, anxiety and emotional trauma, recent physical trauma or too much excitement. In old people it may be because it is just too much effort to bother to eat.

In homoeopathy there are no appetite stimulants per se though things can be improved as the result of appropriate constitutional remedies. If loss of appetite persists and causes real concern or is accompanied by other chronic symptoms then professional help should be sought. For jaded palates in the elderly (or anyone else) then ginseng has a reputation among herbalists for stimulating the appetite and increasing the intestine's ability to absorb nutrients. Gentian is another herb that also improves the digestive system and increases appetite as a result. Both herbs are compatible with ongoing homoeopathic treatment but ask your homoeopath about the advisability of using them and, to be sure of what you are doing, consult a herbalist to determine choice and dosage.

Constipation

We should be able to evacuate the lower bowel at least once every day though twice is even better. It is best to pass motions early in the morning otherwise we have to work with bowels that are storing toxic waste. Yet it is not uncommon to hear people say that they are never constipated even though they only pass motions every other day. The digestive system should be subject to circadian (daily) rhythms. Chronic constipation can be associated with poor circulation and lymph drainage, abdominal pain, bloating and flatulence, shortness of breath, sluggish hormonal function, poor skin, susceptibility to colds and 'flu, alcoholism, loss of motivation and focus, depression and irritability. It might be a symptom of poor diet, wheat and gluten intolerance, candidiasis, a sluggish thyroid gland, taking antibiotics, an emotional trauma or it might simply be a hereditary disposition.

Temporary constipation might be triggered by any of the following: eating things that don't suit you, not drinking enough water, a change of weather, anticipation and anxiety, taking allopathic drugs for an acute condition, getting out of your usual routine, a change of circumstances, travelling or following an accident.

Most people resort to laxatives when the constipation has gone on too long; some wait a day, others might wait for a week (never a good idea!). Laxatives can be a short-term solution that has no side effects. However, it is not good health-keeping to use laxatives too often because they can cause the bowels to become lazy and the chemistry of the gut to become unbalanced.

The following are reasons for constipation and their indicated remedies (use 30 unless otherwise specified or advised by your practitioner):
- < with backache: **Aesculus-hip.** (hard, dry stools which are painful to pass and accompany pains in the sacrum and hips).
- < during a cold: **Ignatia** (pressure and tightness in the rectum even with sharp pains).
- < because there is always a feeling that there is something left to pass: **Nux-vom.** (frequent but ineffectual urging < for having used laxatives long-term).
- < abuse of medicinal drugs: **Bry.** (large, dry, hard motions with a very dry system; tremendously thirsty). **Nux-vom.** (feeling bunged up and irritable).
- < during a headache: **Bry.** (headache with dryness and strong thirst). **Nat-mur.** (looks very like **Bryonia** and it is sometimes better to give **Bryonia** to avoid any aggravation of the head pain which can sometimes happen after **Nat-mur.** in headaches).
- < away from home: **Ambra Grisea** (< because of embarrassment at having to use public or unfamiliar bathrooms). **Lyc.** (hard, small and unsatisfactory stools with a feeling of more to come; often accompanied by bloating and flatulence). **Nat-mur.** (hard, dry, crumbling stools or little balls only passed with great effort).
- < eating wheat (gluten intolerance): **Lyc.** (odorous wind and bloating; tiredness in afternoon). **Nat-mur.** (heartburn, mild nausea, dry, crumbling or pebbly stools, distension, picky appetite and feeling withdrawn).
- < after a physical trauma: **Arn.**
- < before menstruation: **Bry.** (see above). **Kali-c.** (with sore breasts,

water retention and low backache). **Nat-mur.** (see above). **Nux-vom.** (see above). **Sepia** (a sense of weight on the rectum with exhaustion and irritability). **Silica** (stool begins to extrude but then retreats back into the rectum). Constipation before or during menses is often not an isolated symptom; if you have other symptoms as well as constipation then you should talk to your homoeopath.

- • < during pregnancy: consult your practitioner about this.
- • < with rectal prolapse: only treat this if it is a 'one-off' acute and inform your homoeopath; use a 200. The main remedies are **Ignatia** (sharp stabbing pains shoot up the rectum), **Sepia** (heavy, dragging sensation in the lower bowel; may have a sensation of a ball in the rectum making sitting painful). If the chosen remedy does not relieve then consult your homoeopath.
- • < after surgery: **Opium** (talk to your homoeopath about this).
- • < travelling: **Alumina** (often called for in the elderly when travelling enforces inactivity for too long. Dry, hard and lumpy stools which are very difficult to pass: may not have any urging at all or may feel sore and itching in the rectum). **Ambra Grisea, Lyc., Nat-mur., Nux-vom.** (see above references for details).

The main remedies for having to strain to pass a constipated motion are **Nat-mur., Nux-vom., Sepia** and **Silica** (see above). Straining should never be allowed to become a chronic feature. It is damaging not only to local tissues but also puts under severe strain all the tissues and organs of the lower abdominal cavity. The prostate can be pulled out of place causing the typical symptoms of middle-aged men: slowed stream of urine and dribbling. The liver can also be compromised; there are ligaments that hold the liver in place and straining on the lower bowel can pull the liver out of place. This has the knock-on effect of encouraging piles and poor elimination of toxicity. Always consult your homoeopath about chronic constipation. You may be recommended to take psyllium husks (a supplement derived from plantago) which are indicated most frequently in those who have low-fibre diets (those low in grains and green vegetables). Drink more water if more fibre is added to the diet or the constipation will stay. The extra water is needed to swell the fibre in order to push it through the bowel.

Diarrhoea

Acute diarrhoea could be part of a gastric bug (see pages 181–2), food poisoning (see page 181) or it may in fact be a good thing: as a speedy form of elimination after having eaten something inappropriate or as an expression of emotions. It can also be an aggravation, the result of taking an indicated homoeopathic remedy prescribed for a long-term condition. Diarrhoea in babies is common during teething, with a change of diet or circumstance, or in hot weather. However, it can be the result of milk intolerance or weaning a child onto unsuitable food; if this is the case then you should consult your homoeopath. It is a good idea, especially if you are caring for a family, to have Dioralite in the first-aid cupboard. You can buy this from the chemist as a means of preventing the worst effects of dehydration when the loss of fluids causes the electrolyte balance (essential to the proper functioning of the body) to be upset. You can recognise a drop in electrolytes (mostly potassium and sodium) from the symptoms: lightheadedness, confusion, faintness on trying to stand, pallor and profound weakness with a sudden drop in blood pressure. It can be very difficult to get babies to drink water with Dioralite; you must ask for professional help as shock and collapse with dehydration can cause severe damage, not least to brain cells. A teaspoon of salt and sugar in a glass of warm water can be effective. In households with children who throw frequent fevers or have very reactive bowels it is worth keeping **Phosphoric Acid** and **China** (30 or 200) in the first-aid kit as these remedies are often needed after heavy loss of fluids.

1. < after acute diseases: **Carbo-veg.** (foul smelling and windy motions causing some burning of the anus with general weakness; often useful in the very young and the elderly). **China** (frothy, yellow, watery stools that smell foul with coldness of the body and flatulence; the patient is likely to be thirsty and you may see undigested food in the motions). **Phos-ac.** (painless, odourless but profuse, pale and windy stools with general debility). **Sulph.** (diarrhoea < early morning with redness and soreness of the anus; patient may be hot and sweaty).
2. < alcohol: **Arsen-alb.** (profuse, dark and foul stools with burning sensation in the anus). **Nux-vom.** (< in the morning after binge drinking). **Sulph.** (see 1 above).

3. < alternating with constipation: this is a situation best treated by your homoeopath.

4. < after being in a rage: **Cham.** (sour, slimy stools that might be yellow or green mixed with mucus and smelling like rotten eggs). **Colocynth** (after indignant anger from being humiliated; frothy, watery stools accompanied by cutting pains across abdomen which cause grimace of pain and force the patient to double up). **Nux-vom.** (frequent urging with passing of small amounts of diarrhoea with the feeling that there is always more to come).

5. < anxiety and apprehension: **Arsen-alb.** (see 2 above – with restlessness and worried expression). **Arg-nit.** (lots of wind and bloating with persistent diarrhoea like chopped spinach mixed with mucus). **Gels.** (sudden attack of yellow or cream, mucous stools when full of dread; generally weak, tired and listless).

6. < after beer drinking: **Sulph.** (see 1 above).

7. < after breakfast: this is often a chronic state and needs professional help (but see **Sulph.**: 1 above).

8. < after catching a chill: **Arsen-alb.** (see 2 above). **China** (see 1 above). **Nux-vom.** (see 4 above but also note irritability). **Puls.** (rumbling gut with loose motions that change in appearance from one motion to the next).

9. < after too much chocolate: **Arg-nit.** (see 5 above).

10. < after a cold drink especially in hot weather: **Arsen-alb.** (see 2 above). **Bry.** (urging with spurting diarrhoea < making any movement). **Carbo-veg.** (see 1 above). **Nat-sulph.** (noisy gut with sudden explosive, spluttering stools < in the morning; frothy and yellow stools). **Nux Moschata** (most common remedy for diarrhoea after cold drink in hot weather).

11. < after suppression of acute conditions by antibiotics: **Sulph.** (see 1 above).

12. < damp weather: though **Nat-sulph.** (see 10 above) is the most usual remedy for this, consult your homoeopath as this symptom might indicate the need for long-term constitutional treatment.

13. < dentition (teething): There are many remedies indicated for this. If **Cham.** (see 4 above) does not help or is not indicated then speak to your homoeopath. This may be an ideal moment to give constitutional treatment.

14. < drains, after clearing out stinking: **Pyrogen** (disgustingly foul, dark stools with general feeling of exhaustion, malaise and restlessness) is often needed but you should consult the homoeopath as this state can call for other, similar remedies.

15. < eruptions, suppression of skin: **Sulph.** (see 1 above). This is a situation that should be treated by your homoeopath as the reappearance of the skin eruptions is to be expected.

16. < excitement: **Arg-nit.**, **Arsen-alb.**, and **Gels.** (see 5 above).

17. < exercise, unaccustomed: **Arsen-alb.** (see 2 and 5 above). **Calc-c.** (rush of stools after eating soon after exertion which then = emptiness and discomfort in bowel). **Nat-sulph.** (see 10 above). **Puls.** (see 8 above). **Rhus-tox.**(frothy, painless stools with protrusion of haemorrhoids after lifting or heaving heavy object).

18. < fear or fright: **Acon.** (sudden urging to pass watery stools with restlessness and weakness). **Arg-nit.**, **Gels.**, **Puls.** (see 2, 5 and 8 above).

19. < fish, after eating: **Arsen-alb.** (see 2 and 5 above).

20. < fruit: **Arsen-alb.** (see 2 and 5 above). **Bry.** (< stewed fruit with sudden, imperative urging on least movement and gushing stools). **Carbo-veg.** (see 1 above). **China** (see 1 above). **Colocynth** (cutting pains across abdomen which force the patient to double up in agony followed by frothy, watery stools); best to use the 200. **Nat-sulph.** (see 10 above). **Puls.** (see 8 above).

21. < hot weather: **Bry.** (esp. < after a cold drink; see 11 above). **China** (watery, foul, yellow stools < at night and < after eating fruit or drinking milk or beer). **Gambogia** (useful in old people with watery, gushing stools and burning anus). **Podophyllum** (profuse, gushing, yellow or very pale stools, < mornings, that are foul smelling with lots of rumbling and gurgling in the gut).

22. < ice-cream: **Ars-alb.** (see 2 and 5 above). **Puls.** (see 8 above).

23. < loss of fluids, after: **Carbo-veg.** (see 1 above). **China** (weak, thirsty and windy and see 21 above). **Phos-ac.** (mental and physical exhaustion and debility especially at the end of an acute; follows **Arsen-alb.** well).

24. < menstruation, during, before or after: consult your practitioner.

25. < milk: **Calc-c.** (in children: if diarrhoea persists then consult the homoeopath in case of milk intolerance!) **Mag-c.** (colic followed by diarrhoea: milk passes undigested in breastfed children; child is very

sensitive and anxious; does not seem to be doing well nutritionally, consult the homoeopath about this state). **Podophyllum** (< after sour milk).

26. < after onions: **Lyc.** (bloating, wind and greenish diarrhoea). **Puls.** (nausea and watery, green diarrhoea with lack of thirst).

27. < overheated, from becoming: **Puls.** (see 26; also feeling faint and dry mouthed).

28. < sugar or sweets, after eating: **Arg-nit.** (frequent urging to pass small amounts of watery diarrhoea with lots of wind).

29. < weaning: **China** (see 1 above; diarrhoea that threatens to become chronic; the baby gets weaker and more drowsy and breathing becomes quicker and audible: consult your practitioner!)

Abdominal Pains

Pains felt in the abdomen need to be differentiated. On the right side under the ribs are the liver and the gall bladder and the hepatic flexure (where the colon turns the corner next to the liver); below this there are the ileo-caecal valve and the appendix (where the small intestine joins the ascending colon) and, nearby, the right ovary. On the left side under the ribs there are the spleen and the splenic flexure (where the transverse colon turns the corner and begins its descent to the rectum); below this there is the left ovary and then the sigmoid colon, the last turn of the bowel before the anus. In the middle, behind the umbilicus, are the intestines. An apron of fatty tissue called the omentum covers the internal organs of the abdomen like a quilt; swollen glands in the omentum can be painful during fever. It is important to find out if pains are on the left or right, above the navel or below. Wind pains can be anywhere and they can shift about. Liver and gall bladder pains are in the upper right quadrant but can spread across and down. Pains in the right ovary can be mistaken for appendix pains. Aching in the spleen is under the left lower ribs. Pains in the left side are usually from constipation or diverticulitis. Pains in the left lower quadrant might be in the ovary. Pains at the bottom of the abdomen might be either in the colon, the uterus (or prostate) or the bladder.

Appendicitis

An appendix may either 'grumble' or erupt into appendicitis. 'Grumbling' covers nagging pain, intermittent feverishness, loss of appetite and irritability. Recurrent pain should be reported though the homoeopath may suggest remedies to have at hand. In appendicitis there is fever, nausea, vomiting, severe pain which is often worse for any movement and a frontal headache. **This needs immediate attention in case of rupture which can lead to peritonitis, a widespread infection of the abdominal cavity with abscess formation.**

Piles

Piles are varicose veins. Veins have no power to force blood upwards, and when their walls become weak under pressure, blood returning to the liver, lungs and heart tends, through gravity, to become sluggish and fill out the incompetent vessels. This causes local tension, irritation, pain, bleeding or itching. The cause of the pressure is often the liver not functioning as well as it should. The exception to this is when there has been strain on organs above the anus such as happens during pregnancy and delivery or after a long period of constipation when straining to pass motions creates undue stress on the anal sphincter. Some drugs will also contribute to pressure from the liver thus causing the piles.

Piles can be either internal or external. If internal there may be anal protrusion after passing a stool which needs to be pushed back manually. If external the veins can produce either a single lump or a 'bunch of grapes' appearance. There is purplish discoloration because veins carry used, deoxygenated blood. Both types of piles might bleed either with passing the motion or from wiping afterwards. Sometimes, if the piles are chronic and large, bleeding might be profuse and gushing into the pan. The more blood there is, the more pressure from above. Those most susceptible to piles include women who have had difficult labours, men who live adrenalin-charged lives, those who eat too much and unwisely (especially junk food), alcoholics, those whose lives are too sedentary and who are generally constipated, very angry people and the obese.

Piles are generally a constitutional problem that requires a professional prescriber. This is because it is necessary to understand why there should be a pressure build-up in the system. It is never enough to treat the piles without investigating the liver and its associated functions. It is for this reason that the orthodox treatment of ligature, surgery or injection to reduce the piles is extremely unwise. The results usually create a tendency to heart and circulation problems. However, there are a number of remedies that can be helpful for those who suffer intermittently from piles and which are complementary to ongoing constitutional treatment. Consult your homoeopath about their usage.

Aesculus: internal or external piles but both have the characteristic sensation of having sticks inside the anus < while sitting or walking. There can be burning or soreness with prolapse; while passing a motion there are shooting pains up the back or aching into the hips. Useful in older men who have abused their digestion and in menopausal women. Use 30.

Aloe: 'bunch of grapes' protrude > cold water; heaviness and sense of prolapse is constant < after stool; rectum feels open and 'unsafe' as if it would not hold in the stools which are loose and mucousy. Use 30.

Hamamelis: internal or external piles that bleed profusely and feel sore and throbbing. Blood can be darker than the usual bright red as it flows more slowly despite the amount. Use 30.

Lycopodium: aching and tender to touch but > for a hot bath. Often has stools that are hard and solid to start with and then become soft and loose. Use 30 or 100.

Nitric acid: piles bleed easily from fissures which have sharp, needle pains and sore aching that goes on for ages after stool. Patient usually feels miserable and snappy. Use 30.

Nux Vomica: internal piles < for frequent urging with little result; feeling that there is always something waiting to be passed. Piles can itch and burn. Often < for using suppositories or laxatives or after alcohol. Patient is sensitive, irritable and intolerant. Use 30.

Paeonia: piles are present with fissures and terrible pains that force the patient to walk around in agony even long after passing a motion; itching and burning are followed by internal chilliness as reaction; piles might even be ulcerated; think of this if **Nit-ac.** fails. Use 6 every 15 minutes or 30 every 2 hours.

Phosphorus: burning and bright red bleeding with prolapsed anus and piles; stools and piles = general weakness. Use 30.

Pulsatilla: itching and sharp pains in small piles that are < menstruation. Use 30 or 200.

Sepia: characteristic is the sensation of sitting on a ball in the rectum; prolapsed rectum < chronic constipation; pains shoot up the rectum with constriction of the anus; piles bleed or the anus oozes moisture. Piles < during pregnancy or in menopause after history of difficult labours. Use 30 or a 200.

Sulphur: itching, burning and redness round the anus; rectum oozes moisture and is odorous. Piles may be internal or external when they appear in bunches; very sore and tender. May be < for chronic constipation (after years of bad diet) or chronic diarrhoea (from an overactive elimination system). Commonly needed by alcoholics. Use 30 or a 200.

In addition to remedies it is feasible to apply ointment. Homoeopathic pharmacies supply 'piles cream' or ointment which is made with a combination of well-known remedies. If this is not suitable use **Hypercal** ointment which heals broken skin and blood vessels and deals with sharp nerve pains. If there is protrusion and damage to the anal sphincter from straining then frequent use of a combination of **Hypercal + Ruta** ointment is useful in calming and healing the aggravated area. It is always a good idea to wash after passing motions as hot or cold water (depending on the individual) so often helps settle things down.

Diverticulitis

'Diverticulum' refers to a pocket of mucous membrane gut-lining protruding through the herniated (ruptured) outer muscle wall of the bowel. (It is also possible to have a diverticulum of the oesophagus or of the gall bladder.)

Diverticulitis is inflammation of a diverticulum, whereas diverticulosis is the presence of a diverticulum without inflammation. This is an increasingly common condition in anyone over 40 and may never be more than a periodic nuisance. However, trouble arises when the pouch becomes the site of infection. This only happens when the patient's immune system is at a low enough ebb to allow bacteria to proliferate along with inflammation. It can be triggered by faeces becoming trapped in the pouch or when food stuff becomes wedged in there and causes irritation. Diverticula can bleed especially in those who are chronically constipated and pass large motions, or those who have frequent bowel movements with purging. Pains associated with diverticulitis include cramps, stabbing and shooting, burning and pinching. They are most commonly sited in the descending colon just before the sigmoid flexure, the final turn of the gut into the rectum. Any pains here would be felt in the lower left quadrant of the abdomen. If the inflammation is trying to deal with infection then there may be a fever. Bleeding may be intermittent and may not be a sign of any infection. If it is quite bright red then the diverticulum is in the descending colon; if the blood is darker then it is more likely to come from a site in the ascending colon on the right side of the abdomen.

Diverticulosis is not a condition to treat at home; you should consult a homoeopath if the condition causes any acute symptoms. It is also unlikely to be reversed unless the patient is particularly fit and prepared to follow a strict regime. However, constitutional treatment makes sure that the acute flare-ups are reduced to a minimum. If there is frequent or profuse bleeding then be prepared for your homoeopath to suggest that you see the doctor to have it investigated though some practitioners will be content, from their close questioning, to observe how speedily and well the first prescription works. Also be ready to follow some common-sense dietary advice. You may be prescribed psyllium husks to assist with satisfactory elimination.

Crohn's Disease and Ulcerative Colitis

These two conditions are increasingly common and have their origins in emotional stress and miasmatic inheritance. Orthodox medicine is frank about not knowing the causes; this is because doctors do not take sufficient account of the psyche when questioning patients about their bowel symptoms. Diagnosis can be rather hit and miss unless the symptoms are very obvious, because both diseases can be intermittent, similar in their symptom pictures and yet variable. The symptoms of both can be vicious and debilitating and require professional treatment and regular monitoring. However, it is a good idea to discuss the use of acute remedies with your homoeopath so that the patient is able to take some charge of pain relief.

Crohn's is a chronic, intermittent inflammation of a part of the gut wall and is characterised by bouts of diarrhoea, intestinal cramping, recurrent low-grade fever, weight loss and appetite loss. The inflammation occurs in restricted areas towards the end of the small intestine or in the colon (though it can happen anywhere in the digestive tract). When the area swells it creates a blockage through which faeces cannot pass; the body then creates a temporary fistula (tunnel) between the adjacent loops of bowel or on either side of the diseased part. (Sometimes the fistula will break into an adjacent organ such as the bladder.) This allows faeces to pass and gives the isolated diseased part time to heal. Occasionally the area bleeds. Patients also often suffer from joint pains, back pains, gall bladder symptoms and skin conditions. Orthodox treatment consists of using steroids, antibiotics and anti-inflammatories depending on the severity of symptoms; when seriously debilitating and persistent, surgery to remove the section of the bowel is considered. None of this is a cure as Crohn's usually relapses. The most common remedies to relieve the acute symptoms include **Aloes, Apis, Arsen-alb., Arsen-iod., China, Colocynth, Merc-corr., Nit-ac.** and **Terebinth**. Occasionally **Zingiber** is useful when there are bladder and kidney complications. Patients should always seek guidance on indications, potency and frequency of dosage. Cranial osteopathy is of great service when used intercurrently with homoeopathy in this condition.

Ulcerative colitis is restricted to the large intestine. Inflammation and ulceration of the wall of the bowel leads to bleeding, severe cramps, burning or sharp pains. Diarrhoea is persistent and very frequent; blood, pus and mucus are in the watery stools. Acute episodes are sometimes accompanied by feverishness. Occasionally there is only one acute attack but if it becomes a chronic recurrent condition the patient becomes debilitated and at risk of more serious pathology. As there are quite a few reasons for intestinal inflammation the doctor would expect exhaustive tests to be carried out to make a certain diagnosis which, even so, might be frustratingly difficult to confirm. It is not unusual for the patient to be anaemic and look poorly nourished.

When consulting a homoeopath about either condition the patient should expect to give detailed and specific information about the bowel symptoms, other physical symptoms and anything that qualifies the general state such as times of day, appetite changes and environmental conditions that might be associated with flare-ups. Not only will the homoeopath be getting an understanding of the acute disease but also how the patient is between flare-ups. In addition, there will inevitably be questions about emotional history as there is no chronic inflammatory condition without a certain degree of emotional suppression either current or long buried. Cranial osteopathy is a recommended additional treatment.

Coeliac Disease or Intolerance to Gluten

Coeliac disease is a severe, chronic allergic reaction to gluten, a protein in wheat and rye. It used to be regarded as a condition that only affected babies who, as soon as they were introduced to solids containing wheat, became malnourished, sickly, pot-bellied and who did not grow. (In severe cases babies react to the breast milk of mothers who eat wheat products.) Nowadays it is seen as a condition that can affect anyone at any age. No reason is offered as to why adults should suddenly or gradually become susceptible after having eaten wheat products for years but homoeopaths are likely to look for emotional background in case a trauma (or long drawn-out stress) has been sufficient trigger.

In addition, alternative practitioners are likely to be suspicious of the fact that wheat is no longer unadulterated; talk to any alternative practitioner and they are likely to say what a huge and rising increase there has been in gluten intolerance since the last quarter of the twentieth century. In Britain we use Canadian wheat which has been hybridised and genetically modified to produce vastly more gluten in order to make greater quantities of flour. Gluten is extremely hard on the human gut; it causes the walls of the intestines to become smooth and sticky, making it very hard to absorb nutrients and encouraging the system to retain water. The net result is the creation of sticky mucus, diarrhoea or constipation or an alternation of the two and a predisposition to candida and intestinal parasites. It is also responsible for headaches, depression, lethargy, weight gain and sluggish functioning of the body generally and is sometimes bad enough that a doctor might wonder if the thyroid needs investigating. Anyone suffering from this condition needs to adopt a strict diet; there is little chance of recovery unless all gluten is cut out. This means looking at labels on packets and tins; anything with 'GM starch' or 'modified starch' should be left on the shelves. Gluten is in a bewildering number of foods; from gravy mix to chocolate powder, spaghetti to sausages. (People with blood group 'O' seem to be more prone to gluten allergy than others but it is by no means exclusively so.)

The majority of people with a gluten allergy suffer symptoms that only eventually cause them to complain about a failing body after a 'long time of putting up with it'. Such patients are likely to find relief from constitutional treatment. They will need remedies that are known for being indicated by those intolerant to starchy and farinaceous foods (i.e. used to make meal or flour): **Lycopodium, Nat-mur., Nat-sulph.** and **Pulsatilla** are the main ones though **Okubaka Aubreville** should now be added to the list. When these remedies are given but cannot resolve the symptoms then gluten must be suspected and eliminated. One other aspect cannot be ignored: those with gluten allergy (mild or severe) seem to be more susceptible to leaking mercury from amalgam fillings. The patient needs to be prepared to discuss the possibility that old fillings might have to be removed under specialist care.

The Liver and the Gall Bladder

The liver is the post office of the body: it receives and it distributes. It is also part of the waste disposal unit, as it is involved with storing what cannot be used until it can be eliminated, and it cleans up the blood that passes through it; thus it is always central to any detoxification process a patient may be asked to go through. In addition to this, the liver is also a factory for biochemicals and is involved in digestion and hormone activity. Because it is vital to so many functions, the liver is often found to be associated with many different problems. Anyone with a dysfunctional liver/gall bladder should ask the homoeopath about the advisability of keeping **Chelidonium** 30 in the house. The liver may be a key player in any of the following conditions:

• Migraine and headaches with pain in the forehead and above the eyes
• Thick and dark-coloured earwax
• Foul breath (especially if it smells faecal) and furred tongue (and

sometimes cracked tongue)
- Floaters in the eyes
- Excessive mucus in the throat and post-nasal drip
- Poor drainage of mucus from the lungs (despite indicated treatment)
- Frozen shoulder (Large joints in the body can be very susceptible to long-lasting pains from injuries or strains if the liver is dysfunctional.)
- Poor recovery in skin diseases including acne, acne rosacea and eczema (The skin cannot eliminate toxicity from the body if liver function is compromised.)
- Fever
- Abscesses including tooth abscesses
- Chronic constipation or diarrhoea or their alternation
- Heartburn (acid reflux)
- Jaundice
- Gout
- Varicose veins and haemorrhoids (and hiatus hernia if it is a consequence of suppressed piles)
- Diverticulosis
- Abdominal water retention
- Clotted menstrual blood loss
- Atherosclerosis and atheroma
- Fatigue, weight loss and weakness
- Mood changes with confusion, sleepiness and poor coordination (especially in the elderly)

Symptoms that suggest liver and gall bladder pathology include:
- Jaundice; yellow discoloration of the skin and of the whites of the eyes; may manifest as sallow skin with 'dirty' whites of the eyes in a chronic jaundiced condition (such as long-term asthma suppressed by steroids).
- Aching in the right side of the upper abdomen just below the ribs. If accompanied by nausea and a pain in the back at the bottom corner of the right shoulder blade that extends through to the front or round to the side of the body, then it is likely that the gall bladder is acutely inflamed. (Give **Chelidonium** 30 4-hourly and call the homoeopath.) Other liver pains include heaviness in the liver region; burning or stitching. Sometimes there can be a dull pain with aching under the

shoulder blades and soreness of the left shoulder.

- Sharp pains in the left side of the upper abdomen may be referred pain from the gall bladder but if so they are usually accompanied by nausea.
- Dark urine (almost brown and can look like ale) and pale stools (jaundice).
- A sensation of bulk and swelling in the right upper abdomen (hypertrophy of the liver that may occur due to alcoholism or certain drugs' side effects or because of cysts).
- Swelling and discomfort in the left side under the ribs with fluid retention in the abdomen accompanied by distention, difficult breathing and stitching in the liver with bleeding piles. **This suggests high blood pressure in the vessel bringing blood into the liver and it must be reported as soon as it is suspected.** One of the main remedies is **Carduus Marianus** and it can be used in the 30 4-hourly until the appointment.
- Confusion, drowsiness and coordination problems with slurred speech and disorientation; moods can change and be punctuated by periods of anxiety. **This suggests severe toxicity of the liver or a stroke and requires urgent treatment.**
- Episodes of nausea, fluid retention, weight loss and disgust for food suggests cirrhosis which is the hardening of areas of the liver leaving scar tissue. (The causes are various and not always alcohol-related; it requires long-term supportive and 'detoxing' treatment.)
- Nausea, vomiting, dark urine, lack of appetite, feverishness and a disgust for the smell or sight of cooking suggests acute hepatitis especially if there is a sallow appearance. (This should be dealt with by the homoeopath as soon as possible; treatment may need to be continued intensely for several days and the patient monitored for 2 or 3 weeks. While waiting for an appointment give **Chelidonium** 30 twice daily.)
- Coughing up of blood intermittently with any typical liver symptoms suggests that an internal varicose vein has ruptured. **This must be reported to the homoeopath straight away.** If you have to wait for an appointment give **Aconite** 200 for shock and follow within 5 minutes, in the case of alcoholics, with **Nux-vom.** 30 every 4 hours or **Phosphorus** 30 at the same dosage. **If the haemorrhage is more persistent then take the patient to hospital immediately.**

The liver is also susceptible to problems if there are certain types of emotional turmoil. Esoterically the liver is strongly associated with and affected by the person's will; the will to do and to be creative. The liver will begin to suffer (and thus create symptoms) if a person's creativity is frustrated or suppressed. Suppressed anger will also tell badly on the liver. The liver is the physical organ most affected by success or failure in meeting challenges and dealing with conflicts, so if there is any liver pathology the homoeopath is likely, where appropriate, to investigate any causes of problems that might originate in these areas. The more that anger is part of a case the more likely it is that the liver and particularly the gall bladder will be involved in creating symptoms. Homoeopathic treatment would inevitably encourage the voicing of what has been suppressed so that frustration and old resentments can be resolved gently.

The Pancreas

The pancreas is vital to digestion as it produces enzymes to break down food and hormones that maintain the correct sugar balances in the system. Acute and chronic pancreatitis are the two main causes of symptoms:

- Severe sharp pain just below the breast bone which penetrates through to the back; nausea and vomiting; feverishness with sweating may follow; sallow skin; bloating. Both chronic gall bladder problems and alcoholism predispose a patient to pancreatitis.
- **Pancreatitis must be reported immediately as it is sometimes life-threatening.**
- While waiting for treatment if there is a high fever then give **Belladonna** 200; if strong thirst, diarrhoea and weakness give **Phosphorus** 30 every hour; if restlessness, anxiety and thirst for sips of water give **Arsen-alb.** 30 every hour.

The Spleen

The spleen is located tucked away under the bottom ribs of the left side. It is involved in the breaking down and production of blood cells and is part of the immune system as it produces antibodies. The most common problems are either that it swells to cause discomfort or it needs to be removed as it has been ruptured in an accident. It should be the size of a bantam's egg though it does expand naturally in the course of its function; if it enlarges through pathology then it causes an ache deep in the left side which can be felt in the back on the left. This is often part of a general infection or conditions of the digestive tract. If not it might be swollen as part of an emotional condition in which the patient has lost all motivation and aspiration. This should be reported as part of a general symptom picture at an early appointment; a spleen in trouble should not be ignored for long or it will precede susceptibility to deeper pathology. For those who have lost their spleen it is always necessary to mention this early to the homoeopath. Contrary to some orthodox opinion, it is not necessary to take antibiotics on a regular basis if the spleen is removed, but the patient does require constitutional prescribing to maintain an efficient immune system.

14   FEMALE CONDITIONS

Period Pains

Menstrual pains may be intermittent and acute but they are seldom anything but part of a broader chronic pattern. Causes can include a hereditary disposition (a look at the mother's and grandmother's menstrual history is helpful), a history of taking the Pill (in mother or patient) or the morning-after pill, adhesions following an appendectomy, poor posture as the result of a traumatic accident or a difficult birth, termination, the presence of fibroids, hormone insufficiency, poor diet and emotional trauma. Anyone suffering from symptoms regularly should be consulting their homoeopath. There are a host of reasons for any of the conditions in this section and it is really important to have professional guidance, not least as there may be more than one maintaining cause that will have to be eliminated. However, it is reasonable for you to keep remedies that are indicated in the *acute* phase of pain as long as you have support and agreement from your practitioner. The remedies in the list below are described to illustrate the potential of homoeopathy in treating gynaecological distress. (NB If you are starting constitutional treatment then do not be surprised if the remedy that once helped with pains no longer does so; as the body heals, indications for remedies change.)

Apis: stinging pains often due to ovarian cyst. Very tender and sore over the right abdomen with drowsiness and irritability: does not appreciate being disturbed. Pains < before the flow which is scanty. Patient may complain of retaining water. Use 30.

Belladonna: ovarian pains are < on the right: hot and throbbing; bleeding is heavy or gushing with bearing-down pains as if everything would drop out. Blood is hot and bright red. > walking about or standing; < lying down. May have a throbbing headache, dry sore throat and cold limbs. Use 200.

Borax: heavy period comes on too soon with gripping pain going into the sacrum. Very easily startled and hates sudden noise. Feels sick and may have a sore mouth. Use 30.

Bryonia: period comes on too soon with tearing pains in the right ovary << for moving and which go down into the leg. Even deep breathing can < the pains. Bilious and thirsty for cold water. Wants to be at home; very bad tempered. Pains may be < between the periods; at ovulation when the abdomen is extremely sore. Use 30.

Cactus: sharp, piercing pains with pulsation that make the patient cry out; uterus feels squeezed and constricted. Pains cause her to double up in agony. Use 200.

Calc-phos.: useful in younger women and girls who are thin and tend to lack stamina. Stitching pains in the uterus before the flow starts which go through to the back. Restless and peevish with the discomfort. Use 30.

Chamomilla: excruciating uterine pains which make the patient intolerant and very difficult to help: she refuses help while complaining bitterly. This may be a genuine acute rather than a regular monthly period pain as the symptoms can be brought on from being furious. Pains are like labour pains which extend into the back. Use 30 or 200.

China: easily weakened by loss of blood (see **Phos.** and **Calc-phos.**); very useful in restoring strength after a heavy period. Flow is dark red and clotted and accompanied by general distension and congestion in the pelvis. Use 30.

Cimicifuga: neuralgic pains in the groin or across the pelvis from hip to hip or from ovary to ovary that come on with gloom and despair: feels that a black cloud descends on her; tearful and moaning. There can be tension and stiffness in the shoulders. Frequently indicated in those who are approaching menopause. Use a 30 unless your homoeopath suggests differently.

Cocculus: pains with dizziness, weakness and a nausea; feels almost like seasickness. Use 30.

Colocynth: pains in the abdomen (ovarian region) that force the patient to bend double and put pressure on the painful part (might lean over a chair, for example). Cutting, gripping pain with bearing down which comes on in waves and brings on a slight sweat and extreme irritability. Use 200.

Gelsemium: scanty flow with severe pains that radiate upwards into the back, across into the hips and down into the legs. Patient is droopy, hot and flushed, has no thirst and is apathetic. Use 30.

Lachesis: pains in the uterus and ovaries >> once the flow starts. Pains (< on the left but move to the right) may come on with pressure headache, hot flushes, palpitations and feelings of high blood pressure. Thick, dark blood with clots. She feels weak, irritable and easily overheated; she can't stand pressure of any sort especially clothes around the waist. Often indicated in the menopause. Often finds it 'hard to string two words together'. As this remedy always suggests that there is a lot of constitutional work to be done it is best to be guided by your practitioner as to dosage.

Lilium Tigrinum: strong bearing-down pains with sense of congestion in the pelvis. Feels bloated in abdomen. Very depressed but feels rushed and hurried; has to keep busy. Stabbing in the ovaries < left. Heart can feel oppressed during the menopause; fractious temper and inclined to swear or crash utensils about in the kitchen. This remedy usually suggests that there is quite a lot of constitutional work to be done by the homoeopath. Use 30 or 200.

Lycopodium: windy, bloated and inclined to feel faint with violent pains < on the right but which move over to the left. Pains are > for passing stools. Very tired by late afternoon. Use 30 or 100.

Mag-phos.: severe cramps which are > for a hot-water bottle and pressure (crossing arms over the abdomen or clutching a pillow). Pains come on before the flow starts. Blood is dark and stringy. Patient is likely to be 'down', drowsy and disinclined to do anything especially brain work. Frequently indicated in younger women. High potencies work best; use 200, 1M or even a 10M but give the dose in warm or hot water.

Nux-vom.: cramping period pains confused with feeling the urge to pass a motion (which does not happen satisfactorily); uterine spasms which feel bearing down and go into the sacrum. Use 30.

Phosphorus: burning pains in the uterus and ovaries < left. Feels the loss of blood weakening her. Wants to lie down from time to time but is restless and fidgety. Is sensitive and needs reassurance. Use 30.

Platina: bearing down in the uterus, drawing in the ovary and dark clotted blood. Strong tendency to mood swings. Can be indicated by hysterical symptoms during menses with paroxysmal pains in the ovary (< left) and uterus which bring on jerking and shrieking. This is a remedy best prescribed by your homoeopath; it is described here to suggest that such patients can be helped.

Pulsatilla: pains with absence of menses which might be suppressed from emotional stress or from getting her feet wet. Blood flow is thick, dark, slow and stops and starts. No pattern to the symptoms. She is tearful and dependent. Use 30 or 200.

Sepia: bearing-down sensations with dragging pains and exhaustion; late period flow which is scanty or too early and too much. Feels as if the bladder and uterus will prolapse and has sharp pains that stab upwards. In some it may be that the period pains are < since the birth of a child. Indifferent mood and snappy with the family: feels bad about it but can't help herself. Wants to be on her own or going out for a brisk walk. Use 30 or 100.

Sulphur: generally weak, overheated and sweaty with burning and itching in the vulva which might be reddened and sore from passing scanty, thick, dark blood. Patient is tired and wants to flop onto a sofa with a drink. Likely to be thirsty for water as well. Use 30 or 100.

Veratrum Album: dreadful pains with nausea, vomiting and cold sweats leaving her exhausted. Feels faint. This is a frightful condition and is best supervised by your homoeopath. However, in emergency use a 200 and report back to your practitioner.

Xanthoxylum: severe nerve and/or labour-like pains that travel from the ovaries and uterus into the back or down the anterior thighs. Slow flowing bleed with very dark blood. Use 30 or 200.

There are two remedies worth bearing in mind for the aftermath of a long or heavy period: **China** and **Phos-ac. China** has apathy and despondency with picky appetite and strong thirst for cold water. **Phos-ac.** has weakness and debility sometimes out of proportion to the blood loss; it has 'spaciness' and indifference as if there were no energy left to do anything at all. They can be used in the 30 twice daily to restore spent or lost energy. For those who have nervous exhaustion from premenstrual tension there are supplementary remedies that can be considered. For those who have scanty menstrual flow with nervous exhaustion and general loss of libido **Agnus Castus** is very likely to be useful. It can be taken in tincture form, in capsules or in low homoeopathic potency. For those who have nervous systems that are easily jangled by stress and made worse in the run-up to the period, and who have difficulty sleeping and finding energy to get through the day, **Avena Sativa** is indicated as a support remedy. This is also available as a tincture or as a potency. If it is taken in tincture then it works best when given in hot water. **Aletris Farinosa** is another remedy in tincture or potency which is useful in support of those who have heavy, painful periods that come too frequently; they also suffer from a feeling of prolapse, weakness, poor appetite, leucorrhoea and constipation. If you can identify with one of these then discuss the options of form and dosage with your practitioner. If you do not have a practitioner yet then you might consider that **Agnus Castus** is available in capsules from most health food shops and that **Avena** and **Aletris** are available in 2 or 3 doses from homoeopathic pharmacies. These potencies (to be taken up to once or twice per day) are so low that they are close enough to the original herbal tincture to contain some material medicine. These would not interfere with any other remedy which may be prescribed for the general constitution.

Pre-menstrual Syndrome

The symptoms of PMS are the result of hormonal imbalances. The hormones involved are principally oestrogen and progesterone though these are regulated by other hormones secreted by the hypothalamus and the pituitary, glands deep in the brain. Adrenalin can also play a part in the chemistry by flooding the system, especially in those who lead a fast lifestyle or who are stressed. PMS may occur regularly each month or every other month (which suggests that one ovary is malfunctioning) or it may happen intermittently. It can start two weeks after the last bleed at ovulation when oestrogen levels are supposed to drop; if they don't then bloating from fluid retention and breast tenderness come on. It might start only days or hours before the arrival of the flow. Sometimes PMS stands for *post*-menstrual syndrome. The symptoms might only be gynaecological or they may include changes in temperature, appetite, digestion and sleep pattern, headaches, susceptibility to minor infections, swollen glands, joint pains, bad complexion and energy loss. Moods can swing from anxiety to fury, despair to confusion. Because PMS is so varied in its manifestation it is really important to consult your homoeopath for long-term treatment. It is not enough to use the remedies to get over the acute phase each month; though they may do just that, the patient is no nearer a lasting resolution to whatever underlying condition there may be. If the symptoms of PMS are part of a larger picture of fibroids, polycystic ovaries or endometriosis then much deeper prescribing will have to be undertaken. Many of the remedies above such as **Lillium-tig.**, **Platina** or **Lachesis**, which are helpful in such conditions, are almost never more than one layer of a whole case. Nevertheless, it is worth mentioning that treatment that concentrates exclusively on gynaecology is seldom satisfactory. Nothing goes wrong gynaecologically unless the patient has a family history of menstrual problems or a personal history of trauma (which may or may not be known because 'trauma' can stem from an event before puberty or from a difficult birth) or she is in some way 'ungrounded'. Such things need investigation and remedial treatment. It is best if cranial osteopathy complements the homoeopathy.

It is worth mentioning that PMS is often aggravated by food intolerance and by the presence of candida. These can be the cause of continued or worsened leucorrhoea (the 'whites'), a mucous discharge which often stops with the arrival of the period and, if candida is present, causes itching and soreness. While some of the remedies above cover white (or yellow) discharge, it is important to seek professional homoeopathic help as complicated gynaecological symptom pictures are very unlikely to be solved through self-help alone.

Irregular or Absent Periods

The causes are many: dysfunction of the hypothalamus and pituitary glands (which stimulate the ovaries and uterus to function on a monthly cycle), underactive thyroid gland, overactive adrenal glands, polycystic ovaries, a history of side effects after taking the Pill, a history of physical trauma (which might have led to a compensatory body posture that causes compression of the ovaries and uterus) or a hereditary pattern of menstrual difficulties are some of the common reasons. While the first few periods may take a while to settle into a rhythm it is abnormal for women to have anything but a 28-day cycle. Ideally menstruation should go according to the moon; we are made of a little over 70% water and we have natural tides in our bodies over which the moon has a very significant influence. Establishing a regular pattern or investigating the reasons for its absence is very important because too frequent periods are draining to the general constitution and infrequent periods deny the body the benefits of a valuable elimination system. Though supplementary nutritional help may be useful it is unlikely to solve any long-term problems; it is best to consult your homoeopath so that constitutional treatment can get to the bottom of the problem. You may well be advised to have complementary treatment as well from a cranial osteopath.

Leucorrhoea and Thrush

Leucorrhoea is a white or creamy-coloured vaginal discharge. While it is normal for there to be a lubricating discharge, if the discharge is odorous, thick (like yoghurt or cottage cheese) or causes itching then treatment is advisable. If the discharge is bloody or green or brown then you should seek professional advice straight away. The more itching, odour and intensity of discharge, the more likely is it that candida, a yeast infection, is present. Candida takes a considerable amount of time to resolve; be prepared for a long haul though it is definitely worthwhile. Thrush is synonymous with candida: the itching and variable discharge are typical so leucorrhoea may be part of the picture. Occasionally it is the cause of flare-ups of vaginitis which requires professional prescribing.

Fibroids

Fibroids are made up of fibrous muscle tissue and grow on the wall of the uterus. They are non-malignant though they can be a nuisance or a threat due to their size and location; some will grow to the size of a grapefruit or more. They often grow larger during a pregnancy and can diminish in size afterwards. They may be the cause of irregular or excessively heavy periods, bleeding mid-cycle, frequent urging to urinate or pass motions, heaviness in the lower abdomen and even infertility if they block off the Fallopian tubes. Sometimes a troublesome fibroid is present in someone who has not been able to express feelings after emotional trauma (usually long buried). In cases like this homoeopathic treatment either encourages expression of these feelings (and thus removes the need for the fibroid) or strengthens the constitution so that, if an operation is required, removal of the fibroid leads to no further complications. Sometimes a general anaesthetic can bring about a return to a historical moment long buried that will encourage the resolution of grief. (A homoeopath will find it significant that a fibroid should grow on the left or the right of the uterus; information from a scan is useful.)

Endometriosis

The endometrium is the lining of the womb which thickens in response to oestrogen each month in the expectation of pregnancy. If fertilisation does not happen, the unwanted extra blood supply is sloughed off with the endometrium. Endometriosis is a condition in which patches of endometrial cells develop outside the womb. This maverick tissue adheres to the outside of the uterus, the ligaments that hold it in place or the ovaries, though it can be found in other, more distant parts where it causes even greater trouble. When these patches respond to progesterone they 'bleed' in the same way that the endometrium does; this brings on painful cramping. A long-term effect is scar tissue and adhesions forming in the areas. It is one of those conditions that might have been developing for several years before causing any noticeable symptoms. Endometriosis is relatively common (found in more than 10% of women) and more so amongst women who find it difficult or impossible to conceive or in women who have had babies after their early 30s. It is also more common among women whose close relatives suffer or suffered the same problem. Though orthodox medicine is unable to find a cause, homoeopaths work with the knowledge that there are both hereditary (miasmatic) and emotional reasons (sometimes common to several generations of women) for endometriosis. Treatment is long term but far more positive than the hormone drug and surgery options of orthodox medicine which claims no cure. The homoeopath will not concentrate exclusively on the gynaecology but will also ask searching questions about emotional issues and menstrual history of other members of the family if this is available.

Pelvic Inflammatory Disease

PID is a chronic state of infection of the Fallopian tubes. Bacteria that cause pus to block the tubes proliferate after being introduced during intercourse, a miscarriage or an abortion. It is common after the suppression of non-specific urethritis or other sexually transmitted diseases. Orthodox medicine treats PID with antibiotics but this results in further suppression of the body's immune system. Homoeopathy seeks to restore the integrity of the immune system so that it can eliminate the susceptibility to allowing bacteria to grow unhindered. This requires long-term heavy-duty prescribing with a careful assessment of heredity, the patient's health biography and a precise understanding of the presenting complaint. Symptoms include abdominal pain (which may be aching, cramping, burning, piercing or cutting and may change location or be constant), irregular bleeding, scanty discharge, odorous vaginal discharge, intermittent mild fever with nausea, headache and occasional vomiting and a general feeling of frailty and malaise. **There is grave cause for concern if acute flare-ups result in a high fever and development of an abdominal abscess as this can lead to peritonitis; such symptoms must be treated professionally at once!** The homoeopath is likely to work not just on gynaecology but also on the health of the liver and spleen as well, taking into account the efficiency of the bowels and kidneys too, as the elimination organs are of paramount importance.

Polycystic Ovaries

This condition often takes some time to diagnose as symptoms can vary. The first symptoms occur fairly early in puberty. Periods may not start at all or they may come intermittently. There may be scanty or profuse bleeding, no pain or much. Some girls may put on excessive weight while others none at all. Similarly, some will grow abnormal amounts of body hair and others will not. Diagnosis is usually by means of blood tests and ultrasound scans. The cause of the symptoms is fluid-filled cysts on the ovaries (usually both of them) which contain androgens (male hormones) that bring about the abnormal hormone-related symptomatic changes. Orthodox medicine does not offer any certain resolution as it has to rely on synthetic hormones (including the Pill) to counterbalance those present in the system. Such treatment is frowned on by homoeopaths as it offers only a complication of a state that remains unchanged beneath, and can be the cause of infertility and a progression towards other chronic disease patterns. As with other gynaecological conditions homoeopathy seeks to rebalance the body's own hormone system. The homoeopath will be very exacting about the symptoms and how they change the period cycle from the ideal. In addition, the practitioner will frequently ask about changes in body temperature, physical routines (such as times of day for passing water and motions and going to sleep), energy patterns and other details that will subtly show how the whole body is responding. Polycystic ovaries are never a condition without hereditary implications; there is always a miasmatic state, often several layers of it. It may take many months of concentrated prescribing but an otherwise healthy constitution should be able to create a sustainable hormonal balance eventually even if the cysts remain.

Infertility

Infertility can arise for various obvious reasons: absence or irregularity of periods, chronic pathology of the reproductive organs, chronic dysfunction of the pituitary gland, the side effects of synthetic hormone interference (the Pill or the morning-after pill), the traumatic results of surgery or an accident and congenital defects of any of the reproductive structures in either sex. There are other, less well-known reasons: the woman may be 'intolerant' of her partner's semen and either 'kill it off' or physically reject it. Occasionally, emotional reasons, though they cannot be tested through blood or scans, can be sufficient to prevent conception: a history of broken relationships, terminations or of sexual abuse is sometimes enough to be an obstacle. Until these are resolved, pregnancy is delayed. (Very occasionally women who are apparently anxious to conceive realise, after starting constitutional treatment, that they do not truly want children but have been trying for their partner's sake.) The homoeopath is likely to be searching not only about the gynaecological history and general state but also about the patient's past biography of health and emotions.

Contraception

The contraceptive pill is the most popular form of prevention but it has a steep price. Synthetic hormones are sent in to alter the body's own natural rhythms. This seldom happens without side effects which are not always evident till later. Usually the side effects are not enough to be bothersome; the benefits outweigh the disadvantages. Unfortunately, thinking like this can lead to long-term chronic conditions. Increased breast tenderness, aching legs, the appearance of varicose veins, headaches, weight gain, reduction of menstrual blood, loss of libido and skin tone, fluid retention, raised blood pressure, depression and greater susceptibility to infections are some of the changes that result. None should be ignored. These symptoms are the thin end of a wedge of future pathology. Very often the patient does not pick up the bill till the menopause which proves to be complicated, long drawn-out (sometimes several years) and very debilitating. If the patient smokes or drinks then all the risks are greatly increased. Hormone injections and implants carry the same caveats.

Intrauterine devices carry other risks: they are responsible for inflammatory conditions within the uterus and tubes, and can lead to infertility and contribute to PID. The devices also slow-release hormones or copper into the system which can both cause problems. The long-term presence of a foreign object in the uterus can cause structural damage to the organ. White blood cells are sent to the site and create an inflammatory response which is, incidentally, toxic to sperm. What this means is that the uterus is in a constant state of inflammation alert; a condition that is not healthy for the whole. Frequent examinations and insertions of new devices can set up emotional trauma in sensitive women.

Diaphragms and spermicides may be constitutionally safer but they are not without some risk. Spermicides can set up local reactions which cause irritation and skin changes to both partners. The most satisfactory of these methods is the honey cap; a cap that is smeared with runny honey (preferably organic), a contraceptive that has been in use since ancient Egyptian times. Honey is both spermicidal and antibiotic. (See the appendix for the UK contact.)

Many women seek homoeopathic help for Pill- or diaphragm-related conditions and would like to stop using them but feel that they cannot because their partners refuse to use condoms. Homoeopaths are often asked if there is a *homoeopathic* contraceptive but we are doomed to disappoint patients; there is none. Apart from the rhythm method and runny honey we have nothing better to offer.

It is not uncommon for a woman to consult a homoeopath about either menopausal problems or even seemingly unrelated conditions only for her to say that she has 'never been well since taking the Pill'. The long-term results can be expressed by a huge variety of symptoms; anything from 'break-through' bleeding to depression, loss of libido to underactive thyroid. The practitioner will take a thorough history of the period cycle, children born and miscarriages and details of the use of contraceptive methods. This is all to determine how much the present complaint should be attributed to artificial hormone interference. It may well be that it is of primary significance and requires a prescription that reminds the body of what its original hormone cycle was. This can set up reactions such as a vaginal discharge resembling a period, often of dark, thick blood, and other hormone-related changes. This may seem worrying but is absolutely natural.

The same may be true of an acute episode following taking the morning-after pill. Though this is a seriously damaging drug, some feel obliged to take it and then they feel the side effects. The homoeopath does have remedies to deal with this but the result can set up a short-term reaction which might involve an eliminative discharge.

One other point to consider: some schools of homoeopathic thought see the range of hormone drugs that are used for contraception and hormone replacement therapy as seriously deleterious to the constitution and an impediment to homoeopathy working. While there is truth in this, it is not true that remedies do not work at all on patients while they are on hormone drugs. Remedies may be unable to achieve 100% of their full potential for creating positive change in such cases but they can still do a lot. One reason for homoeopaths continuing to prescribe while drugs are being used is to help patients to come to the time when they feel ready to cope without any artificial support.

The Menopause

There are three different times at which the menopause can occur in a woman's life: following a hysterectomy before the normal menopause, premature menopause occurring before the early 40s and natural menopause that can occur from the late 40s to the mid 50s. A surgically induced menopause can have a variety of implications: if only the uterus is removed then the ovaries can continue to be hormonally active giving the patient a sense of cyclical patterns continuing. If one ovary is removed with the uterus then a state of imbalance can occur which may be negligible but may be enough to cause symptoms of 'not feeling quite right'. If uterus and ovaries are removed then the shock of a full menopause may set up feelings of disorientation, though initially women feel immense relief to be rid of the symptoms they had before surgery. It is always advisable for a woman going through the process of gynaecological surgery to have both homoeopathy (to prepare for the operation and help re-establish hormone balance afterwards) and cranial osteopathy (to ensure physical harmony and to complement the homoeopathy) or acupuncture.

Premature menopause is often caused by either hereditary disposition or chronic pathology involving the endocrine glands. For such patients both homoeopathy and cranial osteopathy or acupuncture are recommended.

The menopause is sometimes preceded by the perimenopause: a phase in which the cycle seems to stop or become irregular. This is a very propitious moment to use homoeopathy. It is a time when the homoeopath will take the opportunity of assessing the significance of past history in relation to present symptoms. If main constitutional remedies do not appear to create the positive changes needed then others are sent in to deal with buried layers of such conditions as 'never been well since' (NBWS) the Pill; NBWS the birth of one of the children, NBWS a general anaesthetic, glandular fever, a divorce, radiotherapy, etc.

Many women are encouraged to avoid the menopause by going on hormone replacement therapy because it is seen as a pathological condition.

This is understandable when osteoporosis might threaten to debilitate the patient. However, HRT is an artificial means of prolonging an energy state that should naturally change. It is not natural for endocrine energy to be flowing through the sacral plexus after the time for the natural menopause. Obliging the body to continue functioning as if it is procreative is profoundly disturbing to the whole body. In alternative philosophy, the energy that flows through the reproductive system during the procreative years does not stop at the menopause; it changes. What was once necessary for conceiving and rearing children is now needed in the heart centre. This is the time that would, if we were living in a tribal society, mark the change to becoming an 'elder', imbued with the wisdom of experience. With HRT this is physiologically (and psychologically) prevented. In some ancient cultures the womb is regarded as the 'lower heart' and the energy that has kept it functioning creatively needs to rise to the 'upper heart'. Unfortunately, there is sometimes a physical price to pay: dry eyes, lack of energy, insomnia, poor bladder control, weight gain, poor memory, loss of libido with dry mucous membranes and unaccountable nervousness. Worse than these can be hot flushes, with or without sweating. As homoeopathy is very effective at relieving women of these symptoms, HRT should be the very last resort. Acupuncture is also excellent at balancing a system disturbed by menopausal symptoms.

Osteoporosis

This is a chronic progressive degenerative condition of the bones that raises the risk of fractures especially in the spine and wrists. It mostly affects white people who are thin and have a history of it in the family. The risks are worse for smokers, heavy drinkers and those who have used steroids for a long time. The condition is the result of an imbalance in the calcium-phosphorus ratio in the body, which is controlled by the parathyroid gland, together with a reduction of oestrogen in the body. The longer the condition has been going the less effective homoeopathic treatment is. If it is addressed early then it is possible to encourage the body to slow or even halt the progress.

Breast Problems

The breasts may be a combination of fatty and glandular tissue run through with ducts and blood supply but, to homoeopaths, they are an integral part of the reproductive system and cannot be treated as if they were no more than appendages. Pathology of the breasts is seldom present without a history of other problems either emotional, hereditary or gynaecological and quite often a mixture of all three. Furthermore, to a homoeopath there is significance in whether the left or right breast is affected; the left side of the body is regarded as yin or to do with the feminine or mothering principle, and the right is yang and to do with the masculine or father principle. The significance of this should not be underestimated as the origins of breast pathology so often lie in relationships with other members of the family (especially mother or father or forbears), living or past. The theme of 'nurture' is almost always part of the emotional picture underlying.

Breast pain is most common as part of PMS or at ovulation. Many women put up with it especially if they have 'lumpy breasts' (as in fibrocystic breasts or fibroadenoma) and have been told to expect it. But this is unnecessary. Painful breasts in PMS in an otherwise healthy person is likely to resolve quite speedily after constitutional treatment. If the pain is due to cysts then treatment will focus on hereditary factors as well, as there is always an underlying miasmatic condition. It is not a good idea to have fluid-filled cysts drained; it offers only temporary relief and can, if done too often, aggravate a benign condition into something more aggressive. The remedies prescribed by a homoeopath for breast pains are likely to be indicated on much more than simply 'pain in the breasts before menses' so it is important to seek a consultation. However, if the symptom is the most aggravating problem then it will be central to the choice of medication. It is not unusual for an initial prescription to bring up issues relating to family or to mothering and nurturing.

Mastitis

This is not always only a problem of the breast; if there is fever with it then it is a whole body event. Suppression by the usual antibiotic treatment not only causes defective milk if the patient is breastfeeding but also predisposes her to a future breast abscess. The most common cause of mastitis is inflammation and engorgement of the breast from a blocked milk duct (see 'Pregnancy and Birth'). Always inform your practitioner of this condition so that they can monitor progress.

Breast Abscesses

These are due to pus collecting in the tissues. They can be extremely painful and need careful management. They sometimes require high potencies to resolve them. Abscesses are never simply local problems, wherever they form. They are whole-body events with the liver, the main blood-cleansing unit of the system, a central player even if it is not symptomatically apparent. For an abscess to form there must have been toxicity to be eliminated even if it is the result of a traumatic injury. Always report an abscess to your homoeopath because it is a major opportunity to do some clearing of 'old stuff'. Suppression of an abscess by antibiotics is simply not a safe course of action to take. Either it will return or it will find another site or it will come back in a more malignant form at a later date. It is likely that an abscess would call for one of the following:

Belladonna: the area is red, hot and throbbing with tenderness and sharp pains. (Use 30 unless you know that the patient does well with the 200.) There may be a general fever as well which will be over 102°F. < around 3 a.m. or p.m. (Use a 200 and repeat if the fever rises again.)

Bryonia: the area is very hard, hot and extremely sensitive. Pains are << for the slightest movement. The abscess is more likely < on the right side. (Use 30 unless otherwise directed by your practitioner.)

Hepar-sulph.: extremely painful area which is swollen and reddened and very sensitive to touch. (Use 30 or 200.)

Lachesis: abscess most likely of the left breast with swelling, tenderness and purplish discoloration. The breast is < the least pressure. Patient is likely to be very irritable or anxious and a bit incoherent. The pains are likely to wake her at night. (Use 30.)

Merc-sol.: more likely to be < right side; painful, sensitive area which is swollen and red (can look like **Bell.**) but there is frequent alternation of temperature, strong thirst for cold water and sweats at night which make the patient feel worse. (Use 30 but go up to 200 if there is little change within 8 hours and let your homoeopath know what is happening.)

Phytolacca: abscess more likely on the right side of the right breast. Breast area becomes stony hard. Swollen and tender; also purplish in colour. The glands under the right arm swell and become sore and the muscles of the arm are achy. (Patients who need **Phytolacca** should not eat anything salty or milky. Use 30 but be ready to go up to 200 if there is no change within 6 hours and inform the homoeopath.)

Silica: early stages of an abscess; hard lump with little pain starts and then develops intermittent sharp pains. The patient is likely to feel delicate and in need of support (though she will hate to be told what to do). May be chilly and defensive. (Use 30 but watch for a change in symptoms; you may find the picture change to **Hepar-sulph.** or **Merc-sol.** If **Merc-sol.** seems indicated then give a **Hepar-sulph.** 30 first and then wait for 10 minutes before giving the **Merc-sol.**)

Discharges from the nipples should always be reported to the homoeopath. Sometimes blood or pus exudes and sometimes milk even when there is no pregnancy. Such discharges are not necessarily alarming; there may be a lump in a duct (bleeding) or a small abscess under the nipple (pus). Milk present in women who are not pregnant or just delivered of a baby suggests a hormone problem.

Breast Cancer

A patient presenting breast cancer is not unsusceptible to the homoeopathic healing process. Though most patients want to follow the orthodox route and have all the tests and current treatment available, those who do so while taking complementary homoeopathic treatment have a far greater chance of success. Chemotherapy, surgery and radiotherapy are all highly suppressive of pathology that originally had a historical root cause, nothing of which is investigated by doctors. If the homoeopath works with the patient going through the suppression of the cancer not only will the side effects of the treatment be remedied but the hereditary and emotional causes that underlie the disease will sooner or later be focused on. It cannot be stressed just how important this is. Official statistics never take the resolving of emotional issues into account and the only therapy, alternative or otherwise, that knows what to do about the *miasmatic* aspect of cancer is homoeopathy.

For those who are going through the process of chemotherapy there are a number of remedies that are of use: **Arsen-alb.** (restless and anxious with waves of nausea and griping abdomen); **Cadmium-sulph.** (persistent nausea and vomiting with chilliness and debility which is > resting < lifting anything); **Ipecac.** (constant nausea with vomiting and especially indicated if there is pressure in the head and headache). Ask your homoeopath about potency though **Cadmium-sulph.** is commonly given daily in the 30 and the others work well in the 200 when given as needed (up to 3 per day when symptoms are severe). **Echinacea** as a herbal supplement has been recommended to improve the white blood cell count after chemotherapy; the homoeopath should advise on whether to use the tincture or the health food shop pills.

For those who are being given radiotherapy ask your practitioner about using **Cadmium-sulph.** as it can help with the extreme tiredness, burning and itching of the skin, hair loss and nausea. Another remedy is **Radium Bromide** which is useful when the indications for **Cadmium-sulph.** are indistinct and this is often prescribed by practitioners regardless of symptoms as a way of combating radiation. None of these remedies can interfere with the orthodox treatment; they support the body as it undergoes suppressive therapy. For the itching and burning of the skin after radiotherapy **Rad-brom.**, **Sol** and **Calendula** are all helpful though it is best to ask your practitioner for guidance on dosage.

15 MALE CONDITIONS

Thrush

The symptoms are irritation, soreness and redness of the glans (the end of the penis) and foreskin (if uncircumcised) and these usually occur after intercourse, particularly in new relationships. This is usually regarded as a fungal infection and is sometimes referred to as candida. Smegma (a white deposit under the foreskin) may also be evident. Sometimes assiduous washing is enough but if symptoms are persistent then professional help is necessary. Though fungal infections are not always viewed by allopathy as transmissible through sexual relations, the alternative view differs. It is not the fungal aspect that is paramount, but the quality and intensity of the symptoms that betray the possible link with miasmatic inheritance. Anti-fungal creams prescribed by doctors remove thrush symptoms but not the chronic tendency; persistent suppression of fungal infections can lead to susceptibility to STDs.

The most commonly indicated remedy for a sore, red penis is **Merc-sol.** which can resolve the problem within hours if the 30 is taken at the rate of one every 4 hours for 3 or 4 doses. If this does not clear the problem, see the homoeopath. (A clear description of the symptoms, when it began and what changes have occurred is enough to prescribe on.)

Balanitis

This is inflammation of the head of an uncircumcised penis and is usually the result of a yeast infection. There is pain, redness, soreness and itching with swelling. Symptoms can interfere with body functions. Acute phimosis (see over) may cause balanitis or result from it. It is best to seek professional help quite soon for this, though if the symptoms of **Merc-sol.** are obvious (redness, soreness, itching and swelling), this can be taken while waiting for an appointment.

Problems with the Foreskin: Phimosis and Paraphimosis

If the opening of the foreskin tightens and prevents retraction, this is phimosis; it is common amongst babies and young boys. If the foreskin is retracted back (as if too short) over the glans with a phimotic opening then it is known as paraphimosis which causes swelling and pain. Phimosis is often left to resolve by itself but can be the cause of acute symptoms in which constitutional treatment is required. Paraphimosis can be persistent and circumcision may be recommended; if there is opportunity then the homoeopath may be able to resolve it if given time unless it is a congenital defect. It can take anywhere between 3 months and 3 years to effect the complete change needed. In a person young enough (up to the age of about 10 or 11) it is worth being patient and allowing the homoeopathy to work as the problem is unlikely to be passed on to the next generation.

Circumcision: this should be preceded by a prophylactic dose of **Emerald** 30 and followed by **Arnica** 30 (one dose) and **Calendula** 30 (one twice daily for 3 – 5 days) and **Hypericum** 30 (one each night for 3 – 5 days).

Orchitis and Epididymitis

This is inflammation of the testicle and the epididymis, the bundle of tubes attached to the testicle. The cause may be poor drainage due to injury, a bladder infection, the results of surgery or investigation or it may be a symptom of gonorrhoea or NSU (see pages 239–40). In men, mumps (see pages 76–8) can move to the testicles from the parotid glands and cause painful inflammation. Symptoms can range from swelling with discomfort to pain extending up into the abdomen or into the hips or thighs. The pain is usually aching and there may be heaviness. It can make a difference to the choice of remedies whether the problem is on the left or right. For contusion of the testicle **Arnica** is the first remedy to consider (use the 30 or 200). Otherwise the most common remedy for either of these conditions is **Pulsatilla** especially if it is the left testicle that is affected. Though it is always best to consult the homoeopath, if the symptoms include heaviness, drawing and aching which extends up into the abdomen and all < while sitting then use **Puls**. 30 (one every 4 hours) while you are waiting for help. (The same symptoms can occasionally result from sitting on cold, damp ground or on stone; **Puls**. is still the remedy of choice.)

Hydrocele, Varicocele and Hematocele

A hydrocele occurs when water collects between a testicle and its covering membrane. It is usually painless and harmless unless it becomes so large as to cause discomfort. They can be resolved with remedies but it is often best to complement these with cranial osteopathy as this encourages good drainage and the return to balanced posture in cases where this has been lost. A varicocele is a collection of varicose veins in the scrotum and is the result of downward pressure from the liver and digestive tract. Though **Pulsatilla** and **Hamamelis** are the two most commonly indicated remedies it is more likely that the problem would resolve by combining homoeopathy and cranial osteopathy or acupuncture. A hematocele is the result of contusion to the testicles when bruising causes blood to collect in a pocket. **Arnica** (bruising and dull aching pain) or **Hamamelis** (sore, aching and occasional sharp pains running into the testicle; purplish discoloration may be apparent) are the most indicated remedies though ask for advice on potency and dosage from your practitioner.

Priapism

This is a condition of continuous painful penile erection which is without any desire. It is caused by some orthodox drugs (such as some steroids, chlorpromazine, anticoagulants and drugs for impotence) or other pathology (such as a blood clot or a tumour in the pelvis). While remedies are of service, investigation may be advisable to discover the cause. If small boys are troubled by this problem it suggests that there is a hormonal and emotional imbalance which can become quite disruptive in the household. This requires professional help so that the child can return to a more normal and steady development.

Testicular Torsion

The testicles are suspended by ligaments into the scrotum; blood vessels and the vas deferens, the tube that transports sperm up into the seminal vesicle, are also attached. Sometimes these structures can become tangled causing considerable pain and the blood supply to be blocked off. Where no other help is available surgery is usually the only option. The cause of the torsion might be overstraining while lifting heavy objects, as an emotional reaction or for no obvious reason, though there is always one there. Other symptoms that can manifest include nausea, vomiting, heaviness in the testicle, drawing sensation up into the abdomen and aching into the hips or thighs. There are a number of different remedies that might be indicated including **Pulsatilla** (the typical symptoms will include tearfulness or dependency in a young person or worry and a need for support in older men), **Rhododendron** (pains will go into the hips and thighs) and **Aurum** (comes on with anxiety and depression). There is also one other remedy that practitioners might use: **Ayahuasca**, a vine from South America which is often useful when anything in the body becomes twisted. It is important to get very prompt professional attention for this condition; speak to the homoeopath as soon as possible who may advise going to A & E. While you are waiting a dose of the indicated remedy may be of considerable benefit.

Testicular Cancer

Firm or hard lumps on the testicle or a swollen, hard testicle are causes for a consultation. (Lumps on the scrotum, the testicular sac, are usually cysts that have developed from a hair follicle and harmless.) This is not a condition for home prescribing. It is important, though, to have homoeopathy even if surgery is the chosen option of treatment because the practitioner will be able to give remedies to improve recovery and minimise the likelihood of metastasis (spread) to other organs. Remedies will not interfere with allo-pathic procedure.

Impotence

Erectile dysfunction is not just the preserve of old men. The reasons for it include the following: emotional stress; depression; excessive workload; overindulgence in high living; long-term use of marijuana; an unacknowl-edged realisation that one is with the wrong partner; alcoholism; a trauma such as occurs after surgery to the spine or rectum; certain drugs such as anti-depressants or sleeping pills; diabetes or any condition that disturbs nerve function or blood supply. Impotence can even strike young men when they feel trapped in an early relationship and unable to move on. It can be a problem for some men who reach retirement and suddenly feel 'put out to grass'. Unless there has been irreparable damage to blood and nerve supply, homoeopathy is able to offer treatment that is based on the current constitutional state. While there is no need for physical examination, patients should be prepared to answer queries about libido and the level of dysfunction as part of the whole picture so that an indicated remedy may be chosen. There are no aphrodisiacs per se in homoeopathy; there are only remedies that have a reputation for being frequently indicated by those with problems of libido and impotence. It is well worthwhile following this route as the orthodox alternatives include drugs that can cause side effects and surgical procedures that are less than satisfactory. Homoeopathy is well complemented here by cranial osteopathy or acupuncture. In addition, it is worth noting that herbalists might prescribe Gingko Biloba for impotence. Bach Flower Essences that can be helpful are Elm (feeling inadequate), Larch (fear of failure), Mimulus (shyness) and White Chestnut (unable to switch off from the day). Any or all of these can be added to a bottle of **Lotus** 6 or 30 and one drop taken as required. This is a very therapeutic approach but one that does not interfere with constitutional prescriptions though always inform the homoeopath of what is being taken.

Prostate Problems

The prostate is awkwardly situated; it sits below the bladder and around the urethra. If it swells (hypertrophy or hyperplasia) then the bore of the urethra can be restricted leading to difficult, slow or dribbling urination. Though the condition is benign and common amongst men over 45 it is worth seeking help from the homoeopath. Hypertrophy is not the same as prostatitis which is inflammation of the prostate, usually the result of a bacterial infection though it might occur as part of a viral condition or candidiasis.

Enlarged Prostate

Reasons for the enlargement are varied: hormone changes (the male menopause); a chronically held accident pattern in the musculo-skeletal system; years of straining to pass motions due to chronic constipation; a history of chronic and suppressed urinary infections. The early signs are difficulty in getting the flow to start, needing to get up at night to urinate, feeble stream, dribbling at the end of urination and a sense of not having quite finished passing all the water. Sometimes there is the need to go back to the lavatory to pass more within 10 minutes. This may eventually progress to complete blockage of urine if urging goes unheeded for too long (as may happen on a long motorway drive, for example) which requires catheterisation unless an appropriate remedy is to hand (most commonly needed is **Causticum** 30). The homoeopath would want to know the details of the difficulty in urinating. There are subtle differences in symptoms that can make all the difference between choosing one remedy and another (i.e. 'has to stand with legs apart while urinating' or 'has to sit, leaning back in order to urinate'). Herbalists extol the virtues of saw palmetto as a remedy for prostate enlargement and it is a supplement that many homoeopaths will recommend too. It has quite a high rate of effectiveness at lessening the symptoms though it is only rarely a 'cure'. It is available from health food shops or as a tincture from the homoeopathic pharmacies though it would be best to be advised by the practitioner.

Prostatitis

The symptoms of prostatitis can be similar to a bladder infection with the addition of a strong ache in the low abdomen and a bruised pain in the testicles. A doctor might only be able to diagnose this by a rectal examination but a careful description of symptoms is usually sufficient for a homoeopath to select a remedy. Prostatitis can be either an acute one-off condition or a chronic state. If the latter then long-term treatment may be required to deal with a history of suppressed urinary tract infections so the patient should be prepared to give details of these.

16   BLADDER AND KIDNEY PROBLEMS

Infections of the Lower Urinary Tract

Urethritis: is an infection of the urethra, the tube that draws urine from the bladder. It can be a one-off acute or it can be a chronic intermittent problem. It is more common among girls and women and can be associated with bacteria or fungi (as would be the case in candida). The usual symptoms include inflammation of the urethra, frequency of urging with scanty urine and a variety of pains as it is passed such as burning, stinging, smarting, cutting and stabbing. Sometimes there is a discharge of pus which may have an unusual odour; if this is present then non-specific urethritis or gonorrhoea should be suspected. As far as homoeopathy is concerned recurrent urethritis and discharges of pus are regarded as symptoms of miasmatic susceptibility and require constitutional treatment.

Cystitis: is an infection of the bladder. It is more common in women than in men. The symptom picture includes frequency of urging, acidic urine which may flow in small quantities, burning or stinging pains and aching or cramps in the lower abdomen. The urine may change colour and be dark and have an offensive odour. In women, cystitis may occur with new sexual relationships; it used to be known as honeymoon cystitis (see **Staphysagria** page 234). Older women can become susceptible to cystitis because of lax ligaments that no longer hold the organs of the pelvis in place; they tend to sag causing stagnation of urine in a tilted bladder (see **Sepia** and **Populus Tremuloides** pages 234). The same can be true of those who have had surgery or several children. Men who have urethritis or cystitis may also go on to have aching in the prostate. Men and women can become susceptible to cystitis after catheterisation or examination procedures (see **Staph.**).

Cystitis often calls for one of the following remedies:

Apis: burning and stinging pains especially severe when the last drop is passed; patient is very irritable especially when disturbed but otherwise tends to doze. Urethra feels swollen and may be red and puffy as if stung by a bee. (Use 30.)

Belladonna: tender lower abdomen with accompanying fever. Urine is dark burning hot. (Depending on the degree of fever use 30 or 200.)

Berberis Vulgaris: cystitis with kidney pains that radiate down into the bladder and the legs or through to the liver and stomach; burning in the urethra when *not* passing urine; aching into thighs while urinating. Always feels some urine is left in the bladder. (Use 30.)

Cannabis Sativa: painful urging to pass very little urine which eventually dribbles out drop by drop. Burning all up the urethra to bladder. Urine may be reddish or have sediment or pus. Patient may want to walk with legs apart. (Contact your homoeopath if this remedy does not clear the problem quickly in case there is more to the cystitis than is apparent.)

Cantharis: burning on passing urine which only dribbles or comes drop by drop; scalding urine causes sensations of cutting and burning in the bladder and tenderness and sensitivity in the lower abdomen; can feel as if the intestines are involved. The patient is anxious and restless and can fire up in a fit of anger. (Use 30 or 200 if severe.)

Merc-sol.: burning in the bladder or urethra at the start of releasing urine and for a while after. Urine might be dark, scanty, bloody or cloudy and might smell like ammonia. The patient will be alternately hot and chilly, very thirsty for cold water and have offensive breath. (Use 30; if this does not hold then contact the homoeopath.) It is worth mentioning **Merc-corr.** as this remedy is often needed when **Merc-sol.** does not do what is expected. **Merc-corr.** has very similar symptoms but is far more aggressive and has greenish urine and sweating after passing it. (Use 30.)

Populus Tremuloides: useful for cystitis after operations or in pregnancy or in older women who suffer dyspepsia, flatulence and tenderness in the lower abdomen. Sometimes useful in older men who have similar symptoms but with prostate troubles. The urine is scalding on passing and it leaves an ache behind the pubic bone afterwards. (Use 30.)

Pulsatilla: cystitis after an emotional upset that has left the patient weepy and dependent. The end of the urethra burns when urine is passed; pressure and cramps in the lower abdomen. Spasms of pain in the bladder after urinating. Anger < the symptoms. The patient knows they should drink water but they are not thirsty. End of the urethra can feel swollen. (Use 200.)

Sarsaparilla: cystitis in small girls who suddenly scream as they pass urine; urine dribbles out and scalds; adults feel like screaming but grit their teeth. Urine may look sandy or even have some blood in it. Pains in the urethra can feel as if they are penetrating up into the abdomen. So anxious about the pains that she will avoid drinking. Bladder feels full and very tender. Indicated when the patient is stressed by something that they have not been able to express satisfactorily. (Use 30 though the 3 given every 10 minutes has been effective.)

Sepia: marked sensation of bearing down with heaviness in bladder and lower abdomen < before passing water; with cutting and burning sensations on passing small amounts of urine slowly. Incontinence of urine on coughing or sneezing. Patient is likely to be exhausted and irritable and indifferent to anything that would normally interest her. (Use 30 but go up to a 200 if no improvement within 12 hours.)

Staphysagria: cystitis at the start of new physical relationship, after catheterisation or from suppressed anger after some form of abuse. Pains < when *not* urinating: urging and burning before and after urinating with sensation of a drop rolling along the urethra all the time. Patient is likely to be extremely sensitive emotionally. (Use 30.)

Certain herbal remedies have a good reputation for aiding recovery from cystitis: cranberry juice (try and get organic juice with little sugar added; the taste is tart), nettle juice or tea (which acts as a diuretic and helps flush the urine through) and uva ursi (from the herbalist or health food shops or as a tincture from the homoeopathic pharmacy and useful in problems associated with E. coli; this supplement is reputedly more efficacious if acidic foods such as citrus fruits and tomatoes are cut out of the diet). The old-fashioned idea of drinking home-made lemon barley water still holds good. For those who can dig up couch grass from a patch of rough ground, a handful of roots (about 2 ounces/50g) of this boiled up in 2 pints of water (till reduced to one pint) can provide an excellent bladder cleanse. In addition to any supplements it is always important to drink up to 3 litres of water a day. Indicated remedies should start giving relief within 4 hours. **If not then you must contact your homoeopath to avoid the symptoms threatening to become a kidney infection.**

Interstitial Cystitis

This is a chronic inflammatory condition of the bladder walls. It is puzzling to the medical profession as it is not caused by any particular bacteria and it does not respond to orthodox treatment. Patients may be left without any definite diagnosis for a long time while tests are conducted and therapeutic management tried out. The symptoms include varying degrees of bladder, abdominal and urethral pain (spasms, burning, stinging etc.) before, during and after urination; frequent urging; pus and/or blood in the urine. Both men and women can be affected though more women have the symptoms. The most severe pains are felt when the bladder is filling up though pain may be experienced while just sitting, during intercourse or through the night. Though IC support groups say that there is no psychosomatic element to the problem, in truth there is even if it is buried. In any chronic bladder/kidney complaint there is always an underlying unresolved issue that, if it were unearthed, would involve an emotional outpouring, even if that issue were of only historical significance to the patient's family (i.e. the patient is suffering the symptoms because they have assumed moral responsibility for a problem that stems back to a parent). IC is a condition that must be treated by a homoeopath; for patients the advice is to keep up the treatment despite the frustration of slow progress. A lot of remedial help is needed and much constitutional prescribing to deal with a problem that has very deep miasmatic implications.

Kidney Problems

Never feel that you are being too fussy or troublesome when calling for professional help if the symptoms seem to indicate kidney pathology.

The kidneys are located below the bottom ribs on either side in the back. The kidneys are, perhaps, the most delicately balanced organs of the body and they have an important connection with other vital organs. If in any doubt about their condition always seek advice at once! It is better to be wrong than sorry. If there is any question about the health of the kidneys the patient should stop drinking alcohol, coffee and tea straight away and drink more water (still, not sparkling and preferably warm or hot). Acute kidney problems are often consequent on a neglected or undiagnosed bladder infection or a stone may be blocking the flow of urine. Chronic conditions of the liver, lungs or heart can predispose patients to kidney symptoms. The kidneys are very responsive to what goes on in the rest of the body and they will produce symptoms when other organs are the main focus of illness. *Any* change in frequency and urgency of urination or colour or consistency of urine is worth reporting to the homoeopath (see page 113 on kidney and bladder infections). *Always* report any of the following symptoms:

- Obviously reduced urine output (which may be due to low blood pressure, dehydration, the heart pumping insufficiently or a mechanical block such as a stone).
- Highly coloured urine which contains blood or sediment or is malodorous.
- Bloody urine with puffy face and swollen ankles after a bout of tonsillitis (especially in the young).
- General malaise with puffy eyelids, shortness of breath, frothy urine and retention of fluid in various parts of the body as this suggests a kidney condition dependent on one of a large number of conditions which should be identified through clinical tests. **If this occurs inform the doctor as well as the homoeopath**. Tenderness and pain when the kidney area is touched with cessation of urine and bouts of acute excruciating pain that cause writhing. This suggests the presence of a stone passing in the ureter.
- Frequent urination and a significantly increased thirst are signs of diabetes.

The most common kidney problem is nephritis which can be a complication of cystitis. There are aching and dragging feelings in the back below the ribs on one side or the other. (It is important to tell the homoeopath which side is painful.) There might also be blood in the urine. If the case is severe there might be a fever and general malaise with aching, or the intestines may seem to be involved with gut pains. Anyone who has this symptom picture intermittently should ask their practitioner about keeping **Terebinth** 200 in the first-aid kit as this can halt the progress of the acute disease quickly. Another remedy to ask about is **Berberis Vulgaris** which is often used as a 'kidney support' remedy. It is invaluable for those who have weak kidneys but it needs a professional to advise how to use it most effectively.

Kidney Stones

Stones are calcified mineral deposits which may appear as 'sand', 'gravel', small chunks or as a mass that is wedged in the kidney itself (the so-called 'stag horn'). Sand and small pieces of gravel are sometimes passed with only little discomfort. Larger pieces can cause the most agonising pains as they pass down the ureter to the bladder where they might lodge. The symptoms of passing a stone include excruciating pain in the side which spreads throughout the abdomen and down into the thighs, nausea and vomiting, sweating, fever, shivering and the symptoms of a urinary tract infection, such as frequent urging, and sometimes blood in the urine. Anyone prone to producing kidney stones should be having constitutional treatment but needs to talk to their homoeopath about keeping remedies in store in case of an attack. The main remedies are **Berberis Vulgaris** (radiating pains), **Calc-c.** (colicky pains with feverishness), **Colocynth** (cutting pains which cause the patient to double up), **Dioscorea** (writhing in agony and arching back), **Lycopodium** (pains in the right kidney which go towards the left with bloating and flatulence) and **Sarsaparilla** (severe sharp pains extend from the right kidney downwards into the groin) though **Belladonna** may be needed if there is a high fever with an infection. If a stone has reached the bladder and blocks the urethra then an infection may brew; see the cystitis remedy list above but call the homoeopath for advice.

Damage to the Bladder from Surgery or Catheterisation

Symptoms can arise from catheterisation, cystoscopy (examination of the bladder by camera), or surgery. It is always a good idea to tell the homoeopath if any procedure is going to be carried out so that the patient can be given remedies to take before and after in order to lessen or eliminate side effects. **Staphysagria** 30 or 200 is useful when given to sensitive patients before the examination in order to assist the process. **Arnica** 30 is helpful in limiting any bruising. If a biopsy is to be taken both of these are indicated before and **Calendula** 30 should be given afterwards. **Calendula** is also indicated if any bleeding follows. If there is any burning afterwards that feels as if there is an infection brewing then **Cantharis** 30 may be indicated especially if there is burning in the urethra as well. If polyps or warts are being removed from the bladder (which is never a long-term solution and generally an unwise course to follow unless there is urgency in the case) then it is a good idea to precede the operation with a dose of **Emerald** 30 and follow it with **Staphysagria** 200 and then **Arnica** 200. However, always seek the homoeopath's advice about polyps and warts in the bladder so that you can be fully aware of the implications of their surgical removal.

Sexually Transmitted Diseases

Syphilis and gonorrhoea are regarded as notifiable diseases. This puts homoeopaths in an awkward position as homoeopathy is one of the few systems of medicine that can bring about the cessation of symptoms without suppression. Neither disease has been remotely affected in terms of cure by allopathic medicine; both remain diseases that wax and wane in periodical waves. There is no orthodox cure for these diseases; there is only suppression by chemotherapy with long-term chronic consequences, some of which may seem to have no relation to their origins. Furthermore, if either disease is suppressed before the patient has children, the chronic consequences are inherited in one form or other by the next generation. (See *The Companion to Homoeopathy* part III.) The same can be true of the lesser-known infections such as non-specific urethritis, chlamydia and trichomonas all of which are far more rife today as a direct result of the suppression of the better-known syphilis and gonorrhoea.

None of these diseases should be dealt with by the amateur prescriber. Prescribing for them requires careful monitoring and the experience to follow the subtle shifts of emphasis in the presentation of symptoms. Men rarely need a physical examination if they are detailed in their information about the quality of pains, discharges and sensations as well as moods and any other physical symptoms that might arise. Few homoeopaths are qualified to give a physical examination to women who may prefer to go to their doctor for a diagnosis and take the information to their practitioner for assessment. It is worth remembering that some STD symptoms may be mild enough to be confused with candida or thrush. The following descriptions are to help with recognising the signs.

Syphilis: starts as a small (sometimes tiny) raised red pimple that soon turns into an ulcer, usually on the genitals or any part that is in contact with the infection including the mucous membranes of the mouth or anus. The ulcer exudes a fluid that is highly infectious. Lymph nodes in the vicinity swell. This process is usually painless. The ulceration heals within 1 – 3 months. During this period the patient is highly infectious and often has a raised level of libido, a symptom that ensures the further spread of the disease. The second stage produces a skin rash that looks like measles and is often symmetrically disposed over the body; there may also be reddened palms and soles. There may also be enlarged lymph nodes about the body and sore, red eyes, bone pains, jaundice and biliousness, or kidney pains with a general sense of malaise. Throughout the second stage sores may open up and be highly infective. There is also a third stage for those who recover from the first two or who have had their symptoms suppressed: symptoms can affect any part of the body including the lymphatics, the brain, the cardiovascular system and the bones; it also affects the mind causing such conditions as dementia.

Gonorrhoea: is associated with a proliferating bacterium that is deposited on a mucous membrane of the urethra, cervix or rectum where the body's reaction is to produce mucus which becomes pus. In men inflammation occurs and causes characteristic pains such as the sensations of trying to pass broken glass; the end of the urethra becomes red and swollen and partially blocked. The pus discharge is often green and has a fishy odour. In women the infection takes longer to incubate and may result in few or no symptoms or there may be soreness and a discharge. (Even if there are no symptoms to be ascribed to bacterial infection, women can show latent effects such as inflammation of the Fallopian tubes, endometriosis, pelvic inflammatory disease and infertility.) Infection can also spread through the bloodstream to other sites or deeper into the orifices of the body such as the bladder, prostate, uterus or Fallopian tubes. Problems with these areas are commonly seen among those who have had the disease suppressed earlier. Chronic effects include warts, inflammatory conditions and rheumatic problems.

Non-specific urethritis: this is seen as a less serious threat than gonorrhoea with which it shares characteristics. NSU often has milder symptoms with burning in the urethra while passing water, a discharge of fishy, yellow or greenish pus and frequent urging to urinate.

Chlamydia and trichomonas: both of these bugs may be associated with similar symptoms to NSU and gonorrhoea despite their different names. In homoeopathy it makes no difference which one it is; what is important is the symptom picture which tells us about the body's reaction. It is on this that the prescription is decided.

Genital herpes: is a form of herpes simplex and is associated with a typical process of symptoms which includes feeling low with malaise, tingling and itching around the site, some inflammation and soreness of the area, the appearance of a blister or blisters which may be filled with clear fluid or pus and which crust over and, when the dried scab falls off, a sensitive, reddened area which eventually fades. The most common remedies for this include **Arsen-alb**. (burning, itchy and crusty dry eruption with restlessness and anxiety), **Merc-sol**. (burning, moist, yellowish eruption which spreads out with alternating heat and chills with night sweats), **Nat-mur**. (sore, tingling and itching with eruption that smarts and tends to leak watery fluid that dries to a thin crust, with thirst and a withdrawn mood), **Rhus-tox**. (large, crusty eruption that burns, tingles and itches and turns yellowish with a scab, with restlessness and irritability), **Sepia** (area looks chapped and sore, itches and becomes crusty and scaly; patient is worn out and fed up) and **Sulph**. (eruptions are sore, burning, scaly and moist with a yellowish exudate; the patient is tired and can't be bothered, very thirsty and rather hot at night).

Genital Warts

Genital warts come in all shapes and sizes and are regarded by allopathy as sexually transmitted. This is not necessarily so as far as a homoeopath is concerned. Sometimes warts develop on the genitals just as they might anywhere else on the body because there is a hereditary disposition for them. Though they *are* often part of the picture of an STD they can appear *despite* condoms through sexual contact or simply because the constitution has been given the opportunity (whether or not there is any sexual activity) to put a negative growth out onto the surface of the body. (New relationships are often a signal for the process to begin as the mixing of two energy systems can be the trigger for miasmatic changes.) In both cases miasmatic treatment is called for which should not be self-administered. Allopathy, confused by the variety of papilloma viruses associated with warts, does not recognise that the viruses are the *result* of the general miasmatic disease state that already exists in the body and not the cause; warts come from within! This means that the suppression of genital warts is sheer folly; it leads to the warts turning back inwards and either appearing on an internal mucous membrane such as the cervix, bladder or the bowel or becoming cancerous. This is often missed by medics as the doctor who excises warts is not going to be the oncologist who treats cancer. Homoeopathy has an extremely good track record for dealing with warts, and all that is required of the patient is a precise description of the warts, their location, any sensations in them or in that part of the body, any general symptoms that have arisen, a biographical rundown of the patient's health history and a willingness to follow the prescription to the letter. Anyone seeking treatment for this condition might find not only that the warts change shape, colour, size and texture but that life takes on different perspectives. Miasmatic treatment is, in a sense, extremely liberating.

17   HORMONE IMBALANCES

Hormones are the body's messengers. They are sent out from a deep part of the brain to organise the functions of the whole. The 'master' gland is the pituitary, in the middle of the head, though it takes its cue from the hypothalamus just above it. Every other hormone gland in the body responds to the messages sent out from this command centre. The major glands include the parathyroid, thyroid, adrenals, pancreas and sex glands. All the involuntary activities of the body work according to the body clock of hormone delivery. A lot can go wrong with this clock.

There are disorders of the pituitary that are beyond the scope of this book. Suffice to say that if a pituitary disorder is diagnosed it is important to consult the homoeopath to ask for constitutional treatment in addition to whatever other route the patient may want to take.

Thyroid Malfunction

Broadly, there are two main problems with the thyroid: hyperthyroidism and hypothyroidism – overactive and underactive thyroid. They are very confusing for the patient as well as the practitioner. The medical textbook tells us that a hyperactive thyroid produces too much thyroid hormone and causes a fast heart rate, higher blood pressure, shakiness and trembling, nerviness, sleeplessness, weight loss and insatiable appetite, fast metabolism, bulging eyes and confusion. Hypo-activity produces slow heart rate, weight gain, slow metabolism with constipation, depressive tendencies, dull brain function, excessive sleep and puffy face. Those who are overactive tend to race around trying to do everything at once while underactive people tend to find it hard to do anything with any stamina or enthusiasm. However, blood tests are notoriously fickle and sometimes wildly inaccurate. Doctors tend to go by the blood level readings while homoeopaths go by the symptom picture of each individual. It is not uncommon for a patient to have a diagnosis of hypoactive thyroid and yet have symptoms that belong to the opposite diagnosis – and vice versa. The truth is that the thyroid should never be seen in isolation; it works only because the pituitary sends it messages. The language of the hormone messages is miraculously complex and one blood test never tells the practitioner enough about that particular individual. Blood tests taken regularly over a year, say, quite often reveal no stable pattern, yet drugs to alter the activity of the thyroid are prescribed based on insufficient evidence. It is no surprise to homoeopaths that among the many remedies that restore the thyroid to balanced functioning is the family of iodine medicines, iodine being essential to the health of this gland. The core of any thyroid case is almost certain to be a feeling of 'When is it my turn?' – a sense of having been left out and disregarded. If this is not true in a case then there will be a history in the patient of some kind of trauma in which the connection between the pituitary and the thyroid is compromised: whiplash, a general anaesthetic that went wrong, etc. A consultation with the homoeopath is strongly recommended as well as complementary therapy from cranial osteopathy.

The Adrenal Glands

The adrenals are situated above the kidneys. They control blood pressure, heart rate and are central to our ability to sustain effort. They also help in the regulation of sweating and the levels of essential chemicals in the system. Anyone who develops tiredness, dizziness, weight loss, chilliness and brown staining of the skin should ask the doctor for blood tests as these symptoms suggest underactive adrenal glands. If the patient develops thinning hair, a deeper voice, hirsutism and heightened libido then this too should be investigated as overactive adrenal production is likely. Either condition is susceptible to homoeopathy though Addison's disease (underactive adrenal glands) becomes difficult to deal with when the patient loses faith in their own ability to get better. Both require long-term, deep constitutional and miasmatic treatment.

Diabetes Mellitus

The pancreas produces enzymes to create the digestive process as well as insulin to regulate the correct levels of blood sugar in the bloodstream. If there is a drop in insulin production then the patient gradually develops, sometimes over years, strong thirst amounting to a craving, frequent and excessive urination, increased hunger, weak vision, sleepiness and lack of enthusiasm for physical activity. This is called late onset diabetes. It is often controlled by diet; removing sugars from the menu altogether. A nutritional expert is invaluable here. As the origins of late onset diabetes are usually in the emotions it is important to seek constitutional homoeopathic treatment. The pancreas is known as the 'seat of joy' and most diabetics, at some level, have or have had grief that has compromised their sense of joy. **In rare cases in young people the symptom onset can be more rapid and dramatic and suggests 'early onset' diabetes which must be treated immediately!** The cause of early onset diabetes lies in heredity (even if the actual disease is not manifest in a previous generation) and is helped by ongoing constitutional and miasmatic homoeopathy.

Hypoglycaemia

Low levels of blood sugar is a very common problem indeed and yet it is one of which many patients suffering mildly from it are unaware. Children who come out of school feeling irritable and fractious and who feel better for a Mars bar are usually mildly hypoglycaemic. Those who feel weak, tired, cross, shaky and headachy after working for several hours without a break are hypo-glycaemic. The symptoms can be so severe that the person becomes anxious and full of dread or they give the appearance of being drunk. Older people may suffer from hypoglycaemia through the night; they wake feeling the symptoms. They need to eat something late at night to ensure that symptoms do not catch up with them before an early breakfast. It is important not to feed hypoglycaemic patients with sugar. Sugar is a quick fix that exaggerates the problem. A Mars bar is not a good idea; it is better to eat a piece of fruit or some mixed nuts and follow that up when possible with a balanced meal of protein or carbohydrates and vegetables. Regular eating habits are essential for those severely affected. Hypoglycaemia is often suffered by those with a gluten and/or dairy intolerance. The more strict care that is taken over the diet early on in treatment, the sooner the symptoms will regress. It is important to have constitutional treatment throughout as remedies are able to address such problems as gluten and sugar intolerance as well as the other listed symptoms.

Skin conditions seem to be problems on the surface of the body and therefore apparently little to do with internal functioning but this may conceal the fact that a healthy body will often use the skin to display its symptoms of general distress: a rash, an eruption, a cyst. For acute reactions home prescribing works well but for any problem that is either chronic or intermittent or has emotional or miasmatic implications always seek help from the homoeopath as there is almost always more to it than meets the eye.

Boils

A boil is a skin abscess; if they are large they are called carbuncles. Allopathy sees them as bacterial infections that result from minor skin abrasions that allow bacteria in to multiply. While it is true that staphylococci frequently live on the surface skin, it is equally true that boils develop because of an internal process in which the immune system assisted by the liver, needing to rid the body of toxicity, creates local swelling and heat which leads to pus forming just beneath the surface. If the boil is big enough and there is a lot of toxicity to expel there might be a low-grade fever as well (unless **Belladonna** is called for by a general fever). Pus is no more than white blood cells that have died in the normal process of killing off opportunistic bacteria; when the pus is expelled so are the dead bacteria. Usually the body can cope very well though boils can be painful and long-running. Sometimes boils come to a head and resolve by bursting; sometimes they are 'blind' and are absorbed into the system for elimination through normal channels. Boils are not uncommon in childhood; they should be regarded as part of a child's development as they are a symptom of constitutional cleansing. Occasionally boils result from insect bites. Remedies are useful to assist the speedy resolution. Boils are best left uncovered where practicable. Avoid waterproof dressings; where necessary use gauze coverings. Felons or whitlows (boils around the ends of the fingers) are mentioned among the following most commonly indicated remedies:

Apis: the swelling is puffy and not as hard as other remedies; there is stinging and burning as if stung by a bee. The core has no particular head but might look paler than surrounding skin. The patient is irritable and wants to be left alone preferably to sleep. (Use 30.)

Arsen-alb.: burning pains in a dark red or blackening swelling which make the patient anxious and restless. (Use 30.)

Belladonna: hot, hard, red swelling with no head but which throbs. Occasionally there is a general fever of up to 102°F. Often appears on the right side of the body. (Use 200.)

Calc-sulph.: boil stems from a cut or an eczematous lesion in the skin which festers and eventually swells to form a painful boil with a head with obvious, yellow pus beneath the surface. The pus may exude from time to time but does not resolve the boil. Patient is likely to be grumpy and miserable. (Use 30 though sometimes 200 will do the job more quickly.)

Echinacea Angustifolia: very useful for small boils that result from insect bites that have been scratched. Itching and burning with sore red pimples in a cluster on the surface. Patient is weak and feeble with no wish to exert himself. (Use 30.) **NB The skin can suppurate badly when this remedy is needed and so needs to be carefully monitored.**

Hepar-sulph.: little wounds threaten to suppurate; boils are very painful indeed and the patient is extremely sensitive and irritable. Pus is usually evident and may ooze out with some blood. Local glands might be swollen. Is useful in whitlows but see below in **Myristica.** (Use 30.)

Lachesis: boils are purplish or bluish; likely to bleed and look septic; often appear on the left side of the body. The patient is likely to be very snappy and is best left alone as they are inclined to take offence easily. The tense burning pains are often < at night. (Use 30.)

Myristica: painful boils that form pus; useful when **Hepar-sulph.** or **Silica** do not heal speedily. Main remedy for felons, septic finger ends. (Use the 30 or 200 in severe cases.)

Pyrogen: for septic wounds that form abscesses that are swollen and inflamed. The fever is lower than **Belladonna** and the skin tone of the boil is darker. The patient feels they have 'flu like symptoms and looks tired, flushed and dull. (Use 30 or 200 in severe cases.)

Silica: boils are slow to develop, usually as a reddish gathering with no head to begin with. Particularly useful for boils that form around a foreign object such as a splinter. The skin around is pale and waxy and local glands may swell. The patient is likely to be feeling delicate and withdrawn. (Use 30 but see **Myristica**.)

Tarentula Cubensis: for boils that look purplish, feel extremely hard and painful and look puffy and septic; often on soft, fleshy parts. The pains are burning and stinging and make the patient very restless and anxious. (Use 30.)

Acne

Acne is a condition that needs professional prescribing. It is not just a skin disorder; it is part of the maturing process and therefore has constitutional implications. It has little to do with lack of cleanliness; many sufferers wash assiduously but still produce spots. It is a process of elimination that is fuelled by a change in hormonal activity but symptoms are not the same for everyone. Some people have large red, headless eruptions; others have small, pus-filled spots that itch and bleed easily. Spots appear in different places: some patients have them on the chin, some on the forehead, others all over the face, chest and back. The variations can make the selection of appropriate remedies difficult especially in puberty when the state of the whole constitution is going through so much change that only taking the acne symptoms into consideration is unlikely to prove successful. In addition, puberty is often a time when patients throw up symptom pictures that provide opportunities for life-enhancing treatment. To go for the allopathic option of long-term antibiotics is to store up trouble; to suppress acne only leads to future pathology: a tendency to form abscesses, poor bowel function, slow rate of recovery for acute illnesses, lymphatic congestion and other problems.

In addition to seeing a homoeopath, there are some things that patients can do for themselves. As acne often restricts itself to certain areas, the patient should take note of what significance this might have. For example, acne on the forehead or the mid-chest suggests that the liver is underfunctioning or downright toxic. With acne on the chin there may well be stagnation in the reproductive and pelvic organs (suggesting that girls may have menstrual problems). Acne on the cheeks or across the back suggests that there is congestion in the lungs. Acne all over these areas probably means that there is a lot of toxic material in the system and that there is a hereditary tendency to harbouring toxic waste in the body (which means that miasmatic prescribing will be necessary). The patient should take note of advice given about diet and nutrition (eating junk food and drinking too little water are common problems), about medicinal and hallucinogenic drugs (most steroids can aggravate acne and cannabis slows down the system generally) and about keeping reasonable hours (going against the body's natural rhythms has a bad effect on the metabolism). The more that spots contain pus, the more the body needs to detoxify. Patients with spots that bleed and leave scarring need to go through deep-acting miasmatic treatment as there is much work to be done on genetic inheritance.

Blood cleansing herbal tinctures are sometimes of use though they are not a cure. An all-round combination tincture that can be bought from the pharmacies is **Berberis Aquifolium Ø + Echinacea Angustifolia Ø + Calendula Ø** in equal parts. Five drops in half a cup of water is used as a wash over the affected area; the remainder can be taken internally.

Acne Rosacea

This is a chronic condition of the skin covering the cheeks below the eyes and over the nose and sometimes over the forehead; it is most usual in middle-aged people especially around the menopause but it can affect much younger adults. The blood vessels dilate sometimes giving a rather bibulous appearance; alcoholics are prone to rosacea. Red spots erupt onto the surface repeatedly and the skin feels sore and thickened. Corticosteroids tend to aggravate the problem. Apart from constitutional treatment (which is usually deep and requires time and patience) it is best for the patient to avoid any substances that create heat or speed in the system: coffee and other caffeine-loaded drinks, alcohol (especially wine), red meat and spicy food. Antibiotics only load the system with more toxic material which is hard to eliminate and suppress a process that is the tip of the iceberg. In menopausal women rosacea can be indicative of a hormonal imbalance related to the menstrual cycle. It is worth remembering that the contraceptive pill and other hormone drugs may have a part to play in either the causation or in blocking healing.

Rash around the Mouth (Perioral Rash)

A red ring rash appears around the mouth often with a narrow pale border between it and the lips. The skin is sore and sensitive and may burn especially after contact with certain foods. The trigger is often an allergen: tomatoes, oranges and eggs are prime suspects. In young children who produce this rash it is helpful to have an allergy test. To ensure any allergic reaction does not become worse it is best to call on the homoeopath to treat the underlying miasmatic state. The rash can also be associated with a tendency to herpes simplex (cold sores). Another exciting cause can be an underlying emotional state in which the person is unable to be angry to avoid hurting others' feelings or because anger would be unsafe or ineffective. This too needs professional help.

Herpes Simplex

Cold sores are viral in origin. The virus lies dormant in local nerve ganglia while the immune system is healthy but when this is challenged either by stress, emotions, hormone imbalances or environmental changes (such as strong sunlight) the virus breaks out, having travelled along the nearest nerve line. Herpes is often a familial condition being passed by contagion from parents to children or it is the result of intimacy. The symptoms start, very frequently as part of an ordinary cold, with tingling and/or itching and a red sore that develops a blister or several blistery heads, commonly around the lips, below or in the nose or on the chin. (It can also affect the inside of the lips or even the gums.) At this stage the fluid in the blister makes the cold sore infectious for those who are susceptible. The blisters eventually start to dry out and form a confluent yellowish scab (though it might be grey, black, flaky or crusty). The whole process may take anything from a week to three weeks to resolve. While harbouring herpes is a chronic state which requires long-term homoeopathic treatment to weaken the virus's hold on the system, it is a good thing to find the remedy that most matches the patient's acute symptoms so that the virus cannot cause the usual distress and is unable to cause infection in others.

Arsen-alb.: surface skin goes rough, dry, tingling and burning; reddish blister erupts out of swollen area of upper lip and dries out to a scurfy scab over an ulcerous lesion. (Use 30.)

Cantharis: burning and itching with a raw area that feels like a smarting watery blister that blackens. The patient is very irritable and contradictory. (Use 30.)

Dulcamara: red eruption starts on lips like a nettle sting; followed by a thick, yellowish crusty eruption that is wet and tends to bleed if scratched. Mouth can be distorted by the cold sore. Much < for washing. May come on before a period. (Use 30.)

Graphites: eruption is a patch of dry, rough, itchy skin that tends to crack; gluey, honey-coloured fluid exudes and as the surface dries leaves a granulated deposit. The skin of the lip feels as if drawn tight. Corners of the mouth may be cracked and the breath foul. (Use 30.)

Lycopodium: sore patch especially on the right corner of the mouth (which is cracked) or in right nostril (the wing side) which feels tearing on opening mouth or blowing nose. May take time for the sore in the crack to develop. Eventually becomes moist and crusty. (Use 30.)

Merc-sol.: patch of yellow-brown crusts form on a red eruption which is moist and foul on any part of the lips; lesion might spread and suppurate; accompanied by rank breath and much salivation which can be quite sticky. The patient is likely to be hot and chilly by turns and be very thirsty. (Use 30 but sometimes the 200 is needed to complete the job.)

Nat-mur.: most likely caused by exposure to the sun which <; eruption appears anywhere around the mouth (or end of nose) but favoured place is the middle of the lower lip after a crack develops. The lip can feel numb and tingly then itchy, stinging and dry; there may be a feeling of a dry tongue with slimy coating; the patient is thirsty for water and may have a salty taste in the mouth. The main remedy for those who have a cold sore during a fever. (Use 30.)

Nit-ac.: vicious stinging or sudden stabbing pains in a smallish eruption that might be on the inside of the lip or inside the end of a nostril. (Use 30. Do not precede it or follow it with **Nat-mur.**)

Rhus-tox.: eruption is often preceded by general achiness in the muscles on getting up. Burning, stinging and itching follow initial tingling. Sore is large and crusty over a moist blister and appears around the mouth or on the chin. One of the most common remedies. (Use 30.)

Sepia: patch of sore skin appears anywhere around the mouth, lips or end of the nose; dry, itchy, stinging and crusty. Sore can become wet and scabby especially if it suppurates. Sore is often < before the period or in spring. (Use 30 though sometimes a 200 will be needed to finish the job.)

Lichen Planus

Lichen planus is characterised by a bumpy, scaly rash that usually appears symmetrically disposed on the body, typically on the inside wrists and upper thighs, on the torso or on the genitals. It is usual for mouth sores to be present. The rash has a violet colour and the sores in the mouth can be whitish or blue-white. The eruptions are itchy and lumpy. It can be brought on by exposure to drugs or chemicals; those containing gold, arsenic or quinine are particularly suspect. The mouth sores may be the first sign of its presence and can cause an ulcer-like pain. The condition responds relatively well to remedies but as the origin of the problem lies in the tubercular or leprotic miasms it is best to seek professional help.

Ringworm and Fungal Skin Infections

Ringworm has nothing to do with worms; it is a fungal infection and is associated with a variety of different fungi. A fungal infection can appear anywhere on the body but when it affects the feet it is called athlete's foot. Symptoms can vary. Athlete's foot is characterised by skin that reddens or whitens, cracks and peels between the toes (usually the last two on either side) with or without itching. If the groin is affected then reddened rash areas appear and spread outwards across the inner thighs, edged with a darker 'high-tide mark'. It can be hot and itchy and the skin can become quite corrugated or thickened. If ringworm affects the scalp then it is regarded as highly contagious. Hair might start to thin around the patch and it can be quite itchy. Fungus can also invade the nails causing thickening, distortion, discoloration, crumbling or flaking; this is much the hardest form of fungus to shift by alternative means. Ringworm on the body is usually confined to small areas and appears as a pink, roughened, circular area with a redder rim. It is not usually itchy. Barber's itch is another variation which occasionally affects men with beards or those with heavy facial hair growth. Tinea is a form of fungal growth that causes white or brown areas of skin. They can appear anywhere but are commonly seen on the face as circumscribed areas of pallid or whitened skin. (This should not be confused with vitiligo.)

Fungal infections most commonly arise in those with a family history of tuberculosis – which is most of us; even in those who know of no forebears who suffered the disease. Quite often, beneath this miasmatic influence is another one – leprosy. The remedy **Leprosinum** is sometimes necessary to clear a stubborn case. This means that professional prescribing is necessary. It is this susceptibility that means that allopathic anti-fungal creams offer only temporary relief. In some patients, suppression of athlete's foot leads to a fungal rash in the groin. Using tea tree on any skin problem is ultimately counterproductive as it is another form of suppression albeit 'alternative'. One other aspect to bear in mind is that fungal infections are often triggered while experiencing difficulties in making positive creative changes in one's life; this can particularly happen during times of expected turmoil: adolescence, leaving full-time education, the menopause.

For cracking and peeling skin between the toes **Hypercal** ointment can be effective though it is not a cure. Those with athlete's foot should take shoes and socks off as often as possible and should avoid wearing shoes that encourage heat and sweating such as trainers.

Dandruff and Cradle Cap

These are other names for seborrhoeic dermatitis of the scalp. Cradle cap occurs mostly in babies and children. Scaly skin develops on the scalp causing scabby areas and matted hair. It should be seen as an eliminative process and not suppressed. Olive oil rubbed onto the area can loosen the scabs while constitutional treatment will sort the problem. Dandruff is no less an expression of elimination but is usually dealt with by medicated shampoos; this is definitely not a good idea. Constitutional treatment is necessary even though the condition is regarded as no more than a cosmetic nuisance. Those who have spent a long time suppressing dandruff should expect the scalp to react to remedies by temporarily bringing it back.

Cracks behind the Ears

This childhood problem can be very persistent and reappear despite creams and ointments. It might be part of a general picture of eczema or it might be on its own; it can be bad enough to cause a split in the skin which bleeds or becomes infected. (If it becomes infected, treat it as a wound.) **Hypercal** ointment or **Stellaria** cream (for those with ultrasensitive skin) can be helpful while the patient goes through with constitutional treatment.

Keratosis

This is a condition in which dead skin cells are not sloughed off but plug up pores. This results in roughened areas of skin especially on the upper arms, buttocks and thighs. It is only cosmetically a problem but it does belong to the psoric/tubercular miasm. Body brushing helps, as do fresh air and sunshine.

Sebaceous Cysts

Sebaceous cysts are harmless lumps of matter parcelled up and deposited by the body in odd places: often on the face, ears, feet or scrotum. They are rarely

painful and seldom grow once they are formed; they may disappear spontaneously. They should not be removed surgically but reported to the homoeopath
as they form part of the constitutional picture even if a minor one. If a cyst is
cosmetically a nuisance then it may assume a greater significance in the treatment plan; certain remedies have a reputation for dealing with the susceptibility
to forming them. Wens, cysts on the scalp, are particularly noted as being part
of a hereditary susceptibility and they can grow large enough to cause distress.
Homoeopathic treatment can be frustratingly slow.

Calluses and Corns

A callus is skin thickened as a result of pressure and friction. They mostly
appear on the feet especially across the ball joint of the toes. In reflexology
this area of the feet represents the lungs and heart; this might be significant
in constitutional treatment as those with feet callused in this area may well be
demonstrating a deeper emotional problem. Corns are usually on the mid-
joint or under the ball of the last toes. If they are painful the most common
remedies are **Antimonium Crudum** (very hard and painful, even crippling),
Nat-mur. (burning pain at night) and **Silica** (sore and between the toes). It is
best to start with the 6th potency taken daily. If this is not effective within 6
weeks then see the homoeopath who will study the whole picture. This is
likely to encompass difficulties in resolving old issues of 'hardened thought';
corns and calluses represent 'stuck' issues from the past. **Calc-fluor.** tissue salt
is very helpful in cases of hardened skin and can complement the remedies
suggested above: one twice daily.

Eczema

Eczema is a form of chronic dermatitis: inflammation of the top layers of skin
characterised by itching, scaling, scabbiness and redness. In some it is
inclined to ooze serum and bleed when scratched but in others it remains dry.
It is susceptible in some to becoming infected and in others it might trigger
impetigo. It often first appears on the creases of the elbows or backs of the
knees but other favourite places are the ankles and feet, the neck and behind
the ears or on the face especially around the eyes. Acute eczematous out-
breaks can be triggered by various allergens: chemicals, plants and metal

jewellery; this is known as contact dermatitis. Chronic eczema is never just a skin problem. It has its roots in genetic inheritance. For this reason it is not a condition that should be self-medicated; it always needs professional prescribing.

Though certain remedies such as **Sulphur, Calc-c., Arsen-alb., Graphites** and **Merc-sol.** have unique and characteristic pictures and are well known for healing eczema especially among children, it is rare indeed for just one remedy to restore the body to complete health without intercurrent doses of miasmatic remedies and acute remedies, such as **Belladonna, Hepar-sulph.** and **Arsen-alb.,** when sudden flare-ups occur. With the help of the practitioner it is a good idea to choose a stock of the remedies for local infection. Anyone seeking cure of this deep condition should be prepared for setbacks. Eczema is often used by the body as a means of registering stress and emotions. If it has been thoroughly suppressed by cortisone creams then it is likely to aggravate and sometimes quite badly; the reason is that the skin will need to become an elimination point for the removal from within of all the absorbed toxicity of the chemical creams. This means initially that remedies are likely to appear to make things worse as the skin oozes and even bleeds and might throw up an infection; this is all part of the process of healing though it takes a confident, level-headed approach because of the sometimes distressing symptoms of reaction. The general rule of thumb is: the younger the patient, the sooner the healing. Eczema is always more difficult to overcome after puberty. In eczema with skin that festers easily use **Calc-sulph.** tissue salt twice daily to help prevent cracking and suppuration (unless your homoeopath is using this remedy in a higher potency or has some other reason for not doing so).

There is a well-known link between eczema and asthma. This link is often fostered by the suppression of eczema by cortisone. If asthma is present without any preliminary suppression then there is most likely to be both a miasmatic and an emotional aspect underlying it which will both have their roots in family history. When eczema and asthma are present in a patient they often alternate in their manifestation. Though the skin symptoms are often the more distressing cosmetically, the homoeopath will always concentrate on resolving the internal, asthma symptoms first as lung pathology is more threatening to the economy of the body than skin problems.

There is also a link between allergies and eczema; many who suffer from allergies also have persistent flare-ups of eczema complicated by histamine reactions. This is made more distressing by breathing and skin reactions to stress and emotional upset. The search for an allergen that causes the problem is usually frustrating because foods or chemicals are only triggers while the cause itself lies much deeper in the genetic make-up of the patient. Once again, this needs long-term miasmatic and constitutional treatment from a professional. Success can take up to 3 years and occasionally more. This should be weighed against the complications of allopathic treatment which always leads to eventual pathology of other parts of the body; eczema is too deep a condition for it to be suppressed with any safety. Eczema is often, apart from the hereditary implications, a physical expression of feeling unsafe or unable to express verbally what irks and irritates one most. After all, the origins are often buried in a time when the patient was unable to express anything in words. Asthma is a physical expression of feeling smothered and disallowed to express anger or sadness. Asthmatic breathing as a result of tightening of the muscles of the tubes of the airways is a physical expression of the suppression of eczema.

Psoriasis

This is one of the most ancient of all human conditions. It is a chronic condition characterised by reddening and flaking of the skin. Scales, somewhat pearly in appearance, commonly develop on elbows, knees, scalp or buttocks (though it can affect any part of the body or all of it). It is not necessarily itchy and it can come and go, affected by stress or emotions. Triggers for new sites of eruption can include wounds or rashes (especially following a streptococcal infection). In some people the nail beds are crippled and the nails deformed. If it is on the scalp the flakes of skin are like dandruff. Psoriasis can also be associated with arthritis. Indeed, psoriasis that is heavily suppressed with cortisone creams often hastens the onset of arthritic joints or, eventually, heart conditions and so this form of treatment should be avoided. Like eczema, psoriasis needs professional attention as there are always hereditary links of one form or another. Patients should note that psoriasis is a condition that gives the body a means of physical expression for stress on the surface; away from the important organs. Sometimes the body does not give this up lightly. What the skin represents in psoriasis might be described as hardening and deadening of the shell to avoid the pain of hurt feelings. (Most of the major remedies known for healing psoriasis are indicated by sensitive, vulnerable people.) If it is compatible with any ongoing constitutional treatment, **Kali-sulph.** tissue salt taken twice daily can help.

Erythema Nodosum

This is a condition that is a surface symptom of an underlying internal problem. Tender nodules appear under the surface of the skin of the shins and the area has the appearance of a mild inflammatory rash. It is most likely to be associated with a diagnosis of streptococcal infection or as the side effect of certain antibiotics. There may have been a throat infection just before and joint pains may be concomitant. Young people are most prone to it. However, erythema nodosum may be part of the general picture of sarcoidosis, a condition in which inflammatory cells become active in various parts of the body, particularly the lungs. If erythema is the result of drugs then the homoeopath is likely to prescribe so that the body eliminates the chemical toxicity as quickly as possible. If there is an associated streptococcal infection or sarcoidosis then the homoeopath will prescribe on the prevailing symptom picture. Erythema and sarcoidosis are not for home prescribing as there is a strong miasmatic background (the tubercular and cancer miasms).

Vitiligo

Vitiligo is characterised by patches of depigmented skin which do not tan when exposed to the sun but are extremely liable to sunburn. The skin has a mapped appearance. Vitiligo can be triggered by trauma or stress though its origins, as far as homoeopathy is concerned, lie in the tubercular/leprotic miasm. It may also be hereditary and linked with malfunction of the endocrine system; hypothyroidism and alopecia are commonly associated. It is often very difficult to make any positive changes in the condition if it is of longstanding or linked with an internal pathology. However, there are listed remedies which have been known to help amongst which are **Sepia** and **Thuja**. (Indian homoeopaths have had success with **Tuberculinum** and **Arsenicum Sulphuratum Flavum**.) These remedies or others well indicated should be prescribed by a homoeopath.

Scabies

Scabies is a highly contagious parasitic disease associated with a spider mite that burrows beneath the surface of the skin, creates vesicles filled with fluid in which it lays its eggs and then moves on to repeat the process. The result is a network of tiny passages (not always visible) linking chickenpox-like eruptions that itch furiously; when scratched, the tops come off and spread the hatched contents further. Scabies is notoriously difficult to deal with and patients are often driven to seek suppressive treatment before homoeopathy has a chance to resolve it. There are known examples of cure but the practitioner has to be able to effect it very speedily. **Sulphur** and **Merc-sol.** are front-rank remedies though seldom suffice on their own; it is often necessary to alternate and frequently repeat complementary remedies. In addition it is worthwhile using neem oil as a topical treatment. Those who do have to resort to allopathic suppression should not feel bad about it but should make sure that there is follow-up constitutional treatment as there is a tendency to suffer intermittently from chronic itching and to establish a predisposition to other problems (stiffness, aching, colds, etc.). Scabies is sometimes seen as a disease that only occurs in those who live in squalor; the truth is that the patient suffering from scabies *feels* contaminated and filthy.

Scars

Scar tissue can occur inside and outside the body as the result of eruptions, wounds and surgery. Repairing skin gathers and forms a protective join over the damaged site. This can be a problem cosmetically especially if the scar is on the face. Scar cream from the homoeopathic pharmacy is useful after chickenpox or acne spots. Using **Calendula** (Ø externally and 6 or 30 internally) for wounds is a preventative. Scars that become sore and painful need **Silica** 6 (one twice per day for 10 days). Scars that become thicker than usual and cause a drawing sensation need **Graphites** 6 (one twice daily for 10 days). Both **Silica** and **Graphites** follow and complement **Calendula** well. If any further treatment is needed consult the homoeopath.

19   HAIR AND NAILS

Conditions of the hair and nails are generally to be reported to the homoeopath as part of constitutional treatment. Thinning hair and splitting nails may not be front-rank symptoms but they are worth counting in the general picture. However, there are several problems that are distressing enough to be regarded separately.

Alopecia

Alopecia usually refers to baldness that occurs as the result of emotional stress or a traumatic shock, after an acute fever or after excessive doses of chemotherapy. It may also happen as the result of hormone deficiency in thyroid conditions or even during pregnancy. In alopecia areata a patch of baldness may appear around the back or side of the head or, in men, in the beard area; nails may show surface pitting at the same time. If severe, as it may be in hormone deficiency, several large patches may develop and body hair may also be affected. If the patient is obviously suffering from emotional stress and is lacking energy and motivation as well as hair loss then **Phosphoric Acid** (one dose of 30, twice daily for 3 – 5 days) is the most likely remedy to initiate recovery. Nevertheless, this remedy does not cover any of the usual, more volatile emotional reactions and it is probable that **Phos-ac.** would need to be followed by other complementary remedies to deal with these if the patient regains energy enough to express them. (**Phos-ac.** is particularly well followed by **Ignatia, Pulsatilla** or **Nat-mur.** for all of which it would be best to consult your homoeopath as to choice and potency.) For other causes of alopecia consult the homoeopath.

Hirsutism

Excessive growth of body hair in unusual parts may be familial and hormonal in origin. It is most distressing in women particularly after the menopause or in younger women who may have concomitant period problems. There are remedies that do cover this anomaly but they are best prescribed by the homoeopath because the sycotic miasm is likely to be the underlying cause and this requires constitutional treatment and the correct sequencing of the remedies. Babies born with excessive amounts of black hair that subsequently falls out is a symptom that is worth mentioning to the homoeopath as this also may indicate the prevalence of the sycotic state even if it does not in itself require treating.

Ingrowing Toenails

The first practical step is to use a razor blade to shave the surface off the centre of the nail in order to thin it. This eventually has the effect of causing the sides to lift out of the grooves they dig into. Cutting the toenails straight across rather than shaped with the curve of the toe will also help. If there is infection then remedies that are used for infected wounds will be needed: **Hepar-sulph.**, **Belladonna**, **Myristica** and **Silica** particularly. If there is bleeding and soreness without infection that indicates a specific remedy then a wad of lint soaked in **Hypercal Ø** (which will sting initially) is necessary. If infection is obviously causing serious discomfort cross-check with the abscess remedies (see page 154). For persistent ingrowing nails see the homoeopath for constitutional treatment; on a psychological/emotional level there may well be an underlying inability to make a decisive move possibly because of an unresolved issue in the past or in the family.

20 BONES, MUSCLES AND SINEWS

Bones are living tissue with blood and nerves running through them and, contrary to appearances, they are malleable and responsive to changes; they are susceptible to the healing effects of remedies. Tendons are fibrous tissues connecting muscles to bone or cartilage. Ligaments are bands of fibrous tissue that hold together, support and strengthen joints or that support internal organs in their correct position. Bones, muscles, tendons and ligaments become susceptible to damage from physical trauma, poor nutrition, biochemical toxicity and lack of exercise. They can also be in trouble from emotional stress; bone problems, especially of the spine, usually originate in the sense of having little structure in one's life; muscular conditions may arise out of a reluctance to cope with new opportunities. Ligaments and tendons become troublesome when one finds it 'hard to hold everything together'.

Cramp

Cramp can happen in any muscle group in the body though it is most common in the legs; a sudden contraction and tensing of muscle leads to pain and loss of movement in the limb. The usual trigger is sudden sustained exercise, worse after eating or after a period of rest and without doing preliminary stretching exercises. Cramp can also be the result of lack of calcium or the inability to metabolise calcium properly due to a lack of magnesium. Calcium deficiency is a problem for the malnourished and older people as well as those with thyroid conditions. Too little salt in the diet, dehydration, excessive heat, pregnancy, certain allopathic drugs and alcoholism are also associated with cramp. Cramp can also be a major feature of chronic degenerative conditions; in MS or Parkinsonism it is best if the practitioner assists in making the choice of remedy for acute cramp.

Calc-carb.: cramp in bed at night < for stretching leg out. May be < in cold weather; patient tends to have cold feet. (Use 30: one immediately and repeat in 10 minutes if necessary.)

Causticum: cramp in the calf, foot and Achilles tendon < in bed with very hard muscle; unable to stand with foot flat on the ground; must stretch out limb. All the tendons feel shortened. (Use 30.)

Chamomilla: cramps in the calves < after anger and frustration. Violent pain causes a vicious temper. (Use 200.)

Colocynth: muscle of whole leg may contract and force patient into a foetal position. Leg feels drawn up and stiff; patient wants to hold the leg tight and rub the painful area. (Use 30 unless there is an obvious cause in anger in which case use 200.)

Cuprum: cramp in the calf and sole preceded by twitching. Is often indicated in someone who is feeling temporarily vulnerable, nervous and jumpy. (Use 30.)

Ferrum-met.: sudden cramp in bed at night with a sense of pulsation in the limb which is drawn up. Feels > for moving about gently. Indicated by those who are easily fatigued and hypersensitive to their environment. (Use 30.)

Kali-carb.: cramp in legs of those whose limbs tend to 'go to sleep' and/or twitch. Useful in those who complain that the back and legs 'give out'. (Use 30.)

Lycopodium: cramp of the right leg or starting in the right and then going to the left; < at night in bed. Useful in those who are prone to flatulent indigestion. (Use 30.)

Nat-carb.: cramp in the toes and heels of those who have weak ankles, cold legs and a tendency to flatulent indigestion. (Use 30.)

Nux-vom.: cramp in the legs and feet with numbness especially likely to be < after stress and pressure at work plus reliance on fast food and snacking. Can come on after flexing the thigh. (Use 30.)

Rhus-tox.: cramps in the calves < after exertion, < in bed on waking in the morning; limbs become stiff and need to be stretched. Generally > for rubbing the muscles and moving about gently. (Use 30 or 200 in severe cases.)

Sepia: cramp in the legs in bed at night < during the period, pregnancy or through the menopause especially in those with 'restless leg syndrome'. Legs often feel heavy and achy. (Use 30 or in a severe attack a 200.)

Sulphur: cramp in the calf (especially left) with stiffness of the feet and ankles. Comes after stretching in bed. Limbs feel heavy and feet feel hot. Patient is often overheated in bed and wants to throw the covers off. (Use 30.)

Tissue salt: Mag-phos. is a useful supplementary measure for those who suffer cramp. (One twice daily.)

Growing Pains

Growing pains are most frequently felt in the legs though any part of the body may be affected. Some parents miss the signs as they can so easily be part of a 'can't be bothered' general state of inertia so common through some episodes of childhood. The most common pains are felt in the shins, ankles and knees though the hamstrings, arms, neck and spine can also be affected.

Calc-phos.: the most common remedy for growing pains especially in the legs; < at night while lying down. The patient has probably put on a growth spurt and has grown lengthwise too quickly to be sustained. Likely to be peevish and irritable and impossible to satisfy; restless and argumentative. (Use 30 daily for a week.)

Eupatorium Perfoliatum: growing pains felt in the back and limbs with soreness of the flesh round them. Patient feels that they are brewing a cold or 'flu all the time. May feel intermittently nauseous as well. (Use 30 daily for a week.)

Guaiacum: the hamstrings feel too short; pains and stiffness in the legs.

Pains shoot up the leg from the ankle to the knee. May also have a stiff neck. Patient is idle and inclined to criticise everything; 'can't be bothered' attitude. Appetite goes down but may develop a strong liking for apples. (Use 30 daily for a week.)

Phos-ac.: bone pains as if they were being torn or scraped. Patient is likely to have pressure headaches and be thoroughly enervated. They feel weak especially in the chest after talking and have no inclination to study as the mind goes blank. Condition may have started after a bout of diarrhoea or a heavy period or a protracted period of crying. (Use 30 daily for a week.)

Silica: pains in the neck and spine with stiffness and headache. Child grows thin and gangly and prone to colds or swollen glands; appears to suffer from poor nutrition and can be obstinate and withdrawn. (Use 30: one every day for 2 weeks.)

Osgood-Schlatter Disease

This is a condition in which the bone and cartilage of the knee become inflamed and painful. It is more common amongst boys especially between 10 and 15. Allopathy ascribes it to what amounts to a repetitive strain injury from playing sports. Swelling, pain and inflammation usually affect one knee only just at the point where the tendon attaches the kneecap to the top of the tibia and sometimes pains can extend down into the shin bone. Occasionally it is damaged in which case the orthopaedic specialist may recommend a plaster cast. If Osgood-Schlatter has been diagnosed it is essential that the patient stops all sports activities. Failing to do so can lead to permanent damage to the knee and lower leg. Cortisone injections should be avoided if possible as there are remedies that can deal with inflammation and pain in this condition. It is best to consult a cranial osteopath as well as the homoeopath. As this condition is always associated with growth it is a good idea, unless the homoeopath is prescribing them already, to alternate **Calc-phos.** and **Silica** tissue salts: one each, night and morning.

Torticollis

Torticollis is a form of dystonia, a spasmodic contraction of a muscle that 'locks' it into a torsion, and it affects the neck. The head is twisted to one side and either backward or forward making it difficult or impossible to move the neck freely. It is usually the result of injury, shock, high fever, getting wet or caught in a draught or as part of the symptom picture of ankylosing spondylitis. If symptoms of torticollis come on after other episodes of spinal aching and weakness or inflammation of joints then the patient should see the homoeopath and cranial osteopath as soon as possible and they should see an orthopaedic specialist as well to eliminate the possibility of ankylosing spondylitis, a condition that must be treated professionally. Occasionally torticollis is part of the symptom picture of hyperthyroidism. For acute torticollis the following remedies may be indicated:

Aconite: sudden onset after being caught in a cold wind or chilling downpour. (Use a 200.)

Belladonna: symptoms come on during or as a result of a high fever with the head drawn back; compare with **Lachnanthes** below. (Use a 200.)

Causticum: head is drawn to the right and the neck feels rigid especially after getting caught in a draught (typically happens after a car journey with the window down). (Use 30 twice daily for 3 days.)

Cuprum: onset after a bout of rage and/or loss of sleep especially in someone who has been overworking. Head is drawn to the right and forward. Patient has tendency to be pent up. (Use 30 daily for a few days.)

Lachnanthes tinctoria: torticollis with sore throat and chill in the back. Head is drawn to the right. May originate from quinsy and fever. (Use every 4 – 6 hours.)

Lycopodium: onset after long-term stress involving a loss or threat of loss of self-confidence. Head may be drawn to either side and forward with stiff back between shoulders and sensation of swelling in the neck.

Likely to suffer from flatulent indigestion as well. (Use 30 daily for 5 days. If no better call the homoeopath who may advise using the 200.)

Nux-vom.: torticollis after a fright, shock or catching cold. Head is drawn to the left and pains cause the patient to be extremely irritable. Wants to wrap a scarf round the neck; pains < in the morning. (Use 30 twice a day for several days.)

Rhus-tox.: torticollis from getting wet or from overstraining. Stiffness and aching is > for rubbing and massage and for stretching the neck. Also > for hot shower or bath. (Use 30 twice daily or one 200 once a day for 3 – 5 days.)

Tissue salt: Calc-fluor. twice a day can complement the indicated remedy.

Tennis Elbow and Housemaid's Knee

These are terms to describe bursitis, inflammation of the sac that contains the lubricating synovial fluid to maintain the smooth movement of joints. When a joint is injured or overused a bursa (or 'purse') swells and inflames causing pain and restricted movement. The typical sites are knee, elbow and shoulder. Treating this condition can be frustrating not least because these joints are so prone to everyday abuse: carrying shoulder bags, heaving shopping in and out of cars, playing one more game of tennis. It is often best to continue using or exercising the affected joint gently in order to keep it limber (but see **Bryonia** below). Massage and physiotherapy can be helpful as long as they are respectful of the degree of inflammation and pain. Be prepared for a long recuperation period if the shoulder is affected; sometimes it can take the best part of a year without appropriate treatment. Some osteopaths will direct their patients to put ice packs on the affected part; they do this to encourage the reduction of the swelling. This can be very effective in some cases but in others it is detrimental. Those remedies which do not appreciate this treatment are identified below. (Where the instruction is one twice daily, continue for up to one week but if no better then reassess your choice or contact the homoeopath.)

Apis: often < on the right knee: swelling and oedema with stinging pains; joint feels stiff, heavy and hot. (Use 30: one twice daily.)

Arsen-alb.: bursitis of the joints of the balls of the feet; swelling and burning with restless feet and pains < on walking. (Use 30: one twice daily. Do not use an ice pack.)

Belladonna: useful when the bursitis swells acutely, turns bright red, throbs and sends shooting pains up the limb. (Use 30: one twice daily. Only use an ice pack *after* **Belladonna** has done its work.)

Bellis Perennis: chronic bursitis after an injury where there was sprain, bruising and damage to the nerves. (Use 12: one 2 or 3 times daily.)

Bryonia: swollen, red and hot joints with stiffness and stitching or tearing pains that are much < for trying to move the limb or from jarring. Particularly common on the elbow or knee though feet can be affected too. (Use 30: one twice daily.)

Lycopersicum: intense aching in the joint and extending into the muscles especially of the right side. If the right shoulder is affected it is well indicated if the pain extends into the right shoulder blade and/or the pectoral muscle. (Use the 3 potency: one 3 to 4 times daily.)

Pulsatilla: useful as an intercurrent remedy when the pain and other symptoms seem to cause a tearful and dependent mood. Also for red swollen joints with pains that come and go and cause restlessness. If the knee is affected then > for elevating the leg. Swelling > in the morning; < by the evening. (Use 200.)

Rhus-tox.: hot, stiff, swollen joint after a strain which is > for massage, hot water and moving it gently about. The pains are much < for not moving the joint so < on waking. Ankle joints are easily affected. (Use 30: one twice daily or one 200 daily. Do not use an ice pack.)

Ruta: useful after injury to the bone: joint feels weak, sore and stiff after injury or strain and pains extend into the tendons. Patient feels weary from the pains. (Use 30: one twice daily.)

Silica: weakness of the limb where a joint is affected by bursitis. Sore, tender sinews after a strain or injury. May bring on pins and needles and trembling of the hand. (Use 30: one twice daily.)

Sticta Pulmonaria: swelling, heat and redness of the joint (especially the knee) with drawing or shooting pains. Swelling and redness extends into the muscle from the joint. Characteristic red spot of inflammation over the joint affected. (Use 30: one twice daily. Problem may resolve when catarrh or a cold is instigated by the remedy.)

Tissue salts: Ferr-phos. (for inflammatory stage and pain); **Nat-sulph.** (follows **Ferr-phos.** to reduce swelling); **Calc-fluor.** (for persistent trouble, slow to heal). One twice daily as required.

Fibromyalgia and Polymyalgia

'Myalgia' simply means muscle pain. 'Fibromyalgia' is a term that covers several conditions that have pain and stiffness of muscle groups and can occur anywhere locally or throughout the body. It mostly affects men and can be the result of strain injuries (see chapter 1) but is often associated with stress, too little sleep or poor environmental conditions (e.g. cold, damp). It often has a relation to rheumatoid arthritis which might be in the patient's family. Polymyalgia also has severe rheumatic pain and stiffness of muscles which usually affects the neck, shoulders, lower back and hips but can also attack arms and legs as well. It is suffered by women more than men and usually does not manifest until after the menopause. The patient may say that the pains came on after or with a slight fever or there may be a sense of an ongoing intermittent low-grade fever. The pains of polymyalgia are very tiring and are often accompanied by depressive feelings, a fact often reflected in the indicated remedies. To confirm the diagnosis a doctor would ask for a blood test and would prescribe a long course of low dose cortisone. The homoeopath would discover that the patient had developed the symptoms after long-term stress or worry; polymyalgia is frequently a condition suffered by 'worriers' for which cortisone can do nothing but relieve the pain. This condition needs very careful professional management and understanding as it is usually very distressing.

Scoliosis, Kyphosis and Lordosis

Scoliosis is lateral curvature of the spine. It is occasionally congenital and must, when severe, be treated by wearing a body brace. If it is not congenital then it may begin in later childhood or in the teens. Scoliosis should be treated by cranial osteopathy as well as other alternative therapies. Kyphosis is curvature of the spine that develops a humpback. Lordosis is a forward curvature of the lumbar spine. Any of these may be the result of heredity or compensatory posture adopted after injuries or surgery or it may be the result of the tetanus vaccination which can cause symptoms in the spine similar to the long-term effects of the disease. Cranial osteopathy is helpful for those who find that associated symptoms of pain or organ dysfunction begin to curtail normal life though treatment should be begun early for lasting effects.

Ankylosing Spondylitis

This is primarily a condition of the spine which has episodes of inflammation in the vertebrae. It is accompanied by back pain and scoliosis, kyphosis or lordosis. There is stiffness and lower back pain and in some people other joints such as those in the knees and feet may become affected. If the lower back is affected then the patient is likely to adopt a stoop. (The problem often first manifests as pain in the sacroiliac area.) If the thoracic vertebrae are involved then the attachments of the ribs to the spine can be affected and the patient will have restricted breathing. It is a progressive condition which eventually leads to fusion of affected vertebrae and permanent rigidity of the spine. Early constitutional treatment is vital as allopathy has no cure; a doctor would initially prescribe steroids and physiotherapy though a body brace is sometimes essential. Surgery is sometimes required. A homoeopath is likely to prescribe variously over a period of many months. The prescriptions are likely to include high potency single remedies (which are likely to reflect aspects of inherited disposition and the history of stresses) and daily doses of supportive remedies such as **Calc-fluor.**, **Causticum** or **Aesculus**. Some patients may need to have their amalgam fillings checked as mercury poisoning has been associated in some people as a causative factor. **Calc-fluor.** tissue salt is a vital support of any other treatment being undertaken. Common-sense advice would include a suggested gentle exercise routine (swimming and walking are especially important but jogging is inadvisable) and an embargo on straining the body's frame by lifting heavy weights. Patients who have sedentary jobs need to be advised to get up and move about frequently (especially if there is much computer work involved as the body's posture while peering at a screen all day is particularly aggravating).

21 SLEEP

Different people seem to need different amounts of sleep; there is no hard and fast rule though there are guidelines. It is accepted as normal for babies up to 2 years old to sleep for 13 – 18 hours a day; for toddlers to sleep for up to 13 hours; for young people to sleep for 10 hours; for young adults and middle-aged people to sleep for 6 – 9 hours; for older people to sleep for 6 – 8 hours. It is not unusual for some adults to lead very active lives on as little as 5 hours sleep or for small children to seem to thrive on not much more than 7 or 8 hours. However, there are some groups of people who push their constitutions towards the limit of endurance: shift workers who defy their own body clocks by working at times when the body should be asleep; those who are driven by excess adrenalin and who sustain their routine by drinking coffee; hyperactive children; carers who are on call 24 hours a day; mothers who both work and bring up their children without enough support. With the exception of hyperactive children these people are often victims of necessity or poor prioritisation. Without sufficient good quality sleep when the body most benefits from it (i.e. at night) these people are risking their creative potential. Sleep can be disturbed by many things: anxiety and fear, excitement, nightmares, excessive drinking or eating (especially food that is rich, heavily spiced or laced with additives such as monosodium glutamate), certain allopathic drugs, night hunger, sleep apnoea, poor bladder control, arthritic and rheumatic conditions, circulatory disorders, menopausal symptoms, skin conditions, and liver and kidney disorders. Sometimes restoration of good sleep is achieved by self-discipline and re-establishment of a strict routine. For chronic sleep problems it is much more likely that a homoeopath will be needed.

Insomnia

Some patients report that they do not sleep at all. This is usually not true; what they are experiencing is a reduction in the amount of deep sleep in which their body functions are at their most passive: when muscles are relaxed, blood pressure is low and the heart rate is slower. They doze and slip in and out of sleep fitfully giving them the sense of restlessness and unease. Many complain of insomnia because they wake too early in the morning (around 4 or 5 a.m.); this is particularly true of the elderly. Others complain of waking up 2 hours or so after getting to sleep and then not being able to go off again until 5 or 6 a.m. when the alarm rings; this is common among menopausal women and overstretched businessmen. Yet others say that they feel tired enough to go to bed by 11 p.m. but as soon as their heads touch the pillow, they feel wide awake; this is usual among busy people who try to juggle too many things. Another group say that they fall asleep at inappropriate times in the day while not being able to sleep at night; this is also common among older people as well as those who are jet-lagged. Insomnia requires professional treatment because the underlying causes may either be pathological (e.g. < since a stroke or high fever; < due to thyroid malfunction; < menopause; < from liver toxicity; etc.) or emotional (< since a shock or grief) or mental (< anxiety over a crisis) or miasmatic. Sleep is so vital to a healthy constitution that an objective observer with experience to see the whole picture is necessary. However, there are some circumstances in which self-help can be appropriate. Use the 30 except where another suggestion is made in the list of remedies for sleeplessness below.

- < anger after humiliation: **Staphysagria** (awake all night suffering from indignation and thinking of what could have been said and what ought to be said).
- < anxiety: **Arsen-alb.** (panicky restlessness that forces the patient to get up and pace or make a cup of tea all < around 12 – 1 a.m.); **Cocculus** (< exhaustion with anxious dreams in brief snatches of sleep; easily startled; light-headed and weak); **Sepia** (starts out of sleep after a vivid, scary dream sometimes with a sense of having been called which makes the patient feel anxious, sensitive and irritable).
- < in children: **Arsen-alb.** (restless, anxious and demanding < stomach upset, asthmatic breathing or nightmare); **Bell.** (red face, throbbing

carotid artery and generally hot in upper body with fever or fury); **Calc-carb.** (child wakes crying from a nightmare which they can't describe; sits up and rubs eyes continually); **Cham.** (child is furious and fractious unless carried around < teething, nightmare or digestive upset); **Coffea** (< from overexcitement with talkativeness and restlessness yet can become very irritable if not listened to); **Puls.** (wakeful at night having been sleepy in day with tearfulness and need for company); **Sulph.** (tired and grumpy from wakefulness esp. < 2 – 5 a.m. or wakes at 5 a.m. feeling too hot and sweaty).

- < from drinking too much coffee: **Coffea** (feels wired up and buzzy with fast heart rate and excitement); **Nux-vom.** (irritable and nervy with tiredness but can't fall asleep for activity of brain).
- < cramps in the legs: **Calc-c.** (cramps < stretching out and that force the patient out of bed); **Cuprum** (< in calves, feet or shin with spasms of pain).
- < dark room: **Puls.** (must have company and the light on somewhere near).
- < eating too much or going to bed too soon after a meal: **Carbo-veg.** (feels too full, heavy and bloated with burping and breathlessness). A mug of hot water with lemon juice is complementary and very cleansing to the liver.
- < excessive exertion: **Arsen-alb.** (< from mental or physical exertion with restlessness and anxiety < 12 – 1 a.m.); **Avena Sativa** (nervous exhaustion especially after worries which cause brain fag – use 6 potency 3 times a day for 5 – 7 days); **Lyc.** (sleepy all day and wakeful at night after long period of stress with irritability and bad breath on waking in a.m.); **Nux-vom.** (mind keeps working despite tiredness with sleepiness towards morning < excessive talking, working and drinking); **Phos-ac.** (mental and physical exhaustion with sleepiness and lethargy in the day but feeling hot and sad or desperate at night).
- < fright: **Acon.** (fearful and fretful, waking around midnight with crying and terrified expression – use 200); **Ign.** (wakes terrified, screaming and inconsolable from a bad dream – use 200).
- < grief: **Ign.** (inconsolable with weeping and sense of a lump in the throat – use 200); **Nat-mur.** (tearful, withdrawn and worried but without much verbal expression – use a 30 for 3 nights but if no better

call the homoeopath).

- < becoming too hot in bed (but without fever): **Puls.** (sleeps with arms out of covers, above the head and knees drawn up or sticking out of the bed to cool); **Sulph.** (frequent waking with sweating and sticking the feet out of bed because of hot feet; though might also wrap up in the covers despite being hot).

- < hunger: **Abies Nigra** (wakeful and restless with hunger with sleepiness in the day; patient may suffer generally from dyspepsia and experience a sensation of a lump lodged in the area of the sternum); **Lyc.** (especially indicated in those with sensitive digestion, hypoglycaemia and food intolerances; windy and bloated with abdominal discomfort); **Phos.** (weak and hungry with thirst for cold water; hypoglycaemia). If hypoglycaemia is ongoing then eat a banana or a natural fruit yoghurt before going to bed. If these are not acceptable then have a crisp bread with honey and some warm milk (goat's better than cow's).

- < after influenza: **Avena Sativa** (nervous exhaustion after an acute bout of 'flu – use 6 2 or 3 times a day for several days).

- < after a physical trauma: **Arn.** (feels bruised and achy and that the bed feels too hard).

- < after a late supper: **Puls.** (restless and full, wanting company and light). This can sometimes be helped by drinking a mug of hot water with lemon juice.

- < for thinking about things: **Arg-nit.** (plagued by 'what if?' thoughts; < anticipation); **Arsen-alb.** (worried about what has not been done and what is left to do and how to control events); **Bryonia** (worried about business which feels stress-laden); **Calc-c.** (anxious about not having fulfilled expectations or responsibilities; lies awake making lists); **China** (can't stop fantasising); **Cocculus** (anxious thoughts about the health of others); **Coffea** (can't switch off from exciting ideas); **Lyc.** (anxiety over coming ordeal or from loss of self-confidence; wakes anxious at 4 a.m.); **Nat-mur.** (< grief-laden thoughts or from resentments); **Nux-vom.** (oversensitive to noise, light, etc. while unable to switch off from exciting thoughts from the day); **Puls.** (the same thought keeps going round and round in the head which leads to tearfulness or need for company; the same tune recently heard keeps repeating in the mind); **Sulph.** (dozes on and off and wakes frequently to egocentric worries which they fail to think through so wake in the morning feeling irritable and unrefreshed).

- < too much wine: **Nux-vom.** (headache and hangover).
- < worms: **Cina** (itching anus, irritable, restless and grinding of teeth; child is nervous, inclined to tantrums and bites nails). Use 30 twice a day for 3 days. If this helps but the problem returns then consult your homoeopath as dietary and supplementary measures will have to be taken.

Frequent Waking

Frequent waking may be caused by mental, emotional or physical problems (see 'Insomnia' above). For the most part, wakefulness is only one of a complex of symptoms that requires professional help. It is worth knowing what information will be needed. Sometimes the waking occurs at any time of the night, sometimes it occurs quite specifically at particular times. If there is a regular time factor it is really helpful to the selection of the remedy. For example: **Sulphur** has a habit of waking at 3, 4 and 5 a.m. feeling hot and sweaty; **Lycopodium** wakes at 4 a.m. and dozes fitfully till the alarm goes off and then feels heavy and tired from a sluggish, toxic liver; **Kali-carb.** wakes several times between 2 and 5 a.m. especially from back and joint pains, indigestion or breathing difficulties. If **Nux-vom.** has a bad night it will wake at 3 or 4 a.m. feeling liverish and wide awake from worries. The homoeopath will want to know what time the patient wakes, in what manner and state they wake and what symptoms appear or continue once they are awake. Frequent waking may be part of the picture of, say, prostate trouble (so information about urination will be useful), menopause (circulation, temperature and sweat), asthma (breathing, mucus and posture) or digestion (pains, flatulence, posture, etc.). Despite giving this type of specific information it is unlikely that the homoeopath would prescribe therapeutically solely on the sleep pattern; it is more usual for the patient to receive a constitutional remedy for the general picture and possibly organ support remedies to make sure that kidneys, liver, bowel or whichever organ is struggling is able to maintain optimum functioning while recuperation goes on.

Excessive Daytime Sleepiness

This condition, when chronic, is usually the result of unexpressed anxiety and depression though it can also be the result of taking hypnotic drugs, prolonged sleep apnoea, lack of oxygen or too frequent use of marijuana. Occasionally it can be a sign of brain pathology. For those who work in airless offices or have to go on long drives that induce sleepiness, frequent short bursts of exercise or pit stops are essential; part of the solution can lie in finding ways to change the energy of the situation. However, being in the wrong job is frequently a major factor and might even be contributing to an underlying, hitherto unacknowledged depression. Daytime sleepiness that has no obvious causation should be treated professionally.

Sleep Apnoea

Apnoea or the cessation of breathing during sleep is most common among the elderly who are overweight, the very young or those who have a dysfunction of the brain's breathing control mechanism. Symptoms include long periods without taking a breath, sudden choking and spluttering, snoring and sudden awakening with panicky feelings. The cause of apnoea includes obstruction of the airways by mucus, relaxed tissues of the throat and chest or awkward posture during sleep. In the obese and elderly, eating too late in the evening, smoking and excessive alcohol will all exacerbate the problem and the most frequently indicated remedy is **Carbo-veg.** (especially if they need to sit back at an angle and breathe steadily) which is best given in a 30 before bed. Both **Lycopodium** and **Sulphur** suffer from apnoea; see above in 'Insomnia' for accompanying symptoms. Young children sometimes suffer from apnoea especially if they have a history of breathing difficulties or catarrh production. These children must be treated professionally. They often need either **Kali-carb.**, **Lycopodium**, **Carbo-veg.** or **Sulphur** but it is imperative that constitutional treatment covers the susceptibility to breathing disorders as so often there is a miasmatic aspect to be addressed.

Dreams and Nightmares

Dreams are much sought-after symptoms for homoeopaths; they like them because they may indicate remedies that would otherwise be missed by only noting the mental, emotional and physical symptoms, or they tell them how well the last remedy has done. Not everyone can recall their dreams and some deny having any at all; what they mean is that they cannot remember them. Sometimes it is enough to recall the essence or the general theme of a dream: falling, being chased, losing something. It is always worth mentioning recurrent dreams and it is helpful to the practitioner if the patient relates dreams experienced after having taken a constitutional remedy. Bad or frightening dreams and night terrors are even more important symptoms because they often indicate a state in need of urgent treatment. Night terrors in children are rarely an isolated symptom but they may be the most striking (or even the only) indication of what is wrong. They always need to be treated professionally because night terrors are an expression of, among other things, either birth trauma ('never been well since' (NBWS), Caesarean, breech birth or forceps for example) or the tubercular miasm both of which, if treated thoroughly, will allow the patient to make a marked developmental leap forward. (The process is, so to speak, part of the emerging from the chrysalis that all children must do; nothing short of a rite of passage.) One of the most important constitutional remedies of all, **Calc-carb.**, is often called for in children who suffer terrifying dreams. Sometimes the practitioner finds that this remedy is not immediately indicated and that the propitious moment for giving it must be arrived at by stages. This is another reason that the homoeopath should be involved in treatment.

In adults nightmares can be an expression of a similar process of metamorphosis which, as children, they never had a chance to go through or tried to but were prevented from doing in some way. It is not uncommon for adult patients to relate their dreams of death, dying, dead bodies, coffins, empty houses, dangerous seascapes, being chased by unseen assassins or wild animals, being imprisoned in a prisoner of war camp and of a host of other scary visions. These herald an opportunity for profound and positive change if they are described to a homoeopath who can make use of the images of dreams to cast a light on an evolutionary 'state' that can be appropriately prescribed for.

Night Sweats

Though night sweats are not a sleep symptom (they are a 'time of day' symptom and thus belong to the hormone system) they are common and can be very distressing. They occur because of fevers, hormone changes (menopause, pregnancy, etc.), infections, malarial conditions, liver toxicity and unexpressed anxieties. They are also very useful in selecting remedies. If night sweats are an important part of the symptom picture then it is important that the practitioner knows as much as possible about them. The quality of sweat (whether watery or oily), odour and location are all helpful. It makes a difference if the sweat is on the head or legs only or if it is all over or solely on the chest. Sickly sweet sweat indicates different remedies from sweat that smells acrid, like tea or onions. Drenching, all-over sweats can be exhausting and are *always* of great significance to the treatment. Sweats that stain or stiffen the bed linen are very important to report. The major first-aid remedies in which night sweats can help to determine the choice are:

Arsen-alb.: feverish cold sweat with thirst, exhaustion and laboured breathing.

Calc-carb.: fever with cold sweats < on the head with damp hair and pillow.

Carbo-veg.: sweats on the face < after heavy meal with feeling hot internally but chilly to touch; also < night-time cough.

China: fever sweats follow on from chills then thirst then heat; every movement in bed <; drenching.

Ferrum-phos.: night fever with sweaty hands.

Hepar-sulph.: sour smelling sweat all over which is sticky and makes the patient feel more irritable (usually during fever states).

Lachesis: wakes with hot flush (during throat infection) with sweating around the neck and under arms; may also be indicated in menopause but consult the homoeopath.

Lycopodium: shivery chills followed by cold sweat that smells of onions (part of a severe cold or 'flu picture).

Merc-sol.: drenching sweats in heat alternating with shivery chilliness; sweat is sticky, clammy and can be foul smelling; stains the bed clothes yellowish (usually with fever symptoms but sometimes part of constitutional picture or as a result of mercury fillings).

Pulsatilla: sweating comes on with the pains; otherwise tends to be dry (may be with or without fever).

Sepia: sweats at night with hot flushes during the menopause; sweats < around the groin and makes the patient feel unclean. (This is not a first-aid picture; it is described here to encourage **Sepia** patients to seek help from the homoeopath.)

Silica: sweats < immediately on falling asleep or towards the early hours of morning after a chilly, uncomfortable time earlier in the night; sweats < torso; (with or without fever).

Sulphur: generally hot but night sweat < back of the neck and head or other single parts such as hands or back; comes on in flushes (with or without fever). (This can be part of a general constitutional picture and may not be acute; if so it is a signal that constitutional treatment is due.)

Veratrum-alb.: night sweats with gastric bug with extreme coldness, insatiable thirst and nausea; sweat most apparent on forehead but can be all over.

Cross-check the indicated remedy with the general picture in part III. If there is a similar match to the condition then use 30. If the condition is chronic rather than acute then call your practitioner for confirmation and dosage.

22 MEDICAL TESTS, EXAMINATIONS AND SURGERY

When tests, physical examinations and surgery become a necessity it is useful to be prepared with remedies and information to deal with situations that can arise.

White Coat Syndrome

Fear of doctors and their paraphernalia is an important symptom. It can cause test results to be inaccurate; blood pressure readings are typically susceptible to this. It can also cause patients to lose their sense of autonomy; they become passive and even uninvolved, allowing the professionals to take over and make decisions that might not be in their best long-term interests. It is best for patients to meet doctors and specialists feeling clear-headed, calm and determined to get as much information for themselves as any tests or examinations will give the medics. To be passive is to abdicate self-determination and responsibility for the condition. There are certain remedies that can assist:

Aconite: extreme anxiety with hypochondriasis; full of doom and gloom; restless and jumpy or dull and desperate. (Use 200.)

Arg-nit.: anxiety about the forthcoming appointment with restless pacing and runny, flatulent gut; full of 'But what if…?' questions. (Use 200.)

Arsen-alb.: restless and anxious with hypochondriasis; becomes fussy and demanding and frustrated with being inefficient despite trying to control events. (Use 200.)

Calc-carb.: shows anxiety by trying to prepare overzealously for the interview; worries about whether they will say the right things or leave anything out; may lie awake at night thinking about it. (Use 30 or 100.)

Gelsemium: full of dread but becomes passive with outbursts of irritation when fussed; goes into apathy and torpor; wants to be left alone but shows timidity when dealing with authoritative people. (Use 30 though some homoeopaths will prescribe as high as 10M in such situations. Be guided by what usually works for you or by your homoeopath.)

Lycopodium: puts on a brave face but is fearful of confrontation with authority or those with specialist knowledge; often tends to be flatulent and bloated with disturbed bowel routine in the build-up to a medical interview. (Use 30 or 100.)

Phosphorus: terrified of the technology of medical procedures; << hypodermic needles. (Use 30.)

Rescue Remedy: the Bach Flower Essences can be very helpful either as an alternative or as a complementary addition to one of the above.

In addition it is worth noting that **Lotus** 30 or 200 is a very useful remedy before medical interviews; it is both calming and 'centring' and it helps the patient to focus on the essentials. It is a homoeopathic 'rescue remedy'. It can be combined with flower essences. The following essences can be obtained from health food shops or homoeopathic pharmacies can make up a combination of **Lotus** 30 with the selected essences from the list below. Ask for a 5-ml bottle of **Lotus** 30 combined with, say, Cerato + Crab Apple + Elm + Rock Rose. You will get a bottle of drops from which you might take one drop every 2 – 4 hours until after the appointment.
  • Cerato (for those who face professionals who 'know better')
  • Cherry Plum (irrational thoughts that churn round)
  • Crab Apple (loathing one's condition and wishing the body had not failed)
  • Elm (feeling overwhelmed)

- Gentian (gloom and doom)
- Gorse (negative and pessimistic)
- Larch (fears of being bulldozed into agreeing to what they do not want)
- Mimulus (timid and unable to speak up for self)
- Oak (usually strong but too weakened by circumstance to continue struggling)
- Rock Rose (rising panic)
- Star of Bethlehem (dread of bad news)

X-rays, Ultrasound and MRI Scans

Each of these tests carries its own problems, however important they may be for diagnostic reasons. X-rays do emit radiation and, despite what we are told about 'acceptable limits' of radiation, there are no guarantees that any of us fall into that bracket of people who can remain unaffected by it. As with everything, some people are able to take more than others but there are no tests to tell us if you are one of them. It is advisable to let your practitioner know when the patient is going for an X-ray because they will probably choose to prescribe therapeutically to afford protection as far as that is possible. The most commonly prescribed remedy is **Radium Bromide** 30 which is given immediately before and after the X-ray. Some homoeopaths prefer to use **X-ray** 30, a remedy made by subjecting the rays to potentisation. Yet others will simply give **Arnica** 30 or 200 as this remedy is known to assist in clearing radioactivity from the body. One important reason for prescribing for X-rays is that radiation has a habit, even in small quantities, of attaching itself to the electrodynamic field of the body and, in the words of those who are able to 'see' this (the so-called 'aura'), of 'tearing holes in the energy body'. If the X-ray procedure is preceded by the injection of radioactive dye, a barium meal or enema then the likelihood of radiation poisoning, even in a tiny amount, is greater. One X-ray may be negligible; a dozen are not. (This should also cover dental X-rays; though dental X-rays are taken at separate times over several years, radiation does not diminish over time. Each new X-ray adds to the effects of the last.) CAT scans are also a form of X-ray; more powerful and causing greater risk of being affected by radiation. One of the worst side effects of all this is for the patient to suffer an 'energy leak'; they feel constantly tired and drained of any creative force. Radiation 'poisoning' like this is particularly difficult because it is so 'unseen' and can easily be missed. Mammograms are also less than benign. Not only are breasts bruised by the machinery but they are subjected to radiation. If there is a benign lump (or otherwise) to be investigated the radiation used for the examination can contribute to turning the tissue into being actively negative. No woman should go for a mammogram without protective homoeopathic remedies.

Ultrasound scans are quite different. Cells of the tissue being checked are subjected to a bombardment of sound waves that are reflected back into the machine to record what amounts to an echogram. This is a painless procedure for most of us but for the local cells, ever changing and renewing, it is not; they are, so to speak, bruised. It is thus a good idea to take **Arnica** 200 or **Bellis Perennis** 200 (especially when the ultrasound is taken of the abdomen) before and after scans. This is even more important when considering ultrasound scans on pregnant women. The scan affects the developing cells of the foetus. It is not uncommon for babies who have been subjected to multiple scans to be born with haematomas – areas of unresolved bruising. Many women report that as soon as the ultrasound starts, the baby moves in the womb as if trying to get away from the device. If at all possible scans should be resisted; if not, then they should not be performed before 24 weeks.

MRI (magnetic resonance imaging) scans are different again. One of the reasons they have become more popular is that they are meant to be less harmful than X-rays! They record their images using a giant ring magnet through which the patient is passed. They have the ability to alter a patient's entire electrical field just as iron filings are affected by passing a magnet above them; the patient is, in effect, polarised. Though the immediate effects of this may not be at all obvious, any of the body's functions or emotions might be affected by the subtle shift of nucleic energy in every cell of the body. **Arnica** is also called for but some homeopaths like to use **Magnetis Polis Ambo** (the remedy made from the energy of a magnet); a 30 or a 200 in those who are sensitive.

Before and After Surgery

It is best that the practitioner is involved with preparing the patient for surgery. They will know what remedies are best for the individual. However, the following information may help to focus on what might be required and should be discussed with the homoeopath.

Emerald is a relatively newly proved remedy that has demonstrated its worth when given before surgery to remove tissue. **Emerald** 200 as soon as possible before theatre encourages the body to go through with the excision or extraction (it is useful before birth and tooth extraction as well) as if helping to release what is no longer needed, viable or healthy or what has matured sufficiently to be removed safely.

Eryngium Maritima is useful here purely on a therapeutic basis for the prevention of haemorrhage. If given one a day for 3 days before an operation it can lessen the likelihood of excessive bleeding. (This might be even more useful if the operation is scheduled for any time around the full moon as this is when haemorrhage is statistically more likely to occur.)

Arnica 200 is universally known as a major remedy to help recovery from an operation. It is best given as soon as possible *after* the patient has come round from the anaesthetic (but see **Opium** below). It is not unusual for homoeopaths to prescribe **Arnica** twice daily for several days after an operation. It is best *not* to take Arnica *before* an operation; surgeons have reported incidence of more than expected bleeding. (See **Erygnium** above which does not have this problem.)

Bellis Perennis belongs to the same family as **Arnica**, the daisies. It is more useful for recuperation from an operation to the abdomen where a lot of soft tissue has been damaged and internal organs disturbed. It is not unusual for **Bell-per.** (30 or 200 to be prescribed 2 or 3 times a day for several days or even a week or more.)

Bryonia is most useful when pains after surgery are < for the slightest movement, cough, sneeze or laugh (the latter not likely in a **Bryonia** patient). (Use 30 unless the homoeopath suggests higher.)

Calendula is the first remedy to consider for the healing of operation wounds; it encourages antisepsis in the body and promotes skin repair after surgery and episiotomy. It is not unusual for **Calendula** 30 to be prescribed 2 or 3 times a day till improvement is established. It is also useful to apply **Calendula** in tincture; see **Hypercal Ø** below.

Causticum is very useful when surgery has left the patient with difficulties in passing water. A few doses of **Causticum** 30 can act as a homoeopathic catheter.

Hypercal Ø is a combination of **Hypericum** (which heals damaged nerves) and **Calendula** (which repairs damaged skin). **Hypercal Ø** is invaluable when applied topically as it not only brings about rapid healing but also helps to prevent scarring. It can be applied neat but this is likely to sting so it is often used in solution: 4 drops to a quarter of a cup of water.

Ledum: is indicated for all types of laparoscopic (keyhole) surgery.

Opium 1M is frequently needed after a general anaesthetic when the patient does not come round satisfactorily; it is as if the anaesthesia does not wear off and leaves the patient in limbo. The patient appears dopey and sluggish, not 'with it' and 'out of body'. There may also be constipation as well. A single dose is usual. (Sometimes **Phosphorus** is used in place of **Opium** if the indications are there.)

Rhus-tox. is useful after operations in which muscles are affected. This covers birth as well. It follows and complements **Arnica** where there is stiffness and aching. (30 or 200 may be used.)

Ruta is useful when surgery has left damage to the ligaments and periosteum. It is complementary to both **Arnica** and **Rhus-tox.** and can be given in tandem with (at a different hour) or following the others. (30 or 200 may be used.)

Staphysagria stands alone in its ability to relieve the patient of the trauma of the knife or the surgical procedure. If the patient feels the cut of the operation or feels the indignity of the procedure then **Staphysagria** 200 must be given as soon as possible; without it the circumstance can become a chronic maintaining cause leaving the patient unable to get better generally. This remedy also covers things such as pains felt long after a catheter is withdrawn.

Thiosinaminum is a remedy with a reputation for preventing scar tissue from building up after deep surgery on soft tissue such as happens with abdominal operations. This is important because internal scar tissue can be responsible for causing malfunction of vital organs when the gathering scar tissue (adhesions) pulls on adjacent structures causing wrong positioning and poor drainage. The homoeopath may use this remedy in low potency (3 or 6) daily for quite a long time (up to 6 weeks in some cases).

It is always advisable to consult the cranial osteopath after major surgery to ensure that all vital organs return to their correct position in the body and that lymph drainage is restored to as near normal as possible. High priorities after a serious operation include a balance between gentle exercise and rest with care not to lift heavy objects; a gradual return to a normal routine as soon as possible; a balanced diet including easily digested protein food (such as white fish) and green vegetables; plenty of water to drink to ensure that the kidneys are maintained; allowing as much fresh air as is feasible around any wound that may still be healing. It is important to avoid any *sudden* return to a working schedule; there needs to be a gradual process of return to normal work. It is also not a good idea to drink Indian tea as this is dehydrating. Food loaded with salt, fats or flavourings (such as Chinese food with monosodium glutamate or fast food) should be avoided altogether. When the operation has been exhausting to body, nerves and emotions it is worth considering using restorative therapeutic remedies:

Aletris Farinosa: extreme tiredness with poor appetite, nausea and loss of weight after gynaecological operations especially for prolapse or fibroids. May also be a little light-headed. (Use the 3 several times a day.)

Avena Sativa: useful as a support remedy for debility, nerviness and exhaustion with sleeplessness after an operation especially in the elderly. (Use the 3 several times a day.) Some practitioners will prescribe the mother tincture instead especially if another remedy (see **Kali Phos.** below) is homoeopathically indicated.

China: is useful after abdominal operations (especially after removal of the gall bladder) when the patient feels weak, overwhelmed by the difficulties of recuperation and easily irritated; often accompanied by feeling bloated and windy and very thirsty with little appetite for anything but delicatessen food. (Use 30 twice daily for 3 days.)

Kali Phos.: this is of immense value when the operation has caused weakness, fatigue, sensitivity of nerves, a depressive state, lethargy and a disinclination to get back to normal. Though the patient may not be malingering at all, they are despondent and irritable and easily exhausted; fears about the future prevent them from being positive. Sleep is often affected: very tired but too worried to sleep properly. (Use 30 twice daily for 3 days.)

Phos-ac.: useful when there is marked debility of the mind after an operation; the patient tends to stare blankly into space. Also important if there has been a considerable loss of blood during an operation. Is often given in 6x daily as a preventative or restorative but can be prescribed in 30, 200 or higher when the symptoms are severe; a homoeopath's advice would be useful.

Post-operative Blues

Depression after surgery is not uncommon. It can be the result of the general anaesthetic, of drugs to prevent infection and pain or because the operation removed the pathology on which the patient was emotionally dependent or because the patient had not reached a point where they were ready to heal without it. The two latter circumstances need clarifying. Some patients 'need' their pathology as a way of identifying to themselves and to the world what is wrong with their lives; they feel strangely bereft after surgery has removed this physiological expression which stood in for what they could not otherwise communicate. Other patients, quite ready to take responsibility for their physical health though they may be, are negatively affected if surgery removes the symptoms before they are 'mature' enough; before the physical symptoms have been able fully to express the whole state. The reason for this is that physical pathology is usually an *end* result of unexpressed or suppressed mental, emotional and spiritual pathology which takes time to mature. It is only safe to remove symptoms surgically once they have reached a point where the patient is ready to let them go. (This is part of the reason why **Emerald** is such a useful pre-surgery remedy as it is one that has a profound effect on the 'wounded ego'; it helps people to allow their ego to let go of what is no longer necessary to their lives.) Some people are only ready to do this when an emergency obliges them to go through a traumatic 'rescue' operation (i.e. to remove a threatening blockage; to remove a throbbing, inflamed appendix; to extract a rotten tooth associated with an excruciating abscess). Others have pathology that allows them a degree of choice about when surgery is necessary. However, there are times when choice is determined by other people whose approach is measured by the experience of urgency and expediency. This can lead to the hasty removal of symptoms that were still being 'worked out' in the patient's wholeness. For all these reasons it is essential that the patient suffering from post-operative blues should consult the homoeopath. This is not least because it is not uncommon for those who have had their symptoms removed too soon, to redevelop them either in the same way and place or as different and more threatening pathology. Surgery 'cures' nothing; it mitigates circumstances and allows patients more time to heal themselves. Post-operative homoeopathic care is not limited to healing wounds and soothing pains; it is also about making sure that the patient can make the most positive use of their experience and find a way of not returning to the state that brought about the need for surgery in the first place.

Blood Transfusions

Blood transfusions are sometimes a necessary evil and they do save lives. Nevertheless, taking on the blood of other people does have the consequence of potentially taking on their miasmatic susceptibilities. The homoeopath must always be informed if there has been a blood transfusion either in the past or during a recent operation. It is almost always necessary for the practitioner to consider 'cleaning up' afterwards.

Chemotherapy

Having chemotherapy does not preclude homoeopathic treatment. The homoeopath should be willing to accept the patient's choice of making use of allopathic medicines and tailor the treatment accordingly. There are remedies that are extremely effective at reducing the side effects of a heavy-duty drug regime and these include **Ipecacuanha** for nausea and sickness and **Cadmium Sulphuratum** for stomach pains and prostration. Otherwise, constitutional treatment, while not limiting or interfering with the drugs, can strengthen the patient generally and promote the best possible chance of recovery. Some consultants are averse to this choice believing that their work is being interfered with but this stems from their lack of knowledge about the workings of homoeopathy.

Radiotherapy

Much the same as was said about chemotherapy can be said of radiotherapy. It is extremely important that the patient is given remedies to counteract the side effects of radiation treatment. So powerful is the radiation that, while it may blast the rogue cancer cells, it can damage other, healthy cells locally and thus predispose them to becoming cancerous. Unfortunately, radiation has a habit of shifting location indiscriminately, carrying the energy of the recent pathology with it; hence breast cancer can metastasise speedily to the spine, the liver or the lung in those easily affected. By consulting the homoeopath, who is likely to prescribe one of the radiation remedies, the risks of long-term side effects and metastasis due to radiation are limited considerably. One of the most useful remedies to restore the integrity of the skin after radiation treatment is **Calendula** which is complementary to the radiation remedies.

MRSA

The hospital superbug that has proved so resistant to antibiotics is one of the reasons for people – certainly older people – fearing to go into hospital. While it is true that hospital wards leave a lot to be desired in the way of cleanliness, the real reason for MRSA being so prevalent is the general ambience of fear, indignity and loss of individuality that pervades all National Health hospitals. People in hospital these days, despite the caring nature and vocational professionalism of nursing staff, lose their self-respect very quickly. This lowering of spirits is bound to encourage conditions that engender disgust – both with the situation and with the body. (If it were not MRSA it would be another bug; if they find a miracle cure for it then another bug will certainly crop up in its place.) MRSA is a fancy acronym for a strain of staphylococcus, a bug that is often found on the skin or in the nostrils. When a debilitated patient succumbs to it the danger is that septicaemia may set in. If it is successfully suppressed by drug therapy it often leaves the patient depressed, weak and lacking in motivation, making recuperation from the treatment as difficult as from the original condition that took them into hospital. If the homoeopath is involved then progress can be much swifter and far less damaging. There are symptom pictures arising from MRSA that are covered by remedies though it is not unusual for the practitioner to have to monitor progress in case the first picture shifts subtly into another. Remedies such as **Calc-sulph., Pyrogen, Staphylococcus, Silica, Hepar-sulph., Echinacea** and **Gunpowder** all have a reputation for getting the body to respond eliminatively. While these may be prescribed on the physical symptoms, there may be an underlying mental/emotional picture that needs addressing as well. If there is a feeling of suppressed anger and humiliation from going through the hospital's hands then the homoeopath may give a single dose of a remedy such as **Staphysagria** 1M. It is not unusual for heavy-duty multiple prescribing, that might seem to go counter to homoeopathic philosophy ('the minimum dose') to be needed in dealing with this blight but it is a measure of the depth and strength of the patient's negative state in MRSA as to how necessary it is. On no account should tea tree oil be used as this is as suppressive as antibiotics. **Hypercal Ø** also has a place in the treatment of MRSA. When the wound is exposed **Hypercal** can be applied safely in solution (4 drops to a quarter of a cup of water); air reaching the lesion is a positive thing.

23   PREGNANCY AND BIRTH

Nausea in Pregnancy

There are a large number of listed remedies for nausea and vomiting in pregnancy and you may find that, if the symptoms do not clearly point to a particular remedy, you need to consult your practitioner. The symptoms usually start shortly after conception and continue until the 12th week; sometimes the symptoms are more severe and persistent and will last all the way through the pregnancy. **In either case, if the condition is marked by profuse vomiting then it is absolutely essential that the treatment is supervised by a professional because dehydration and weight loss will have serious consequences.**

When assessing the indications of remedies remember to take food cravings, thirst and appetite as well as mood into account. (It may be sufficient to use 30 for any of the remedies below; if the indicated remedy does not help then ask the homoeopath for advice on higher potencies.)

Arsen-alb.: nausea and vomiting with restlessness, anxiety and thirst for sips of cold water. May crave (rye) bread or bacon or constantly want refreshing things.

Asarum: soon after conception she becomes *ultra sensitive* (especially to noise) and 'floaty'. Nausea, belching and flatulence come on after eating. Empty retching with watery saliva.

Bryonia: nausea and faintness with the slightest movement: must remain still. Strong thirst for cold water. Food lies like a stone in the stomach. Retches solid food. Vomit is bitter and acid. When hungry can't think of any food that would satisfy. Wants to stay close to home.

Chelidonium: nausea and vomiting > from eating a little or drinking very hot drinks. Tummy feels tender and she is generally 'liverish'. Lots of flatulence and bloating. May crave cheese which then <. Irritable and a bit unreasonable; doesn't want to talk or explain.

Cocculus: nausea and vomiting make her feel as if 'seasick'; light-headed and weak-kneed; unsteady. Nausea may be accompanied by yawning. Loathing of all food. Refreshing things can > temporarily.

Colchicum: nausea and loathing from the slightest smell of food: makes her feel faint and disgusted; cannot bear to cook. Wants sparkling water or fizzy drinks; *may become dehydrated*. Feels she will collapse from prostration; short attention span when trying to read or listen; intolerant due to being oversensitive.

Ipecac.: constant nausea and vomiting; very pale face with profuse salivation. Stomach feels slack and sinking. Despite the nausea the tongue looks smooth and clean with no furring. **Risk of dehydration!**

Kreosotum: nausea and vomiting < morning with switching from ravenous appetite (especially for smoked meat or fish) to virtual starvation. Becomes 'hormonal' in mood; cross and dissatisfied; very irritable and suddenly looks older. **Risk of weight loss!**

Lac Defloratum: cannot bear milk or dairy food. Nausea and vomiting whether she has eaten or not. May suffer headache and constipation as well. Becomes listless and despondent; may say 'I wouldn't care if I were dead'. Nausea < travelling by car.

Lactic Acid: affects women who are thin, pale and weak. Nausea < on rising and > after breakfast. Heartburn with hot belches. Stomach feels heavy. (Suggest that the patient takes warm water and lemon juice to alleviate the acidity.)

Lycopodium: hungry but small amount of food = fullness and flatulence. Passing wind >. Nausea with acid indigestion. May crave chocolate, sweets or cakes or have a sudden craving for olives. Easily confused. (Try warm water with lemon juice.)

Nux Vomica: flatulence, heartburn, nausea and tender abdomen > from vomiting little bits of mucousy food which only comes on several hours after eating. Wants coffee which <. Acid belching. Wakes at 3 a.m. and cannot go back to sleep. Likes stimulants and spicy food. Flashes of irritability which end in tears.

Pulsatilla: food lies like a stone in the stomach with bitter taste in mouth; nausea and vomiting follow an hour or so after eating. Despite symptoms, can have gnawing hunger which she doesn't know how to satisfy. Not thirsty till later stages of the pregnancy. May start craving soft boiled eggs. **Risk of dehydration!**

Sepia: feels faint with the sickness; sinking sensation in stomach. Fed up and cast down and often ready to blame husband or children for their shortcomings. Feels > for fresh air and exercise but may feel that she has not got the energy to get up and go. Likes lemons and hot water with lemon juice that temporarily >.

If none of the above make any significant difference then ask your practitioner about using **Symphoricarpus Racimosa** 200.

Heartburn in Pregnancy

Heartburn may or may not accompany morning sickness or it may be a problem on its own. It may continue right the way through pregnancy. Sometimes it is the result of lax tissues; the ring muscle between the stomach and the oesophagus might be slack or pulled out of alignment by the increasing weight and thus allow acid to leak up into the throat and mouth. Cranial osteopathy can help here. The following remedies (use 30) might be indicated:

Capsicum: burning all the way up into the back of the mouth; belching < ; wants spicy or strong, stimulating things to eat or coffee (which <); mood can be contradictory, capricious and she feels < for losing her shape.

Carbo-veg.: belching with foul tasting acidic fluid coming up; stomach may burn; general aversion to food but may intermittently want coffee, salty or sweet food. Patient is likely to get breathless and feel weak.

Lactic Acid: heartburn with excessive salivation, hunger and thirst.

Merc-sol.: heartburn especially < at night with excessive thirst for cold water and salivation; breath smells and there might be a metallic or bloody taste; gums may go spongy; there may be a craving for bread and butter and/or fatty food and she may want lemon which can >; she finds it hard to maintain an even temperature.

Nat-mur.: heartburn with strong thirst for cold water, dryness of mouth, throat and skin and a craving for salty or savoury snacks (can't be bothered much with main meals); constipation with crumbly or ball-shaped stools; she may feel withdrawn and emotional. Suffers palpitations on lying down at night.

Nux-vom.: sour belching with retching but craving for spicy or tasty food; stomach might feel bruised and food seems to lie in a lump; tends to hiccough; tends to be constipated with large, hard, dry stools that are hard to expel; piles may start; irritable and snappy.

Pulsatilla: heartburn with revulsion from fats, bread, water or salty food; no thirst but has a dry mouth; feels as if there is a stone lying in her stomach; tends to be constipated though no two stools are alike; likely to be tearful and in need of support.

Tissue salt: Nat-phos. (morning sickness) and **Nat-sulph.** (generally bilious and glum) are useful supports in heartburn; one dose 3 times per day of the appropriate remedy.

Constipation during Pregnancy

Constipation can predispose the patient to piles due to the added pressure on the lower bowel. It may accompany and complicate heartburn (see above). Other remedies (use 30) include:

Bryonia: very large, dry stools; whole constitution feels dry with a strong thirst for cold water; disinclined to stir herself and is worried about how everything will work out.

Lycopodium: first part of the stool is large, hard and difficult to pass followed by softer stool; windy and bloated; anxious that everything is going well.

Platina: passes a few small, black, ball-like stools or sticky clay-like stools; urging preceded by anal itching; may have mood swings between laughing immoderately and weeping.

Sepia: no urging but with a feeling as if there is a ball in the rectum < sitting; lax muscles and dragged down feeling – rectum may feel prolapsed; sensitive and weepy; fed up and just wants to get the pregnancy over and done with.

Tissue salts: alternating **Kali-mur.** and **Nat-mur.** can help relieve the discomfort of constipation: one each spaced out in the morning and again in the afternoon.

Braxton Hicks Contractions

Named after a nineteenth-century doctor who first described them, these are contractions of the uterus that can occur from any time after the third month of pregnancy though they usually do not start till after halfway through. They are practice runs for labour and quite normal. They last anywhere between 30 to 60 minutes and are random though they can be triggered by an active baby, lifting and carrying or strenuous exercise. Unlike the true contractions of labour, Braxton Hicks are not rhythmical nor do they increase in intensity and regularity. These 'dummy' contractions can become uncomfortable or even painful towards the later stages especially if the patient does not drink enough fluids (very typical of those who need **Lycopodium** or **Pulsatilla**). Drinking plenty, gentle exercise and taking warm baths can ease the discomfort. If the contractions are followed by a vaginal discharge or they are more frequent than 3 or 4 a minute and there is a low back ache then the homoeopath, midwife and/or doctor should be informed at once.

Ultrasound Scans

These scans are routine. The first one is done at the first appointment at the antenatal clinic. The next is carried out at 18 to 20 weeks and the last is at around 30 to 34 weeks. Scans before 10 weeks are done using a vaginal probe as these high-frequency machines can detect ectopic pregnancy or foetal abnormalities. Hand-held machines that scan the surface of the abdomen are used for later scans. If there are any concerns about the health of mother or baby then the doctor is likely to recommend more frequent scanning to monitor progress. Even more sophisticated scanning devices are being developed which provide 3-D images and will become a common feature of the antenatal clinic.

Though scientists are at pains to reassure patients that scans can do no harm to developing foetuses it should be noted that many mothers-to-be complain that their babies become restless and distressed by the procedure. It is certain that the developing foetus is bombarded by sound waves. Many homoeopaths are in favour of prescribing **Arnica** for the 'bruising' effects. It is very sensible and not uncommon for a patient to be asked to take **Arnica** 30 or 200 before and after a scan.

Bleeding and Miscarriage

Bleeding during pregnancy is not uncommon but is always a symptom to be reported. Occasionally it is the result of a 'false' period and once it has gone there is no further loss. Sometimes the blood might appear 'old', thick and brown. This is usually the body's way of clearing any old debris that might have remained from the last period. A third reason is that the placenta has developed over the cervix so that bleeding occurs through the opening to the uterus; this is known as placenta praevia. The bleeding is bright red and painless. Placenta praevia almost always requires a Caesarean section in case the baby is deprived of oxygen through labour and the delivery. Another reason for haemorrhaging in pregnancy is miscarriage which is more common than is sometimes supposed. The majority of miscarriages occur in the first three months of pregnancy though others may occur up to 20 weeks. Early miscarriage is usually a natural event being the result of a foetal abnormality though later on it might be the result of a medical problem in the mother. Occasionally it may be the result of a profound shock or trauma. Repeated miscarriages are almost always the result of a congenital problem carried by the mother; in homoeopathic terms this is often miasmatic and requires professional treatment. Homoeopathy has a good success rate in helping women with frequent miscarriages to conceive and come to term. (Do remember that a homoeopath never prescribes to make any one specific desirable thing happen; every prescription is based on the whole symptom picture with the intention to promote safety, welfare and a return to internal balance. It is the patient's own restored good health that makes a full-term pregnancy possible.)

Early signs of miscarriage include spotting of blood leading to a heavier discharge with contractions and cramps in the lower abdomen. The process of discharging the contents of the uterus may take several days, long enough for the doctor to recommend a scan. It is advisable to contact the homoeopath as well so that remedies can be used to promote the safety of mother and baby if it is a false alarm, or to encourage a thorough process of elimination so that the uterus does not require further interference from a D and C (a procedure for the removal of all debris).

To cope with the emotional turmoil that a miscarriage can engender it is worth noting the following remedies:

Aconite: for the fright of finding the signs of bloody discharge. (Use 200.)

Arnica: for those who react by feeling stunned from the 'bad news' and then go into denial: 'No, I'm fine, I can cope with this.' (This can be helpful to husbands as well.) (Use 200.)

Ignatia: when the symptoms are accompanied by bouts of sobbing, lump in the throat and nerviness. (Use 200 or 1M.)

Pulsatilla: when the patient is needy, tearful, frightened and better for support and reassurance. (Use 200 or 1M.)

Staphysagria: when grief is mixed with unexpressed anger due to the invasive procedures and anything that might have been said carelessly that has caused feelings of humiliation or of having been abused. (Use 200.)

Though these remedies are best prescribed by the homoeopath, patients are not always in the frame of mind to contact anyone when emotionally upset and caught up in hospital procedures.

Pre-eclampsia

Statistics tell us that one in ten mothers-to-be suffer pre-eclampsia which makes it common enough for it to be routinely tested for. This condition is of unknown origin and is characterised by raised blood pressure, fluid retention (especially in the face and hands) and protein in the urine. It is more likely to happen in those who have had it in a previous pregnancy; who are carrying twins; who already have high blood pressure or a pre-existing condition of the blood vessels. Because it can lead to premature detachment of the placenta from the wall of the uterus, or convulsions and coma in the mother it has to be treated promptly; treatment involves bed rest and drugs to lower the blood pressure and may necessitate a stay in hospital. Pre-eclampsia can be a reason for Caesarean section delivery. The symptoms may continue for several days after delivery. As there are usually describable symptoms it is worth telling the homoeopath as well as following the advice of the doctor.

Fear of Delivery

This is a very common fear. See the homoeopath who is likely to prescribe one of the remedies known for anticipation and anxiety when facing an ordeal. The remedies are usually part of the first-aid kit: **Acon.**, **Arg-nit.**, **Arsen-alb.**, **Gelsemium**, **Lycopodium** or **Nat-mur.** The most commonly used for this ordeal is **Gelsemium** with its mixed sense of dread, heaviness, apathy and confusion.

Itching during Pregnancy

Occasionally women report that they suffer itching all over without any sign of a rash, particularly at night, and that their sleep is disturbed by it. Ask your homoeopath about **Dolichos**, the only remedy listed for this. The reason for the itching is that the pregnancy is putting a strain on the liver; the complexion may even be a little sallow. **Tabacum** is also a remedy for such itching though there is likely to be nausea, vomiting and a state of feeling wretchedly miserable to go with it. The homoeopath should also be consulted if there is itching of the genital region.

Stretch Marks

Stretch marks are difficult to combat and there is very little in the way of treatment that can guarantee successful removal. There are common-sense guidelines: drink plenty of water through the pregnancy; eat a balanced diet so that the body's biochemistry is at its optimum; use a body brush for exfoliation; take plenty of gentle, routine exercise including stretching. Save your money and leave the special creams on the shelf. They are a snare and a delusion. In homoeopathy **Calc-fluor.** tissue salt is usually prescribed for this problem. **Calc-fluor.** is the first remedy of choice to improve the elasticity of tissue. Taking it is regarded as a preventative measure; stretch marks should not lead to lax flesh after the delivery. It is worth asking the homoeopath for guidance on dosage though one, once or twice daily is the usual.

Breech and Other Abnormal Positions

Babies sometimes adopt a position that makes a normal delivery awkward or impossible. There may be physical reasons: a short umbilicus; the cord is round the baby's neck; fibroids on the uterus wall; twins, etc. It is important that the midwife and doctor are in charge of monitoring progress. Breech presentation is when the baby's buttocks or feet are facing down rather than the head. The midwife may well report this some time before the due date and choose to wait and see if there is any change over the following days or week or two. If not, a Caesarean section may be recommended though natural breech births do occur. In homoeopathy, breech presentation is sometimes considered a sign of the baby's reluctance to be brought into the world. This is easier to tell if the homoeopath knows the mother and her circumstances thoroughly. The most commonly prescribed remedy for this situation is **Pulsatilla**, a remedy normally associated with those who are clingy and needy of their mothers. **Ayahuasca** may also be indicated in some cases especially where there is great fear in the mother. It is important that the mother has professional help as potency and monitoring of changes should be considered professionally.

Labour and Birth

There are certain remedies that are very useful to have at hand during labour, birth and post-partum. Confer with your homoeopath about a birth plan and he or she will be able to advise on remedies that could be needed. The following remedies (with their main indications) are the most commonly useful. (Those in brackets are optional while the rest are usually indispensable. Potency and options should be discussed with the homoeopath well before the due date. While **Chamomilla** is one of the most common extreme pain remedies it is not the only one and the homoeopath should be able to suggest any others that might be needed based on the patient's constitution.)

Aconite 200: fear and shock

Arnica 200: bruising

Arsen-alb. 30 or 200: anxiety with chills and restlessness; pains cause her great anxiety

Belladonna 200: fever or local heat, swelling and redness with sharp pains

Calc-carb. 30 or 200: general state of fatigue, sweat (around the head) and chilliness (especially cold feet); cramps in calves < stretching legs

Carbo-veg 30 or 200: for 'blue' babies; weak, chilly, exhausted and blue from lack of oxygen. Useful for mothers in same state.

Caulophyllum 30: feeble contractions with severe pains that lead nowhere. Exhaustion and false pains

Causticum 30: useful after birth if unable to pass water (homoeopathic catheter)

Chamomilla 30 or 200: unendurable, excruciating pains with furious temper; unreasonably demanding

Gelsemium 30 or 200: lack of progress with rigid cervix while patient looks uninvolved and dulled

Ignatia 200: anxious, trembling and tearful; heavy sighs and sobbing;

feels faint; wants to take deep breaths between contractions

Ipecac. 30 or 200: profuse haemorrhage (sometimes with nausea)

Kali-carb. 30: sharp pains with the feeling that the baby will be delivered through the anus; low back pain going into buttocks

(Lyc. 30): general state of anxiety with bloating and flatulence; pains cross abdomen from right to left

Mag-phos. 30: spasms of abdominal pain with cramps in the legs; bends forward and holds abdomen

(Nat-mur. 200): patient retreats emotionally; looks grey and thin; very thirsty; contractions are feeble

Nux-vom. 30: violent pains with downward pressure which = urging to pass a motion; sensitive and cross

Opium 1M: dazed, out-of-body state after anaesthetic or shock; flushes of heat to the face; constipated

Phosphorus 30: weakness, pallor and rush of heat up into the head with feeble contractions; thirsty

Pulsatilla 200 or 1M: needy, dependent and tearful; hot, dry, no thirst and craving for fresh air or a fan; wants to walk about to > the pains; symptoms constantly shifting emphasis

Rhus-tox. 30: sprained muscles after birth with stiffness, aching and restlessness > hot bath and massage

Sepia 200: feeling of a ball in the anus; heavy, dropping out sensation; apathy and indifference; fed up

Sulphur 200: contractions stop; hot flushes; faint and hungry; thirsty; wants to be fanned

In addition to the above it is worth having **Hypercal Ø** in case of an episiotomy or a tear. The tincture should be diluted: 4 drops in a quarter of a cup of water and used to bathe the lesion.

Caesarean Section

If a Caesarean section should be necessary there are several remedies to talk to your homoeopath about. **Emerald** is a remedy that has a reputation for assisting with 'extractions'; it is very helpful in preparing the body for the removal of what it no longer needs to hold onto. (It is best in the 30 or 200.) If an epidural is chosen for the procedure, **Ledum** 30 (for puncture wounds) helps with any pain and **Lumbricus** 30 (for pain and other side effects) follows well. If there is any aggravation from the surgeon's cut then the homoeopath would give **Staphysagria** (probably 200). If there is any likelihood of excessive bleeding then it is sensible to have **Phosphorus** 200 at hand. For excessive blood loss after an operation **China** 30 or 200 is used.

Meconium

If there is meconium (foetal excrement) in the waters it usually suggests that the baby has been in distress. Sometimes meconium is swallowed during further distress and causes a blockage of the airways. Overdue babies may be particularly prone to this. It is one of the reasons for the baby to be removed for immediate treatment; the meconium must be suctioned out as quickly as possible. It is really important for the homoeopath to be told of such distress and any resulting symptoms because birth trauma of any sort can often be a life-long cause of chronic patterns of symptoms – including the tendency to asthma. It is also advisable to take the baby to see a cranial osteopath.

After the Delivery

Arnica 200, twice a day for 3 to 5 days will alleviate any bruising. If the bruising feels more internal and there is bearing down, chilliness and aching in the lumbar region then use **Bellis Perennis** 200 instead especially if the patient is thin and spare. If she is rather ungrounded by the birth then a dose of **Oak** 30 (one dose is usually sufficient) can help her to come to terms with the reality of her new role. If an episiotomy was necessary and she still feels the effects of the cut she needs **Staphysagria** 200 (a single dose). This might also be true for a Caesarean section. After a Caesar it is sometimes difficult for the mother to feel bonded with the baby. This is an important reason to see the homoeopath who will prescribe on the presenting picture that includes this aspect (**Ayahuasca** is the main remedy). If an epidural was given then it is usually necessary to prescribe for the after-effects which can include pain at the site of the needle and other back problems. (A session of cranial osteopathy is highly recommended after having a baby but is essential if an epidural was used.) The main remedies for this are **Ledum** (for puncture wounds), **Hypericum** (for nerve pain) and **Lumbricus Terrestris** (for any pains from damage to the spinal column). The 30 of these is often adequate though the homoeopath should advise on dosage and indications. Bleeding after birth can continue for some time. If it is heavy the homoeopath must be informed; **China** or **Phos-ac.** may be indicated. If it is prolonged then further constitutional treatment will be necessary. Sometimes there will be blood loss whenever the baby feeds; this will indicate either **Silica** (pains in back and breast with the blood loss during the feed) or **Calc-carb.** (slow or scanty flow of milk with sweating on the upper body and feeling cold). Scar tissue from episiotomy or tearing is also a good reason for seeing the homoeopath; there are several useful remedies that might be indicated including **Calendula**, **Silica** and **Graphites**.

Breastfeeding and Milk

In some mothers lactation may start before the birth though in others the milk is scanty or does not come through at all; it may start well and then tail off; the baby rejects it for some reason or it makes the baby unwell. As breastfeeding is so important and can be so fraught with emotions it is best for the practitioner to be involved to give the necessary support. The remedies most likely to be needed in breastfeeding problems include:

Belladonna: milk absent due to milk fever; mastitis

Borax: problems with thrush and thick milk that tastes 'off'; pain in the opposite breast while feeding

Bryonia: hardness of breasts, mastitis; dryness; soreness; < from feeling the cold

Calc-carb.: absent or scanty milk or excess; rejection of milk; thin, watery and even bluish

Calc-phos.: child refuses milk; tastes salty; mother weakens and becomes achy and irritable

Cham.: severe cramps as baby feeds which make her furiously irritable; milk goes sour or bad

China: mother is weakened by every feed; almost feels that she is giving away too much; < if menses start while breastfeeding

Nat-carb.: child vomits all the milk; baby is easily startled; belches a lot and vomit smells acidic

Phos-ac.: mother becomes weaker and more 'wall-staring' as she has never recovered from the delivery; baby vomits most of the milk; mother's hair tends to fall out while breastfeeding

Phytolacca: pains while breastfeeding spread all over the body; breasts are tender, swollen, hard and heavy

Pulsatilla: mother is tearful every time she feeds the baby; milk might be too profuse or suddenly dries up

Sepia: continued bearing down pains < breastfeeding with exhaustion and indifference; 'fed up' and irritable. Mother 'can't understand why baby won't feed properly!'

Silica: sharp pains in the breast and/or uterus while breastfeeding; blood or vaginal discharge flows with each feed; child refuses milk or vomits after each feed; may seem that the child does not thrive on milk

Urtica Urens: the tincture (Ø) is very helpful if it is apparent that the milk is deficient in nutrients. Five drops of the tincture in water each day can improve the quality of milk quite quickly.

Breast Pains during Breastfeeding

Cracked nipples are especially trying and can spoil the pleasure of breastfeeding. Frequent use of **Hypercal Ø** ointment is helpful to keep the skin around the nipples supple and free from trouble (see **Calendula** below). The following remedies are often indicated:

Calendula: nipples are cracked and even ulcerated; she cries with the pain every time the baby suckles. Even if other remedies may be better indicated on the one symptom of cracked skin, use **Calendula** cream or ointment (or **Hypercal**) topically.

Castor Equi: cracks so deep and painful that she cannot bear anything to touch the breasts; breasts are swollen and sensitive and even jarring them as she comes downstairs is agony. (Use 6 or 30 quite frequently.)

Chamomilla: sore, hot, red and swollen breasts with cracked nipples; extremely irritable; nothing goes right. (Use 200.)

Graphites: sore, cracked and blistered looking surface of the nipples; she feels the cold and wants hot drinks; tearful, fidgety and inclined to feel rather morbid. (Use 30.)

Lycopodium: nipples are raw, fissured and bleed; she is usually windy and bloated as well. (Use 30.)

Merc-sol.: nipples are sore, itchy and cracked; she feels hot and chilly by turns; feels sweaty at night.

Phytolacca: nipples are sensitive, cracked and may tend to become inverted; breasts swell, harden and become lumpy especially < right; pains in the breasts extend into the armpit and may come on with a stiff neck. (Use 30.)

Pulsatilla: breasts become sore, lumpy and achy; she weeps at every feed; she is inclined to be over warm and want a window open. (Use 200.)

Ratanhia: fissured nipples < touch and > cold water compress; pains (sharp and contractive) are < night-time; more likely to be indicated in thin, nervous women who become melancholy when alone; often useful after **Sepia**. (Use 30.)

Sepia: cracks develop across the crown of the nipple; usually tired, fed up and dragged down; irritable with family and tearful. (Use 30 or 200.)

Sulphur: cracks appear around the base of the nipple and tend to bleed; burning pain; pain while breastfeeding extends from nipple through to the back. (Use 30 or 200.)

Mastitis

Mastitis is sometimes referred to as milk fever. The breast swells and becomes lumpy, hard and painful. It might also become hot and red or have red streaks. Sometimes there is a general fever. Orthodox treatment is with antibiotics but the drugs are not good for the baby who will take them in through the milk. Suppression of mastitis is bad for another reason: it often leads to chronic complications such as lumpy painful breasts and a tendency to the later formation of abscesses which might appear in the breast or, much later, as tooth abscesses; this might particularly affect those who have teeth with root canal fillings. The main remedies for mastitis during breastfeeding are:

Belladonna: more likely < right side with bright red, hot and painful breast; fever may not be general but if so can be over 103°F. (If the problem is local use 30 to begin; if general then start with 200.)

Bryonia: < right side; breast is hard and painful < the slightest movement; patient is very irritable and wants to be left alone; is also very thirsty for cold water. Compare with **Hepar-sulph.** which is chillier and more sensitive to noise and draught. (Use 30 to begin but be prepared to move up to 200.)

Hepar-sulph.: more likely < right side; local pain with swelling and < any touch. Patient becomes very irritable and tense, chilly and wanting to be left alone. (Use 30 to start but may need 200.)

Lac-can.: pains and inflammation in both breasts. Most characteristic symptoms: pain alternates in sides from left to right and back and < from the least movement (see **Bry.**); so bad that the patient has to cradle the breasts on going up and down stairs. Patient is likely to be weak and very worried about her health: thinks something really serious is wrong. (Use 30 first but go up to 200 if the symptoms do not ease within a few hours.)

Lycopodium: < right but pains can cross to the left; pains are stitching and leave the breasts feeling sore. Often accompanied by flatulence and bloating. (Use 30 but ask your homoeopath about using 100 if no response within 12 hours.)

Phosphorus: stitching pains < left breast; breast may feel burning and sensitive with cracked nipple. Patient is thirsty for cold drinks. Usually anxious or too debilitated to think. (Use 30.)

Phytolacca: very heavy and stony hard breasts especially < right side. Pains feel as if they spread right through the body particularly when the baby suckles. Sore pain can extend into the armpit. (Use 30 but if little relief is had after 6 hours use 200.)

Pulsatilla: swollen, sore and inflamed breasts < left with low-grade fever; must have fresh air; patient is tearful and dependent and is not as thirsty as she was. (Use 200 but see **Silica** below.)

Silica: lumpy breasts < left with sore nipples and sharp stitching pains; low-grade fever. (Use 30. **Silica** and **Pulsatilla** work really well together. Often **Silica** is used to support **Pulsatilla**: i.e. **Puls.** 200 or 1M then **Silica** 6 twice or 30 once daily.)

Sulphur: burning swollen breasts with general intolerance of heat and a strong thirst. (Use 30.)

Thrush in the Mouth

See 'Thrush' on page 214. Sometimes the thrush will not clear completely until the baby has had a dose of **Calc-c.** to strengthen the general constitution; talk to the homoeopath about this.

Weaning

The right time for weaning is different in every case. The ideal moment is when solids have become a routine part of mealtimes and the baby feels no deprivation for not having milk. Cow's milk is not ideal for the human gut; it is too rich in grease and salt and it can have been adulterated with the hormones and antibiotic drugs with which cows are treated and then pasteurised till there is actually very little goodness left in it. If milk has to be supplemented then it is best to use goat's milk which is far more easily digested; it is the closest substitute to human milk that we can get and is available in most supermarkets. (Unfortunately it is also pasteurised.)

If the mother is still lactating fully when she decides to wean she has the problem of stopping the flow. There are drugs that are used to suppress milk production. They are not safe and should be avoided at all costs. It is not unusual for women who take such drugs to suffer chronic breast pathology; sometimes considerably later so that it appears that the problem is unrelated to the suppression. The mother should ask the homoeopath for advice as there are remedies that help. The best-known remedy to ease off milk production is **Lac Caninum**; if appropriate it causes the pituitary to reduce the amount of prolactin and it will also deal with any pain in the breasts. Allow the practitioner to select the potency.

Post-natal Blues

Patients and doctors do not always agree on what this condition is. Doctors expect up to 50% or more of mothers to suffer a short period of negative emotions and 10% to go through what they regard as a mild form of depressive illness. However, for many mothers 'depression' is a term with which they are not comfortable as the symptoms they go through are far more varied and complicated than the word would suggest. Most women in this condition might not describe all that they feel because either they are in a thoroughly withdrawn state or they believe they will not be taken seriously or they feel 'silly' about their symptoms.

Though depression can be part of the problem there are many other less expected symptoms that any homoeopath would place high on the list of indicators when considering a prescription. Though the causes of post-natal illnesses remain unclear, it is obvious that hormones play a vital role, as can nutrition and family history. The women most likely to suffer are those who have had previous episodes of post-natal illness or depression; who have a family history of it; who are single parents; who have been through an unexpected pregnancy. It is more likely to be prolonged when there is sleep deprivation and poor nutrition. Sleep deprivation usually indicates that treatment is needed by both mother *and* baby; poor appetite and self-neglect can lead to unbalanced biochemistry that leaves the mother's system struggling. The range of symptoms can include any of the following:

- Headaches, nausea and dizziness; fainting and shortness of breath
- Hypochondriasis: fear of failing health or a fear that the baby will never do well or is, in fact, unwell
- Overwhelming tiredness; this can be both physical and mental
- Mental confusion; feels either ungrounded or 'wall staring'
- Fearful that something dreadful will happen; something beyond her control
- Obsessive thoughts; cannot clear the brain of repetitive thoughts of 'What would happen if…?'
- Cannot clear the mind of the memories of the awful experience of childbirth; plays them over and over
- Fearful that she may harm her baby or that she might hurt another of her children
- Obsessively anxious about objects that might be dangerous such as scissors
- Feeling empty of all emotion; cannot respond naturally to husband and other children (even the new baby)
- Complete lack of libido
- Panic attacks with sudden episodes of palpitations, light-headedness and dread
- Violent thoughts

None of these symptoms is unknown to homoeopaths; what is important is the individual's experience of them. Any woman with post-natal symptoms should first consult a homoeopath before assuming that they require a psychiatrist, antidepressants or some counselling. Drugs may settle some of the mental symptoms but they do nothing for the underlying problem which will sooner or later re-emerge – after another pregnancy or even years later at the time of the menopause. There are many remedies that might be indicated, amongst which are common ones such as **Sepia, Nat-mur., Calc-c., Nux-vom., Pulsatilla** and **Ignatia** but the choice is best left to the practitioner; not least because the treatment of post-natal conditions can lead to deep constitutional prescribing from which more is achieved than the removal of the original symptoms. Successful treatment here can mean far deeper bonding with the baby, restoration of balanced emotions in both the patient and family and a reduced risk of the same state arising in future pregnancies.

Jaundice in Babies

Jaundice in newborn babies is not uncommon. It is also relatively easy to heal with remedies. If possible it is best to call the homoeopath for advice. The most common remedies include **Nux-vom.** (diarrhoea, colic, sore abdomen and ineffectual urging to pass a stool); **China** (bloating and trapped colicky wind which makes them draw up their knees, watery, foul liquid stools and drowsiness); **Chelidonium** (pale or bright yellow pasty stools with tender abdomen, listlessness alternating with episodes of whinging irritability). With all three there is a sallow tinge to the skin which can get more pronounced. Sometimes **Bryonia** is indicated (sallow skin with irritability and distress whenever moved with dryness of skin and mucous membranes). If symptoms come up while mother and baby are still in hospital, it is best to give the indicated remedy in 30 and tell the practitioner as soon as possible. If it is awkward to give the baby remedies then the mother can take the remedy herself just before feeding the baby; in this way the infant will get the healing effects through the milk.

The Role of the Husband

Husbands, even if they choose to be present at the birth, are often relegated in the burst of activity around a newborn baby. This may not seem to matter in the excitement of the arrival but men can feel overshadowed by or even jealous of their offspring, even while being proud of their wives and ecstatic about the baby. Some men might feel embarrassed at their inadequacy in handling the baby; others feel overemotional. The following remedies may be of help:

Arnica: extraordinary tiredness after excitement leaving the person feeling 'bashed'. (Use 200.)

Cocculus: dizzy, weak and disorientated from interrupted sleep; may feel a bit nauseated. (Use 200.)

Ignatia: he has contradictory feelings which veer between feeling emotional, overexcited and oversensitive and silent and brooding. (Use 200.)

Lotus: useful when things get fraught; a very calming influence when too much is going on. Especially useful if added to a bottle of Rescue Remedy and taken one drop twice or 3 times a day.

Lycopodium: often needed before the birth as this is an anticipation remedy; he feels tired, irritable, windy and bloated and inwardly worried about coping with the imminent changes to his life; would really like to enjoy fatherhood from a distance as he has a sense of inadequacy. (Use 30: one twice daily for 3 days.)

Nux-vom.: fraught by being caught between the demands of work deadlines and domesticity; becomes irritable and dyspeptic; wants coffee and other stimulants to keep him going; can be quite emotional as well; likely to be adrenalin-driven. Use 200 unless he is under constitutional treatment with the homoeopath.

Oak: for the husband who is managing to keep things going and playing a supportive role but is exhausted and tense (particularly in the shoulders). (Use 200.)

24 VACCINATIONS

Babies are expected to be immunised against diphtheria, whooping cough and tetanus as well as polio and haemophilus B in the second, third and fourth months; the immunisation for measles, mumps and rubella is then given at twelve months. For those already convinced of the inadvisability of these injections, suffice to say that it is sensible to keep a full first-aid kit and to build a trusting rapport with the homoeopath. This will ensure a secure health 'umbrella' as homoeopathy is fully capable of meeting the remedial needs of anyone suffering from any of the childhood diseases or those for which immunisations are recommended.

For other people, the debate about artificial immunisation will concern them. The essential thing is to become well informed about the alternative view. Orthodox medical literature tends to insist on the dangers of inaction and the dire consequences of not being protected against and of suffering from childhood diseases that are *a natural part of growing up.* (They rarely mention tetanus as it is a disease that cannot be stamped out by science nor do they say that diphtheria is actually a negligible threat which was on the wane before the vaccine appeared.) Many parents accept that measles, mumps and rubella are, for the vast majority, mild, acute conditions with few complications but they are more concerned about whooping cough, tetanus and polio. (I discuss tetanus and whooping cough elsewhere in the book.) Polio is a condition which is only contracted in climates which are warm and humid. It is extremely unlikely ever to be contracted in swimming pools as the chlorine would ensure prevention. The only circumstance in which polio is contracted in a northern European climate is from the nappies of a child who has been immunised against it in the previous 10 to 11 days.

Artificial immunisation against *any* disease is deleterious to the patient's general health; no vaccines are safe as all of them are capable of interfering with the activity of the immune system in general and the thymus gland in particular. The thymus is an essential part of a child's own immune system and integral to the production of T-lymphocytes and the establishment of a lifetime's immune system as well as the whole process of maturation. Another reason why artificial immunisation is so damaging is that vaccines are *material* doses of not only disease matter but also poisonous chemicals such as formaldehyde, hydrochloric acid, aluminium and mercury; some also contain antibiotics to which the child might be allergic. Furthermore, the vaccines are cultured on some strange material: cow's brain cells, monkey's kidney cells, chicken embryo and human foetal cells. For further information on the enormity of this appalling practice of artificial immunisation look on the internet: **www.vaccine-info.com**. (For a fuller understanding see *The Companion to Homoeopathy*, chapter 16, 'Artificial Immunisation and Vaccine Damage'.)

If anyone is immunised and suffers side effects it is absolutely essential that the homoeopath be involved in treatment immediately; do not wait for the symptoms to become chronic! The most common initial side effects are fever, rash and malaise. These may be manifest within hours, days or even anything up to 4 months afterwards. After a few days most doctors would not consider the vaccines as having been responsible for the symptoms. Let the homoeopath be the judge of that. Sometimes a child will react mildly or not at all to the first two inoculations and then suffer considerably from the third. No child who already has the symptoms of eczema, asthma or allergies or who has a history of febrile convulsions should ever be artificially immunised; most enlightened doctors would agree with this.

Despite all the advice against vaccination some parents simply cannot trust the alternative approach. They would prefer to vaccinate and then treat any side effects. Other parents find their way to homoeopathy *because* of the side effects, a checklist of which follows.

The diphtheria, whooping cough and tetanus (DPT) jab: if the child develops a rash, runny nose, thick mucus, congested breathing, restlessness or screaming fits then suspect this even up to weeks later. Later symptoms to emerge include glue ear, asthma, allergies and learning difficulties. Major symptoms may not occur after the first dose or even the second thus lulling the parents into a false sense of security. If they do develop it is imperative to refuse any further vaccines; DPT has been shown to be associated with anaphylactic shock and cot deaths. See *A Shot in the Dark* by Harris Coulter and Barbara Loe Fisher (Harcourt Brace Jovanovich, Orlando, Florida 1986).

The polio vaccine: this is associated with fever, fitting, coordination and spatial awareness problems, headaches, paralysis and allergies. (It has also been linked to certain types of cancer.)

The meningitis vaccine: this is responsible for fever, headaches, disorientation, persistent crying, diarrhoea, vomiting and muscle pains.

The measles, mumps and rubella jab: this has resulted in fever, febrile convulsions, tonsillitis, chronic conditions of the bowels, muscle weakness and rheumatic pains, cerebral palsy, epilepsy, autism, behavioural and learning difficulties.

BCG, the TB jab: this is associated with fever, rash, swollen lymph glands, abscesses, asthmatic breathing, congested sinuses, rheumatic conditions and TB itself.

The hepatitis A and B jabs: these are both capable of inducing compromised liver function. The hepatitis B jab is usually insisted upon for those who work in the health services as a precaution in case of contact with infected carriers. It is associated with a host of side effects including fever, swollen lymph glands, headaches, chronic fatigue, muscle pains, abdominal pains, hypersensitivity, water retention, palpitations, rashes and more. Anyone who is obliged by their employer to suffer the jab should report *beforehand* to the homoeopath who will ensure as far as is possible that the side effects are limited.

The pneumococcal disease vaccine: this, the latest addition to the canon, is likely to cause its own side effects though it is too early to say exactly what we should expect to see symptomatically. The effects of pneumococcal disease on those with poor constitutions, weak immune systems and hereditary susceptibilities are extremely serious and life-threatening; septicaemia and meningitis are both possible consequences. However, constitutional treatment from the earliest stages of life and development will ensure maximum natural protection against such eventualities.

The influenza jab: this is particularly recommended by doctors for school children, professional people and the elderly. It is essential that people know that it can be responsible for the very condition it is meant to prevent as well as for bronchitis, pleurisy and pneumonia; conditions which are not considered as side effects of the jab as treatment for them is different from that for ordinary influenza. The usual side effects of the jab include fever, muscle pains, headaches, dizziness, confusion, loss of coordination, tinnitus, depression and tiredness.

25 COPING WITH DIFFICULT CHILDREN

The following paragraphs are for parents who are being tested (sometimes to the limit) by their children. The descriptions of the problems are intended as guides to help identify the nature of the condition that needs resolution. Apart from the use of **Ignatia** and **Pulsatilla** for emotional scenes on the first day at nursery or a new school (and both children and parents can find this really hard) there are no suggested remedies for these very deep problems. They all require professional help and often not just from the homoeopath. Parents often feel extremely helpless when they discover that a child is in need of the kind of help that is completely beyond them to give. As parents we feel that we should be able to sort out all our children's troubles; but there are some that are outside our scope. Parents of children in serious crisis should also be asking for help from their homoeopaths for themselves in order to remain steady and grounded as the family goes through the process of healing; not least because whatever successful healing takes place in the child is often reflected in some fashion in the parent.

Tantrums

The 'terrible twos' can begin at any age. Parents can be severely tested by a toddler or an older child who screams, throws things, stamps feet, slams doors, lies on the floor drumming heels or headbanging or who uses abusive language. This is such a common story for homoeopaths that most have experience in treating the problem. The usual background to it is miasmatic and this requires deep constitutional prescribing. Some children will appear to react with a tantrum when baulked and frustrated yet the underlying reason for the behaviour is actually rational if unacceptable. Others will react furiously for no apparent reason at all; the behaviour appears completely irrational. Yet others will appear to be cold and calculating in their anger; they are highly manipulative and seem worryingly capable of malice. To be able to differentiate these states to the homoeopath is really important as the differentiation determines the choice of remedial action. One of the *results* of treatment is that the child goes through an episode of development, though occasionally one of the childhood conditions such as chickenpox or impetigo might be part of the process. This should not put parents off; it is absolutely the right kind of progress.

Mealtime Trauma

Children often become extremely difficult over food. They may play with it, throw it about, refuse to eat it altogether or be extremely 'faddy'. There may be several reasons for this.

- The child may equate eating with a symptom such as pain while passing a stool or 'tummy ache'.
- The child may not like hot food (typical of **Silica**).
- The child may be suffering from buccal thrush.
- The child may have difficulty chewing due to teething or because of a strain pattern in the cranial bones caused by a difficult birth (a condition that will need cranial osteopathy).
- The child may refuse food but drink quantities of watered down sweet drinks and milk; they are hungry but do not like chewing and prefer to fill up on liquids (typical of **Pulsatilla**).
- Some children have different 'body clocks'; their appetite does not conform and one day they eat large amounts while the next they eat nothing (typical of **Sulphur**).
- The child may find the mother's approach to feeding too forceful; feeding fads can raise aggressive feelings.
- There may be some emotional reason for the child to use food and eating as a way to manipulate the mother: resentment of a sibling's arrival, sibling rivalry, difficulties in the parents' relationship, etc.
- If a pattern of behaviour is apparent do not let it remain without consulting the homoeopath. This is especially true of emotional causes as these can lead to parents feeling the loss of authority in situations

where it is necessary. If remedies seem to hold for only a short while then suspect a food intolerance or allergy; either ask your practitioner about allergy testing or consult a qualified kinesiologist. Cranial osteopathy can also be invaluable here as the osteopath should be able to identify the focus of symptoms: the liver or the colon, etc.

Potty-training and Bed-wetting

There is no set time for potty-training though if the mother is worried it is sensible to seek help. Some children have no difficulty while others can still be in nappies at night when they are four or more. Some have no problem with their bowel habits but continue to wet the bed beyond the age of ten. A very common problem is for a child who may have been doing well with training suddenly to refuse to sit on the potty or the lavatory; the reason is often because it is painful to pass a hard stool (which is typical of **Silica**). Other children are not slow to use their bladder and bowels to manipulate their parents for emotional reasons. Talk to the homoeopath about any developing pattern of bowel and bladder behaviour so that it becomes neither a chronic habit nor a successful gambit. Cranial osteopathy is also very useful here; if there is anything obscurely the matter with the kidneys or bladder the osteopath should be able to identify it.

Behavioural and Learning Difficulties including ADD and ADHD

Deteriorating behaviour in young children may be the result of emotional trauma which has no other outlet or it may be because the child is having difficulty with learning – or both. The emotional problems may originate at home or in the school (bullying for instance). If learning difficulties are the underlying cause then it is often harder to fathom but just as vital to understand. The homoeopath can help with both areas though in the case of learning difficulties it may be necessary to call on the advice of other experts as well. Though it is a bold claim, learning difficulties usually stem from a combination of genetic and miasmatic inheritance, mercury in amalgam fillings and vaccine damage. The problems are exacerbated by intolerance to sugar, dairy products and gluten as well as artificial food additives. Dyslexia (reading difficulties), dyspraxia (coordination difficulties) and dyscalculia (problems with numbers) and any other learning difficulty that becomes worthy of a label are not diseases; the labels simply describe the person's way of doing things. It is not the difficulty that is treated but the person; remedies are prescribed as a reflection of the effects that the difficulty has on the patient's psyche. All too often the child feels socially and educationally at a serious disadvantage but with alternative help is able to find other ways of learning that ensure good social integration. There are certain signals that can help to determine whether a child has learning difficulties. The child:

- avoids eye contact
- has a short attention span
- finds it hard to follow instructions
- finds it hard to get or keep all their school equipment together
- loses items of clothing frequently; forgets where they were last seen
- copies things down incorrectly
- refuses to read
- refuses to write or has spidery or illegible writing
- holds their pencil awkwardly and writes with strong pressure
- rests their head on one arm at desk level while writing
- chews the tongue while writing
- reverses the order of letters or numbers
- chews collars or cuffs persistently
- sits restlessly in the chair
- is excessively ticklish
- is easily distracted by slight activity in the class or outside
- seems to shine on the sports field but does relatively poorly in class or vice versa
- becomes transfixed while watching television; almost 'out of himself'
- seeks to make friends with much younger or older children but not with their peer group
- suffers frequent headaches, tummy aches or sore throats with coughs and swollen glands
- suffers strong antihistamine reactions
- was unable to breastfeed satisfactorily due to latching on difficulties
- has a history of 'bottom shuffling' rather than crawling on hands and legs with delayed walking

- is hyperactive especially after sugar or food and drinks that contain artificial additives
- becomes abusive and truculent

Though none of these signals on their own constitutes a basis for a diagnosis, if a child displays four, five or more of them then it is vital to seek professional opinions including those of the homoeopath. Others who can help are educational psychologists and occupational therapists. Investigation of the various available training programmes for those with learning difficulties can be rewarding. See the list of addresses at the end of the book.

Attention Deficit Disorder (ADD) and Attention Deficit and Hyperactive Disorder (ADHD)

Theseare conditions that are associated with learning difficulties. They may be a feature of autism or Asperger's syndrome. They are often the result of a nervous system that has not kept developmental pace with the rest of the body; foetal and infant reflexes that should have been superseded by mature reflex reactions by six months are still in play and cause havoc with adrenalin production and, often, histamine reactions. Likely causes include mercury in vaccinations or leakage during pregnancy from the mother's amalgam fillings through the placenta. Other heavy metals may also be implicated: that is lead and cadmium. Not all children are affected by heavy metals and this can be to do with the degree to which hereditary disease patterns are prevalent. This is a homoeopath's natural hunting ground. Blame may also rest with the appalling quality of food that is consumed by us today, with all the chemical toxicity and genetic modification for which the body is absolutely not prepared. Cranial osteopathy should also be considered because the overstimulation of the sympathetic nervous system by adrenalin needs to be checked. Acupuncture should be considered if cranial treatment is unavailable. Fish oils and nutritional supplementation have been shown to be of considerable benefit. Early signs of ADHD include:
- persistent startle reflex reactions
- fearfulness
- restlessness

• irritability at any form of restriction
• sudden tantrums which leave the child exhausted
• frequent episodes of staring vacantly

Because of the extraordinary academic pressures put on pupils (and their parents) to succeed in achieving qualifications, there is often a reluctance on the part of school managers to identify pupils with either ADD or ADHD. Parents often have to take things into their own hands; this is doubly important if the child is threatened with being prescribed Ritalin because of their disruptive behaviour. This is a drug that has serious side effects and later consequences; though children on Ritalin often seem to integrate well into class they may go into depression, suffer sleep problems, have bladder symptoms and go through growth retardation. When Ritalin is withdrawn in the late teens, the reaction can be such that all the old symptoms return, causing the patient to throw up the years of learning and 'drop out'. Ritalin is a stimulant of the central nervous system and affects the body in a similar way to amphetamines (see below).

There are various alternative systems of treatment that have varying degrees of success depending on the individuality of the patient; parents will find that they have to search for what best suits their child. Homoeopathy and cranial osteopathy enhance any of the treatments that are listed in the back of the book under 'Useful Addresses'.

Autism

Autism is a condition that is manifest uniquely in each individual who is diagnosed though there are common characteristics that indicate it. The causes of what amounts to behavioural dysfunction are still debated by medical orthodoxy but for many the prime suspect is mercury poisoning. Mercury is one of the most poisonous substances on earth and yet it is used in vaccines, dental amalgams, pesticides and in the manufacturing industry; it is consistently dumped in rivers and lakes thus polluting fish. It has statistically increased some 6000% since the early 1970s when multiple vaccines became the norm though even unvaccinated children may be affected if amalgam has leaked during pregnancy and crossed the placental barrier. It is important to have expert advice on different strategies of treatment. Though many parents rely on chelation therapy (the use of chemical supplements that bind heavy metals to them in the process of eliminating them from the body), they would be well advised to start or continue constitutional homoeopathic treatment. Many of the symptoms listed under the previous heading might also apply to autism; autistic people also have learning difficulties. Other indicating characteristics include:

- difficulty in interacting with others
- showing little or no sign of facial expression
- unable to share in moments of emotion, humour, grief, etc.
- no eye contact
- showing no sign of developing peer relationships
- slow in developing speech
- little or no sign of verbal exchange
- the repetitive use of words, phrases or gestures
- lack of initiative in playing
- having fixed ideas and obsessive repetition of particular activities
- lack of reaction to pain, touch, smell, taste, etc.

Asperger's Syndrome

Asperger's syndrome shares with autism some behavioural characteristics: repetitive patterns of behaviour, limited interest in and adoption of only a few activities as well as difficulties with social interaction. It differs in that there are few or no impediments to progress with language, cognition or coordination skills. The condition may have no effect on academic learning though subjects find it hard to put their learning to natural social interactive use. They can appear to be rudely matter-of-fact and abrupt. They are often extremely sensitive to their environment and suffer from overstimulation of any of the 5 special senses; hence they fear and reject change. It is often harder to diagnose Asperger's than autism or ADD/ADHD as the obvious problems do not stand out as early as symptoms of the other conditions do. It is important to differentiate the diagnosis as the methods of handling the difficulties are different and require different support. The origins of Asperger's are not related to mercury toxicity or, as far as is known, to vaccine damage. There is no allopathic cure though there are drugs that are prescribed for coping with associated symptoms including Ritalin (better known as a treatment for ADHD); the supplement St John's wort, which has a reputation for easing depression, has also been found to be useful. A lot of patience and under-standing of homoeopathic thinking is needed by parents seeking alternative remedial help. The earlier treatment is begun, the better; progress can be very slow and measured only in subtle changes. The more the treatment is aimed towards creating balance rather than searching for any chimerical cure, the better the patient will do. In some cases this can lead to complex prescribing strategies.

Obsessive/Compulsive Disorder

OCD is a condition that may manifest quite early in childhood or at any time up to middle age. In a child patient it may be part of a complex symptom state or it might be the focus of the case. The following symptoms can identify the problem:

- frequent hand washing (fear of contamination and disease)
- repeating actions several times as if in an established ritual (fixed routines ease thoughts of self-harm or aggression towards others)
- counting things (fear of shifting reality)
- checking things in sequence; looking in cupboards, behind doors, under the bed in a particular order (fear of fearfulness)
- touching objects usually in a particular order (some have linked this to intrusive and inappropriate sexual thoughts)
- repeating mantras or prayers (fear of retribution and malign fate)
- putting objects into particular order (fear of the loss of control)
- hoarding things and secreting them (fear of a hostile environment that threatens survival)

OCD is often left undiagnosed because patients tend to be secretive and only show their symptoms in 'safe' places such as the home. When their activities are prevented by anyone, patients can become either depressed or aggressive. Early onset of the symptoms might be preceded or accompanied by nervous tics. The origins of OCD are so far a mystery though it is recognised that there is a hereditary link. This is borne out by the fact that four of the nosodes, **Carcinosin, Syphilinum, Medorrhinum** and **Psorinum**, are listed as possi-ble remedies for this condition which suggests that there is a miasmatic influence. Another factor to be borne in mind is that researchers have found that many sufferers have very low levels of serotonin, the hormone that modulates emotions, sleep patterns and appetite. On a biochemical level it may prove beneficial to investigate causes of low serotonin. These might include drugs used through the pregnancy, gluten intolerance (as gluten can cause types of depression) and, controversially, predisposing unresolved emotional events, even those long buried in family history. It is important to tell the homoeopath of anything that could be of help in the selection of remedies. Art therapy or counselling should be considered.

Self-harming

Though self-harming can sometimes be a feature of OCD, it is always a cri de coeur and needs urgent help. Urgent because, once discovered, it will be found to have been going on for a while before. The person may have cut, burnt, bitten, punched or hit themselves or used an object to inflict pain; head-banging is not uncommon even in some very young children. Chemical medication is not advisable as the origins of this distressing condition lie in heredity and miasmatic influences which are the triggers in confused and damaged psyches. The homoeopath needs a full biographical history of the patient to determine how best to prescribe. Art therapy and counselling are often very helpful here as well.

Anorexia and Bulimia

The core of anorexia and bulimia is lack of self-esteem. Anorexia is an obsession with weight and image, food and diet. Bulimia is obsessional binge eating and drinking with addictive behaviour and self-induced vomiting or purging with laxatives. Both conditions may be found in the same person. They may be the main symptomatic focus or they may be part of a larger canvas of symptoms such as appear in OCD, ADD, ADHD, depression, post-traumatic stress syndrome and panic disorder. Symptoms of anorexia include:
- obsessive counting of calorie intake
- strict and excessive exercise routine
- restriction of food; starvation
- use of pills to control weight

• self-induced vomiting
• hiding food
• fastidious focus on body image with dramatic loss of weight

Symptoms of bulimia include:
  • binge eating and drinking
  • addiction to junk food
  • self-induced vomiting
  • feelings of self-loathing, guilt and shame
  • self-harming
  • mood swings

The underlying influence that dictates *how* a person symptomatically acts out their distress response to unresolved emotional trauma is miasmatic. The events that set off the behavioural patterns will have been of the kind that leaves the person humiliated, ashamed, guilty, abused and grieving. Both the trigger and the causal origin are susceptible to remedies. In dealing with anorexia and bulimia the homoeopath often has to play detective, as the emotional picture can be of such depth and hold such anguish that time to build up trust between patient and practitioner is a prerequisite. Skilled prescribing can encourage the gentle easing of tension and subtle release of emotional burdens where parents might be the last people to whom the patient would be able to speak openly by dint of their very closeness. Parents can nevertheless be of great help in the process of healing by providing unobtrusive practical support and, for the homoeopath, family history. Cranial osteopathy is often highly beneficial in relieving the stress (which can be enormous) on the digestive system and eliminative organs as well as the endocrine system.

Signs of Drug and Substance Abuse

How does a parent tell, except by intuition, if a child is using drugs? If drugs are a problem, cautious questioning or confrontation will be useless. It is better to look for signs and symptoms that cannot be hidden. By becoming certain a parent may be able to find appropriate help without antagonising the offspring. Not all drugs and substances have the same signals. Most addictions cause changes in personality and behaviour; users become secretive, sensitive about themselves but insensitive towards others close to them and wary of being found out. They also become untidy and careless, sometimes losing any interest in their appearance. They tend to disappear into their own rooms for longer than usual and avoid family contact. Communication is limited and may be abusive. Silent disapproval is far more effective than angry confrontation but doing nothing is not an option. While offering constant reassurance of your continued love:

- Become acquainted with the 'enemy' and find out what drugs are about and what long-term effects they cause. An abusing teenager will have more respect for this approach.
- Find out as discreetly as possible if any other parents of local young people are having similar problems.
- Show concern for the young person's health but play down the emotions; they antagonise and scare them.
- Find a way of opening up the problem to the whole family (as long as both parents are in agreement) so that it becomes a shared responsibility which is much more likely to affect the young person's thinking.
- Be prepared to hear some home truths because young adults tend to look for blame outside themselves and they can generally find some reasons for their behaviour that hit home.
- Enforce your moral standards and domestic boundaries; children of any age do best when they know where these boundaries lie and it confuses them when they are only enforced in anger after a period of 'putting up with it'.
- Find out what is available locally before marching the 'offender' off for treatment; Yellow Pages, support groups, PTAs or any other likely group may be of help and be open with the information; an abusing teenager will spot surreptitious activity a mile off.
- Involve the homoeopath. Remedies and an empathetic ear are non-threatening and can be very efficacious.
- Seek help from the homoeopath yourself; you will need all your strength of character and determination to combat the problem and the process is exhausting and ungrounding – do not neglect your own health in your quest for healing for your child.

Marijuana

Though marijuana has been relegated to the status of a class C drug, this is no reason to be complacent about the devastating effects it can have. Marijuana is not safe despite its widespread use; it is less so nowadays as it is far more potent than it was in the 1960s. It is addictive and it causes physical damage to the lungs, the immune system, the reproductive system and brain function. Symptoms of its use are:

- dry throat with coughing
- frequent eating between meals especially snack and junk food
- bloodshot eyes (note the obsessive use of dark glasses) and photophobia (wants the curtains closed)
- poor concentration, defective short-term memory and physical clumsiness
- anxiety or panic attacks
- aberrations in menstrual cycle

Amphetamines

'Uppers' or 'speed' are taken as stimulants which lift mood, prevent sleep and suppress appetite. Symptoms are:

- highs: person is excitable, talkative and as if adrenalin-driven; appears euphoric but the witness senses something is not quite right
- periods of deep depression, tiredness and unrefreshing sleep
- confused thinking

Barbiturates

'Barbs' or 'downers' are relaxants; Valium is one of them. They suppress panic and induce calmness and sleep. They are very addictive and cause physical and mental symptoms:

- increased number of hours asleep but with no positive effect
- irritability and self loathing with suicidal thoughts
- confusion and inefficiency
- mood swings between anxiety and being laid back

Cocaine

Used by those who lead 'high-octane' lives; who need to stay alert and 'with it' for long periods; it enhances excitement. It is dangerous as it causes lung disease, heart and circulation trouble, epilepsy and depressive illness. It can also trigger tumours of the pituitary gland. Signs of its use are:
  • the user is never at home; always out and about partying
  • persistent sniffing and rubbing the nose; loss of smell
  • dry throat with irritating cough
  • reduced appetite and some weight loss but with more energy
  • irritability and tendency to be easily startled

Ecstacy

This is a so-called 'designer drug' which means that it is manufactured synthetically in a laboratory. It is often used in conjunction with alcohol and other drugs at parties. Symptoms are:
  • frequent headaches with blurry vision
  • loss of appetite with frequent bouts of nausea
  • dizziness and loss of focus
  • dark rings under the eyes
  • anxiety, disorientation, irritability, may = irrational fears and paranoia

Inhalants

Solvent abuse is the inhalation of fumes given off by chemicals intended for the manufacturing industry. Signs of its use are:
  • constant sniffing, sneezing, nosebleeds and profuse mucus
  • headaches
  • sore and runny eyes
  • breathlessness and torpor
  • halitosis
  • abusive behaviour
  • personality changes: drowsiness alternated with upbeat mood
  • inefficiency, laziness, lack of coordination and inability to keep time
  • lack of physical sensation that can lead eventually to paralysis

26 TRAVELLING ABROAD

Taking remedies with you on holiday is a sensible precaution. For a continental holiday take the most typically useful remedies: **Aconite, Arnica, Arsen-alb., Belladonna, Hypericum, Nat-mur., Nux-vom., Pulsatilla, Rhus-tox., Silica** and a bottle of **Hypercal Ø**. If there are young children going too then take **Chamomilla** and **Merc-sol.**. If elderly people are travelling and there is a lot of motorway driving, take **Causticum** in case of 'motorway bladder'. This is the inability to pass water due to having held on so long to find a lavatory that the muscles controlling the bladder have gone into spasm preventing the release of urine. In Europe you should be able to purchase any other remedies from any local pharmacy; the French firm, Boiron, make excellent remedies which will either be stocked or can be ordered within 24 to 48 hours.

If you are going anywhere where there are endemic tropical diseases then you will need a few more remedies. **Baptisia, Bryonia, Chelidonium, China, Ledum, Veratrum Album** and **Zingiber** are all useful. **Baptisia** is indicated by prostration, torpor, foul breath and malodorous stools, sore muscles and dark, almost drunken looking expression; it is needed in gastric conditions. **Chelidonium** is indicated in hepatitis-type conditions of the liver. **Zingiber** 3 taken daily is often helpful in preventing water-borne diseases that affect the gut. If you do not have **Zingiber** you can buy root ginger, cut off 3 or 4 thin slices, pour boiling water over them, leave to stand and then drink; this will have a similar effect to taking the remedy in potency. (It is sensible, in hot climates, to avoid drinking any water other than bottled water and it is necessary to avoid any dairy products including ice cream that does not come out of a sealed wrapper and out of a freezer.) In addition, **Medusa** for jellyfish stings and **Apis** for insect bites may be needed.

Protecting the Remedies

Line the box of remedies with aluminium foil to protect them from mobile phones. If you are flying put the box in the middle of your suitcase. The case may be X-rayed by airport security; though it might stretch credence somewhat, it is a good idea to put a few doses of X-Ray 200 in a packet inside the box. This appears to prevent any radiation damage though you will need a fresh dose for future flights. Your practitioner would be able to supply this remedy or you can purchase it from the pharmacy. If you need remedies while you are travelling then it is best to put them in a trouser or skirt pocket wrapped in a single layer of foil; this should not set off the metal detector alarm and so avoid the necessity of the security staff using any electronic equipment to test them. Alternatively, you can buy a photographer's lead-lined film envelope to put your remedies in. This can safely be passed through the X-ray machine.

Inoculations

The official recommendation for tropical disease inoculations would leave us feeling like a pin cushion and often quite unwell. For the majority of countries outside Europe hepatitis A, polio and typhoid are the usual jabs; the typhoid vaccine is regarded even by the medical profession as useless. Diphtheria and tetanus are also fitted into the jab protocol these days though this has more to do with marketing than health. Malaria tablets are recommended for mosquito-infested areas though these are not a good idea as the drug seriously undermines liver function and can cause other side effects. (**China** is the main remedy for malaria.) Inoculation against yellow fever is obligatory in many tropical or Third World countries only if one is travelling from an infected country; if you flew, say, from Egypt to Indonesia you might be asked for a certificate. There are actually very few countries (mostly in Africa, such as Cameroon, Gabon, Ghana) where a certificate of vaccination is obligatory and sometimes even these may not insist. Some insurance companies will insist on vaccination before issuing cover but there are others which are less strict; it is worth making enquires or searching the internet.

For homoeopathic cover of the main diseases you should consult your practitioner. For those who do not want to rely solely on the first-aid kit there is an additional option: there are homoeopathic equivalents to the allopathic vaccines. Prescribing potentised disease material (or vaccine material) may not be 'good homoeopathy' but it is effective. **Malaria** 30, **Hepatitis A** 30, **Typhoid** 30 etc. are remedies which have successfully been used prophylactically for many years. (Dr Dorothy Shepherd was one of the first to do so when she used **Diphtherinum** 200 in an epidemic in London in the 1920s.) The beauty of these remedies is that they do not have any danger of side effects and they hold their efficacy as prophylactics only for a limited time thus avoiding a permanent state of 'on guard' immunity which is so taxing (and toxic) to the ecology of the body.

Travel-sickness

The most common remedies for travel-sickness (which can be used in the 30) are the following:

Arg-nit.: nausea and vomiting with nervous agitation, belching, bloated abdomen and diarrhoea; < drinking or eating; < alcohol. (< flying.)

Bryonia: main remedy for nausea on taking off in a plane; nausea and faintness with strong thirst for cold water; wants to be absolutely still and left alone.

Cocculus: nausea and retching with salivation and dizziness < from raising head up; > keeping head low. (< sea, car or plane.)

Gelsemium: nausea with hot head and a feeling of emptiness in the stomach; < the dread of every manoeuvre of the aircraft.

Kali-carb.: anxiety felt in the stomach, felt like a lump; patient is rigid with tension and anxiety; weak back and shaky legs; hypersensitive to odd noises in the aircraft.

Nux-vom.: useful for those who have had more alcohol than food and feel queasy as a result.

Petroleum: nausea from every manoeuvre of the aircraft, ship or car; < the smell of petrol or diesel; profuse salivation while nauseated.

Tabacum: intense and miserable nausea with a sinking feeling in the pit of the stomach and faintness; complexion goes green; all << tobacco smoke.

For some people dealing with travel-sickness is just a matter of preparation. You can try cutting out sole-shaped pieces of brown paper and fitting them into your shoes; this has proved invaluable for some. Others sit on a newspaper; this often works for children who are carsick. I mention these methods as they have worked for me and my family, although I do not know how! Advise people who suffer any form of motion sickness that looking straight ahead is the best position or lying prone if there is room. Reading or playing a game is the worst.

Jet Lag

Confusingly, different homoeopaths have different means of dealing with jet lag; no one solution works for all. Most people experience the symptoms after travelling from west to east, towards the sun, but others suffer the reverse. Some people only suffer jet lag if they have flown over areas heavy in nuclear radiation such as the Nevada desert in America or the southern Pacific. The best policy is to discuss symptoms with the homoeopath who will select an indicated remedy.

The main remedies include **Arnica, Cocculus, Gelsemium** and **Radium Bromide**. To limit the symptoms travellers should drink plenty of water throughout the flight.

Phlebitis and Deep Vein Thrombosis

Water retention in the legs during a flight can lead to swelling and discomfort while people are confined in a small space. If this is a risk then **Calc-carb.** 30 should be considered. It can be taken through a long flight at the rate of one every 3 or 4 hours. If the swelling becomes hot, throbbing and painful then use **Belladonna** 200 instead. DVT is a serious condition which can be prevented. Consult the homoeopath who will make suggestions. One of these may be **Crataegus Ø**; given long term at the rate of several drops each day it can ensure that plaque on artery walls is emulsified safely. If DVT is a real threat during a flight that cannot be avoided then keeping a dose of **Lachesis**

30 or 200 at hand is sensible but make sure that you have understood its use by speaking to your practitioner.

Pain and Popping in the Ears

Ear pain during take-off and landing can be excruciating. The main remedy is **Silica,** best given in a 200. If this does not help or irascibility is a strong feature then **Chamomilla** 200 should relieve it.

Risk of Infection from Air Conditioning

If you sit in a cold draught from the plane's air conditioning then use a **Causticum** 30. It should prevent stiff neck and shoulders, earache and a cold.

Fear of Flying

Fear can range from anxiety to abject terror. For symptoms of anticipation and anxiety use **Arg-nit.**, **Lycopodium** or **Gelsemium** (see chapter 2, pages 68–9). If the symptoms seem not quite to fit any of these examples then ask your practitioner about **Triple A** which is a combination remedy of **Arg-nit. + Anacardium + Ambra Grisea.** For those who suffer heart-stopping terror of flying, the most useful remedy is **Opium**; speak to the homoeopath about this as it is often best given in a very high potency (10M).

Some Handy Tips

- Always drink plenty of water. Headache from driving too long without drinking enough water is > for **Bryonia** 30 or **Pulsatilla** 30.
- Have frequent 'pit stops' when driving, not just to prevent tiredness: it is better for whole system. Driving non-stop for more than 4 or 5 hours is bad for one's general health.
- The most common remedy needed by children when abroad is **Pulsatilla**. If you forget to take any or it fails to work for whatever problem it is obviously indicated for, then give the patient beer to drink, common sense dictating how much. Beer temporarily > patients in need of **Pulsatilla**.

- If you have run out of antiseptic cream or **Hypercal Ø** you can use runny honey which has antibiotic properties.
- Do not get onto a boat or a plane with an empty stomach; a banana or a fruit bar may be enough but it is best if your digestive system has something else to work on apart from any anxiety.
- To avoid using chemical-based suntan lotion ask the pharmacy for **Red + Sol** cream. This is a combined cream with the remedies **Red** and **Sol** which should be in 3x potency.

Part III

THE FIRST-AID KIT

1   FIFTY REMEDIES FOR THE FIRST-AID KIT

The remedies marked with an asterisk are some of those which are most frequently useful. Their abbreviated names are also shown.

1. ***Aconite (Acon.):** sudden onset of an acute condition when there is shock (accident) and anguish (nightmare/trauma) or sensitive irritability with mental/emotional tension (as with a cold). 'Intensity' is a key word. Especially useful for symptoms < by cold wind. Symptoms < midnight. Useful in croup, fever, dentition, surgery, neuralgia.

2. **Allium Cepa (All-c.):** for spring colds and summer hay fever or allergies with profuse watery nasal discharge and burning and watery eyes. Lots of sneezing and burning in the nose and sore top lip. Cold, damp weather < and patient feels < in a warm room. Fresh air and exercise > but wants to stay well wrapped up.

3. **Antimonium Tartaricum (Ant-tart.):** coughs, asthmatic and bronchitic conditions where patient has lots of rattling mucus. Heaving breathing from abdomen; despondency. In severe cases: bluish tinge to complexion. Symptoms < night. Being too warm, getting cross, milk, getting chilly all <. Feels > for being propped up and must sit up or forward to cough. Every spell of cold wet weather brings on catarrh which < chest. (Follows well after **Arsen-alb., Bry., Carbo-veg., Hepar, Ipecac., Kali-carb., Phos., Sepia, Sil.** and **Sulph.**)

4. **Apis:** for stings, allergic shock and histamine reactions (hives); patient is restless, irritable and sleepy; wants to be left alone. Stinging and burning pains. Parts affected look puffy, swollen, red and hot. If breathing is affected, patient has short panting breaths. < around

3 p.m. Useful in headache, throat, skin and menstrual problems especially on the right side. (Followed well by **Nat-mur.**)

5. **Argentum Nitricum (Arg-nit.):** for attacks of anxiety, fears with bowel reactions; eye, throat and abdominal conditions; splinter-like pains. Patient paces up and down worried about 'What if....?' questions; gut reacts with wind, bloating and profuse diarrhoea. Eyes: gummy with thick, yellow pus and corners; red and swollen. Generally < from sugar, any mental stress, thinking too hard.

6. ***Arnica Montana (Arn.):** for shock (including bad news) and trauma that leaves the patient stunned; patient wants to be left alone; says he is all right though he is not. Bruising and sensations of bruising (physical or emotional) and soreness of muscles. Use after operations and dental work.

7. ***Arsenicum Album (Arsen-alb.):** useful in colds, coughs, 'flu, fever, headaches, asthmatic or bronchitic problems, stomach bugs etc. with dry mouth and thirst for sips of cold water, chilliness yet wanting coolness round head; the patient is restless, anxious and demanding. < after midnight. (Followed well by **Carbo-veg., Lyc., Phos., Sepia** and **Sulph.**)

8. ***Belladonna (Bell.):** for fevers, abscesses, cough, headaches, ear, tooth and tonsil infections with redness, heat and throbbing; radiant heat concentrated either in the head or upper body or in the affected part; all < 3 p.m. (and 3 a.m.). Dryness of membranes; throbbing of arteries and dilated pupils. Sharp, neuralgic pains. < from sun, after getting overheated, a haircut or washing hair or a fit of rage.

9. **Bellis Perennis (Bell-p.):** for injury to internal organs especially after surgery or damage to nerves from severe injuries especially to the spine and joints. Essential for trauma to the breast. For those used to physical labour who have sore muscles and restlessness. Useful after surgery. (Follows **Arnica** well; sometimes superior to **Arnica** in those who are of lean build and wiry. Better to give this remedy before 6 p.m. as patient may otherwise wake early in the morning.)

10. **Berberis Vulgaris (Berb-v.):** primarily a kidney and liver remedy;

pains in the kidney region radiate down towards the bladder and groin < while urinating; pains in the joints with kidney and bladder symptoms. Colic (kidney or gall bladder) pains with a bubbling sensation in the back, often with back stiffness. Important remedy to keep for those with susceptibility to urinary tract problems. Useful when other urinary remedies need 'support' from a complementary remedy. (Complementary to **Apis, Cantharis, Dioscorea, Lyc., Merc-sol., Puls., Sepia, Sil.** and **Sulph.**)

11. **Bryonia (Bry.):** covers many conditions in which dryness and strong thirst are prevalent with << from any movement. Headaches, lung conditions, colds, cough, muscle and joint problems, fever or diarrhoea with wish to be left alone, undisturbed yet irritable and worried about neglecting work. This is the 'bear with a sore head' remedy. Do not give before or after **Calc-c.**! If indicated around **Calc-c.** then give **Hepar-sulph.** 30 between. (**Hepar-sulph.** is also < movement, irritable and wants to be left alone but pains are sharper and more likely to be localised to a small area such as tonsil, ear or boil and the patient is less robust.)

12. **Calcarea Carbonica (Calc-c.):** needed by children who are either pale, chubby and plodding or thinner patients who tend to have swollen glands and fevers; both tend to have sweaty heads when ill. Useful in colds, coughs, ear and teething problems, cramp, glandular swelling etc. when characterised by sweaty head and chilly extremities, exhaustion and sensitivity. Sleep is often disturbed by bad dreams or worries. Useful to support **Belladonna** or if **Bell.** fails when well indicated. Do not give before or after **Bryonia**! (See **Bryonia** above.)

13. **Calendula (Cal.):** prevents sepsis and heals cuts, abrasions, lacerations, burnt skin (also after radiotherapy); prevents excessive scar tissue. Also useful after episiotomy or tears. Especially indicated if patient is chilly after a wound. Use both in tincture and in potency. This remedy can be used in mother tincture; it is very comforting to apply a hot compress of **Calendula** to a wounded part. Add 10 drops of **Calendula** mother tincture to a cup of hot water, soak a wad of lint in the solution and apply. See **Hypericum**.

14. **Cantharis (Canth.):** burns and scalds or cystitis; raw, smarting pains on the skin or urethra. Burns tend to blister with redness beneath. Constant desire to pass water which comes out in drops; cutting pains as water is passed. Urine can be bloody; kidney pains. Anxious, fretful and very irritable. Urinary symptoms < coffee drinking. (See **Berberis**.)

15. **Carbo Vegetabilis (Carbo-veg.):** most usual in the young and the elderly but for anyone who is weak and debilitated with lung or digestive conditions with shortness of breath, exhaustion and chilliness but > for cool air or being fanned. Upset digestion with belching, flatulence and nausea < fatty food. In asthma there is blueness around the lips, spasmodic coughing; unable to take a deep breath. Useful to round off an acute where there is cough, phlegm and exhaustion.

16. **Causticum (Caust.):** after a burn or scald with burning, rawness and soreness. Also in cough, throat and chest conditions marked by rawness and stiffness; voice is weakened; muscles and tendons feel stiff and weak. Earaches or sore throat after being in a draft or air conditioning. Useful in those who tend to have rigid fibre. Symptoms < cold dry weather and wind or draughts. > for warmth and staying in bed. Physical stiffness with mental tiredness. The homoeopathic catheter; 'motorway bladder'.

17. ***Chamomilla (Cham.):** primarily a pain remedy; pains are unendurable; patient is furiously angry and impossible to satisfy; rejects what he has just asked for; wants to be carried about during the pains. Hates cold wind; being looked at. Useful in teething, earache, diarrhoea or sore throats of infants or menstrual colic. One pale cheek, one red in teething and ear complaints. (Antidotes **Pulsatilla** and **Nux-vom.** both of which might appear like **Chamomilla** at times. **Chamomilla** is *very intense* so if in doubt about the indications go for the other remedy; there is often no doubt whatever about **Chamomilla. Hepar-sulph.** can be confused because of the irritability but **Cham.** is far more demanding while **Hepar-sulph.** wants to be left alone.)

18. **China Officinalis (China):** in conditions following dehydration or

fluid loss such as menstruation, haemorrhage, vomiting or diarrhoea. Food poisoning after bad fish, fruit, meat or water. The patient is weak, pale, thirsty and sensitive. In digestive upset is flatulent and bloated; only hungry for delicatessen-type food. May crave smoking which <. (In those who need **China** avoid giving juicy fruit, milk or blood-heating foods like peppers.)

19. **Cocculus Indicus (Cocc.):** needed after loss of sleep from nursing others or for motion or morning sickness. Patient feels light-headed or dizzy with a hollow head feeling; with or without nausea. Weakness with trembly, aching knees. Travel sickness > lying down; morning sickness especially with painful wind.

20. **Coccus Cacti (Coc-c.):** throat irritation (sensation of dust) with paroxysmal coughing. Cough is followed by bringing up masses of thick, clear, slimy mucus which is difficult to clear away; cough may cause internal heat and dark red face. Whooping cough. (May be indicated after **Spongia, Phos.** or **Rumex.**)

21. **Corallium Rubrum (Cor-r.):** the 'minute gun cough'; intermittent violent coughing preceded by a gasp and < eating or taking a deep breath. Cannot bear being too chilly or too hot. (Followed well by **Sulph.**)

22. **Cuprum (Cupr.):** violently painful, spasmodic cramp; < calves, shin, soles or abdomen during menses or diarrhoea. Chesty cough in violent spasms leaving no breath; whooping cough. Cough causes cramp in chest muscles; cough > cold drink. Watery eyes from cough or vomiting. Useful in contractions after birth. Symptoms come on from stress and overwork. Patient responds well to gentle massage.

23. **Drosera Rotundifolia (Dros.):** persistent spasms of coughing < lying down at night (or after midnight) with sensation of a tickle in the throat; whooping cough. Barking, hacking cough < talking, laughing or drinking something. Patient is irritable and restless; easily discouraged.

24. **Eupatorium Perfoliatum (Eup-perf.):** influenza with soreness of the skin and deep aching pains in bones; < and starts in low back. Thirst

for cold water; the pains precede chilliness all > for sweating. Headache and nausea with weakness; patient wants to remain still and covered but is restless. (Often followed well by **Nat-mur.**)

25. *****Ferrum Phosphoricum (Ferr-phos.):** early symptoms of colds, ear, throat and chest infection and fever; does not have enough energy to produce **Belladonna** symptoms. Flushed face with sweaty hands. Also useful in teething and nosebleed. Patient is quiet, weak and sensitive. Only useful early on in an illness; give when you cannot decide between other remedies like **Acon., Bell., Gels**, but then be ready to see symptoms change. (Followed well by **Bry., Kali-mur., Kali-sulph.** or **Arsen-alb.**)

26. *****Gelsemium Sempervivens (Gels.):** cold or influenza with weakness, doziness and chills up and down the spine; face looks heavy and flushed with droopy eyelids. Headache at the back of the head < lying down. Also dread of performing or seeing medics; chilly shivers before an ordeal such as an examination. Useful in influenza, sore throat, cold, dentition and fever. (Followed well by **Bry.** or **Puls.**)

27. *****Hepar Sulphuris Calcareum (Hepar-sulph.):** hypersensitive to pain, draught, noise and touch when ill: abscess, cold or influenza, ear, throat or chest infection. Splinter pains feature in ear, throat conditions and boils. Very irritable and does not want to be touched; every draught causes shivering. Hard to get any verbal information. (Often followed by **Silica** in abscesses; **Spongia** in croup; **Puls.** in catarrhal stage of colds.)

28. *****Hypericum Perforatum (Hyp.):** any wound or injury with nerve pains that are worse than expected; cuts, stings, bites, puncture wounds and lacerations and crushed parts especially those rich in nerves (fingertips and toes). Anti-tetanus. Can be used internally in tincture and potency as well as externally. Is mixed with **Calendula** to make **Hypercal** tincture which should be used as antiseptic in any wound. (See **Calendula** above.)

29. **Ignatia Amara (Ign.):** emotional upset, grief; deep, heaving sighs and sobbing alternating with brooding or alternating moods all <

disappointment. Sensation of a lump in the throat or heaviness in the chest which comes and goes. Confusion of emotions. Insomnia from sadness. Cigarette smoke < chest and headache. (If followed by a cold, **Nat-mur.** may be needed to deal with remaining symptoms.)

30. Ipecacuanha (Ipecac.): continuous nausea and vomiting accompanying asthmatic conditions, cough, pregnancy. Chest feels tight with incessant cough with rattling in the chest which is hard to raise. Eyes and face redden with effort of coughing or vomiting. Generally < warmth; > resting and fresh air. > nausea during chemotherapy. (Followed well by **Ant-tart.** in catarrhal coughs.)

31. *Kali Bichromicum (Kali-bich.): mucous discharges are thick, sticky, ropy, yellow or yellowish green; < after a cold or chest infection. Headaches < from nasal catarrh and sinusitis especially felt in bones over the eyes; loss of smell. Patient feels > in the open air but wants to be wrapped up. (Easily confused with **Puls.** or **Kali-sulph.** in catarrhal conditions. **Puls.** follows well and can be alternated with it if there is a **Puls.**-type mood and **Puls.** will not complete the job on its own.)

32. Lachesis Muta (Lach.): for throat conditions < left side and with swollen, dark red or purplish mucous membranes; unable to protrude tongue; cannot bear anything round neck. Cannot swallow liquids. Symptoms start on the left and then shift to the right side. Patient sounds confused or feels vindictive. Abscesses with purple skin and painful tightness. Should be considered in any dark red or purplish swelling. (Followed well by **Lyc.** or **Nat-mur.** If **Lach.** seems indicated but there is thirst and > for warm drinks then use **Sabadilla.**)

33. Ledum Palustre (Led.): puncture wounds of nails, splinters, injections, stings, mosquitoes etc. Anti-tetanus. Area is swollen, pale and painful with little or no bleeding; pains may creep up the limb which may go cold and stiff. Particularly useful for black eye. Painful part feels > cold water. Bites are itchy and lumpy.

34. Lycopodium Clavatum (Lyc.): useful in upper respiratory tract conditions and digestive disorders. Nose is snuffly, throat is sore < right and > warm drinks; chesty cough with rattly mucus < night.

Most patients tend to be windy, bloated and full; cannot finish the meal. Symptoms < 4 – 8 p.m.; pains or symptoms start on the right side and move to the left (opposite of **Lach.**). Digestion: easily affected by beans, cabbage and gluten in wheat products. (**Lyc.** should be kept by those susceptible to kidney and bladder problems. See **Berberis.**)

35. ***Mercurius Solubilis (Merc-sol.) or Mercurius Vivus (Merc-viv.):** useful in ear, nose and throat, teeth and gums and skin conditions. Cannot stabilise temperature, switches between hot and cold; very thirsty for cold water though has excessive salivation; foul taste (metallic) and halitosis; swollen glands < right side. Abscesses and ulcers. Sometimes **Merc-sol.** does not work despite indications; one of the other mercury remedies may be needed. **Mercurius Iodatus Flavus (Merc-iod-flav.):** useful in sore throat which starts on the right and moves to left (like **Lyc.**); constantly wants to swallow; swollen glands on the right side of neck; tongue is coated yellow with a red tip; jaw muscles feel stiff; light-headed on getting up; may be windy. Back of throat may be ulcerated. **Mercurius Iodatus Ruber (Merc-iod-rub.):** left-sided sore throat with pains spreading over to right (like **Lach.**); left neck is stiff and has swollen glands; inside throat is dark red; foul taste and sensation of a lump in throat < swallowing; ears feel blocked; cheekbones ache; rheumatic aches in various limbs.

36. **Natrum Muriaticum (Nat-mur.):** colds, cold sores, headaches, eye problems; blinding headaches with hammering pain and watery eyes and photophobia; herpes or cracks on the bottom lip < feverish colds; sneezing with egg-white mucus; usually craves salty foods and feels emotionally withdrawn. One of the few remedies which covers cold sores that come on with a fever. (Use **Bry.** in severe headaches as there is less likelihood of an aggravation before improvement. Always let the homoeopath know if you have used **Nat-mur.** as it is often followed well by a nosode. If **Nat-mur.** is indicated but frequently disappoints then change to **Winchelsea Sea Salt** from Helios Pharmacy.)

37. **Nitric Acid (Nit-ac.):** useful in blisters, ulcers, cold sores and fissures that appear anywhere near the orifices of the body: lips, urethra or anus; pains are sharp, needle-like; ulcers may be small but exceedingly

painful; bleeding piles with aching long after initial sharp pain; miserable, anxious and irritable. (Do not prescribe next to **Nat-mur.**)

38. *Nux Vomica (Nux-vom.):** useful in upper respiratory tract, digestion, headache, menstruation and irritable nervous tension. Colic with sore abdomen and spasms of pain (menstrual or digestive); headache < alcohol or sun; stuffed up nose with sneezing and snuffles; cannot blow enough out. Bowels – cannot expel all that seems to be there; nausea and vomiting with spasms. Chilly with burning fever. Very sensitive and irritable. **Nux-vom.** is a remedy that has a reputation for antidoting the effects of other remedies so be sure that the healing effected by a previous remedy is well and truly holding and that the picture is now different before moving on to **Nux-vom.** (A night-time dose works best; if taken in the day, avoid mealtimes.)

39. Phosphoric Acid (Phos-ac.):** exhaustion and 'wall staring' especially after disease with loss of body fluid; weak and debilitated after diarrhoea and vomiting or menstrual flooding or heavy sweats. Dark rings under eyes; frequent calls to urinate at night; feels apathetic and indifferent.

40. Phosphorus (Phos.):** needed by those who are weak, nervous and want sympathy and encouragement; usually feisty, gregarious and impressionable but illness has shaken their resolve. Thirsty for cold drinks (which they may bring up) and hungry for salty food. Tends to colds, coughs, bronchitis, pneumonia, nosebleeds, nightmares and conditions with heavy bleeding (i.e. menses). (Frequently indicated by those who have bursts of stamina followed by periods of exhaustion. Followed well by **Sulph.**)

41. *Pulsatilla (Puls.):** for almost any condition that is accompanied by weeping, dependency, clinging and changeable moods; however, **Puls.** can be very irritable as well especially with anyone other than the person to whom the patient is temporarily attached. Patient is dry but not thirsty unless there is a craving for milk which replaces hunger; milk should be avoided! Either hot or chilly but > for fresh air and being outside. Mucus is thick, yellow or green < first thing in the a.m. and evening. (Well supported by tissue salts and followed by **Silica.**)

42. ***Rhus Toxicodendron (Rhus-tox.)**: injuries, strains, skin eruptions, rheumatic problems, sore throat. Restless, cannot get comfortable; back strain; muscles are stiff < first moving though > gently moving about; > lying on hard floor; > rubbing the part. Herpes: itching, red and swollen; burning in blister. Influenza with swollen glands, sore throat, restlessness and muscle symptoms. (**Arsen-alb., Calc-c., Lyc., Puls.** and **Sulph.** follow well in colds or influenza.)

43. **Rumex Crispus (Rumex)**: useful in upper respiratory conditions: coughs, bronchitis; intense tickling in trachea < slightest intake of cold air; cough < 11 p.m., 2 a.m., 5 a.m. Rawness and burning in upper chest under clavicle. Tends to be low in spirits; frowns.

44. **Ruta Graveolens (Ruta)**: injuries to bones and joints and their protective covering; also dislocation, bruises and damage to cartilage. Soreness, aching and restlessness with profound tiredness. Lame after injuries. Eyestrain. Complements **Rhus-tox.** and **Arnica** and follows or alternates well with both. Is followed well by **Ledum**.

45. **Sepia**: menstrual disorders, energy problems, bladder weakness. General tiredness with sense of sagging; bearing down sensations with weakness; stress incontinence; cystitis with bearing down; headache < menses; generally > for fresh air and exercise or a 'workout'. Very irritable and tends to take it out on husband or children. (Patients who are often in a **Sepia** state may need **Arsen-alb., Nux-vom.** or **Puls.** for acutes or **Sabad.** for throat problems.)

46. **Silica (Sil.)**: needed by those who are chilly, weak and lacking in grit; ailments exhaust the patient. < from draughts, cold wind and damp. Upper respiratory tract infection; swollen glands; ear infections; pains are sharp and stabbing or like a pin. Ears blocked with cracking or popping noises. Slow development of abscesses; hastens suppuration or absorption. (Though a chilly remedy, **Silica** patients are often hot in the acute and go round on cold days in their T-shirts when well or before going down with a problem.)

47. **Spongia Tosta (Spong.)**: upper respiratory tract; cough; croup. Cough causes anxiety and gasping: dry, barking with sense of

breathing through a dry sponge in top of chest – sounds like a saw cutting wood; heaviness on chest with heat and weakness. Cough > drink of cold water or eating something. (Often follows after **Acon.** and **Hepar-sulph.** Always mention the use of these remedies to the homoeopath as a nosode (**Bacillinum** especially) may be required to follow for the constitution especially if there is still any lingering cough.)

48. **Staphysagria (Staph.):** ailments from being angry without being able to express it appropriately: cystitis, sciatica, colic, toothache etc. or fit of shouting and throwing objects about impotently. Cystitis after sex in new relationship; irritable bladder, burning in bladder while passing urine; bladder feels as if it will not empty. Needed after surgery or a visit from someone who causes offence (mother-in-law for example); whenever there is a sense of abuse or one's space or person having been invaded.

49. ***Sulphur (Sulph.):** useful for those who look unkempt, exhausted and who tend to 'flop down'; standing makes them feels weak. Very thirsty for cold drinks. Tend to have loose motions < on rising. Skin looks dry or unhealthy; itching eruptions. Hot at night; sweaty and sticks feet out of the covers. Useful when given after an acute illness to round off the treatment and remove any last symptoms.

50. **Veratrum Album (Verat-alb.):** diarrhoea and vomiting with profuse watery stools, severe cramping in the gut, excessive sweat < on the forehead and intense thirst for cold water which is vomited quickly; patient is totally exhausted. Face is pale and bluish. Feels 'out of it'; does not respond to questions. Very useful in the traveller's first-aid kit. (Use Dioralite to restore electrolyte balance.)

2 PUTTING TOGETHER AND MAINTAINING THE FIRST-AID KIT

Tissue Salts

The 12 Biochemic tissue salts are very low potency (6) remedies that are regarded as support or drainage remedies that work on the cellular level. They can help prevent the worst of an acute condition that is brewing and they can encourage the resolution of symptoms once the illness is progressing. They are referred to and recommended throughout the text. The remedies are made by New Era and are available at most health food shops or through the homoeopathic pharmacies. The twelve tissue salts are: **Calc-fluor., Calc-phos., Calc-sulph., Ferrum-phos., Kali-mur., Kali-phos., Kali-sulph., Mag-phos., Nat-mur., Nat-phos., Nat-sulph**. and **Silica**. For a far more comprehensive understanding see *The Biochemic Handbook; A Guide to Using Dr Schuessler's Biochemic Tissue Salts* by Dr Colin Lessell (Thorsons, 1984, ISBN 0-7225-0891-3).

Tinctures

It is important to keep **Hypercal Ø** (mother tincture) as an antiseptic; this is a mixture of **Hypericum** and **Calendula** both of which can be obtained separately. **Calendula + Salvia Officinalis Ø** (mouthwash and sore throat) and **Euphrasia Ø** (eyes) are both invaluable. They are all available at the homoeopathic pharmacies. For combinations ask for the required size of bottle (3.5, 5, 10, 20, or 100 ml) with the ingredients in equal parts; i.e. a 20-ml bottle of **Calendula + Salvia Officinalis** mother tinctures in equal parts.

Choice of Pills and Potions

When you order the remedies from the pharmacy you will need to say what type and size you want. Pills come in lactose or sucrose (milk sugar and not for those who are milk intolerant). The sucrose pills (called 'dragees') come in small or larger sizes. Lactose pills come in either flat, hard tablets or fat, soft tablets that melt quickly. Dragees are the most economical. For tiny babies granules, like sugar crystals, may be preferred. The dose is administered from the bottle cap.

If you are ordering topical medicines make sure that you know whether you want cream or ointment. Creams are easier to apply but some people are intolerant of lanolin; aqueous cream can be substituted as a base cream. Ointments are thicker and stickier and last longer on the skin.

What Else Do You Need in the First-aid Kit?

Keep micropore plaster for superficial wounds as well as lint, porous fabric plasters and bandages for deeper cuts. Use lint and plaster rather than the waterproof ready-made plasters as these are pre-medicated and prevent air getting to the wound. Lint and plaster are more time-consuming to apply but better for speedy recovery. (Having washed the area with **Hypercal** solution put the woven side of the lint on the wound and drop **Hypercal Ø** on it so that it soaks through.) Use **Hypercal** cream after the bleeding has stopped. 'Burns cream' and 'Scar cream', available from the pharmacy, are also useful as topical applications. Rescue Remedy is excellent for everyday problems where you cannot see a clear picture; a dose can afford you time while you assess what else to do or it can support the action of chosen remedies.

Lotus

Lotus is a remedy that has been proved relatively recently. It has a reputation for being similar to Rescue Remedy though it works on the physical body as well as the psyche (see appendix for website). It is regarded as a remedy to balance the four elements: Earth, Water, Fire and Air. Throughout the book it is mentioned as a remedy that can be used in conjunction with the flower remedies and suggestions are made for particular circumstances. One can order **Lotus** 30 from the pharmacy in the form of a 3.5-ml bottle of 'medicating potency'. This is the remedy in liquid form that can be added to a combination of any flower remedies of your choice. (One drop of the **Lotus** with one drop each of the chosen flower essences in a half tumbler of water to be sipped throughout the day.) Otherwise a bottle of **Lotus** with your chosen combination can be made up for you at the pharmacy.

Maintenance of Remedies

Always keep your remedies out of direct sunlight, away from mobile phones, CD or DVD players, digital phones and computers. It is best if they are in a cool dark place away from strong chemical smells. They should not be kept in the fridge. They are susceptible to radiation of any sort so it is important to store them in a metal box; if this is not possible then line their container or the bottom of the drawer with aluminium foil.

Though all medicines should have a warning to keep them out of the reach of children, in the case of homoeopathic remedies do not fret if a child does help himself. If a remedy is not indicated for them it will not cause any reaction unless taken regularly over a period of weeks. If a child eats the contents of a whole bottle, remember that this is the equivalent of taking just one dose; in homoeopathy we are dealing with physics (i.e. energy) and not chemistry (material doses).

Handling Remedies

Touching a remedy which is for you is no problem as long as your hands are not impregnated with strong scent, soap, oils etc. If you are giving anyone else a remedy then do not touch it; give it from the bottle cap or in a spoon.

When administering remedies to tiny babies it is best to put the chosen pill in a small amount of water (thus causing the water to be impregnated with the remedy energy) and give them a teaspoonful. The water only has to touch the lips to be effective. (Don't forget that **Magnesia Phosphorica** is best administered in a glass of hot water.)

When applying cream or ointment start by putting only a small amount on a small area in case the patient reacts badly to the base. If there is no obvious reaction then apply it over the whole area being treated.

Antidotes

Remedies can be rendered ineffective by peppermint, menthol, eucalyptus, camphor, tea tree and other aromatherapy oils. Proprietary mouthwashes can also negate them. If a patient has just been chewing gum or just had a mint then wait before giving a remedy. It is better to use toothpaste that contains none of the mentioned oils though if the patient separates teeth cleaning and taking the remedy by at least half an hour there should be few problems. (Though it is an acquired taste, fennel is the best variety of toothpaste as it is good for teeth. Avoid fluoride products and fluoride treatment at all costs as it is toxic and suppresses the activity of the throat glands.)

Some remedies are used as antidotes to deal with the excessive or confusing effects of others. If you find that a condition you have been treating has called for too many remedies and you are not clear what is going on, it is likely that the patient has had too many remedies that were not quite on the mark. Give a single dose of **Nux Vomica** 30 and let your practitioner know what has been going on. (If a patient has had too much **Arnica** he will feel deathly tired, achy and sore; give a single dose of **Arsen-alb.** 30.)

A Last Word

If you, the prescriber, are confused, tired and worried by what you are trying to sort out take a dose of Rescue Remedy, sit down in an upright chair with both feet on the ground and breathe deeply for a few minutes. If this becomes a typical scenario for you, see your homoeopath and keep a bottle of **Lotus** 30 + White Chestnut + Oak + Scleranthus + Red Chestnut (flower essences), one drop as required, which should afford you some clarity and perception in a crisis.

APPENDIX

USEFUL NAMES AND ADDRESSES

Pharmacies

Ainsworths
36 New Cavendish Street
London W1G 8UF
Tel. 020 7935 5330
www.ainsworths.com

Buxton and Grant
176 Whiteladies Road
Bristol BS8 2XU
Tel. 0117 973 5025
www.buxtonandgrantpharmacy.co.uk

Galen Homoeopathics
Lewell Mill
West Stafford
Dorchester
Dorset DT2 8AN
Tel. 01305 263996

Helios Homoeopathic Pharmacy
97 Camden Road
Tunbridge Wells
Kent TN1 2QR
Tel. 01892 537254
www.helios.co.uk

Helios Homoeopathic Pharmacy
8 New Row
Covent Garden
London WC2N 4LJ
Tel. 020 7379 7434
www.helioslondon.com

Flower Essence Remedies

English Flower Essences from
Healing Herbs, are available online
from www.health4youonline.com or
they can be obtained from the Helios
Pharmacy.

Contraception

Honey Cap Contraception
Dr Shirley Bond
127 Harley Street
London W1G 6AZ
Tel. 020 7935 4367

Homoeopathic Organisations

Alliance of Registered Homoeopaths
Millbrook
Millbrook Hill
Nutley
East Sussex TN22 3PJ
Tel. 08700 736339
www.a-r-h.org

The National Association of
Homoeopathic Groups
11 Wingle Tye Road
Burgess Hill
West Sussex RH15 9HR
Tel. 01444 236848
www.patient.co.uk

The Society of Homoeopaths
4a Artizan Road
Northampton NN1 4HU
Tel. 01604 621 400
www.homeopathy-soh.org

British Homeopathic Dental
Association
www.bhda.co.uk

Homoeopathic Colleges

Here is a selection of the many
colleges now open. Many of them
run student clinics which are open to
the public.

The Centre for Homeopathic
Education
1st Floor, 243 Upper Street
London N1 1RU
Tel. 020 7359 7424
www.homeopathycollege.org

College of Practical Homoeopathy
760 High Road
North Finchley
London N12 9QH
Tel. 020 8445 6123
and at:
186 Wolverhampton Street
Dudley
West Midlands DY1 3AD
Tel. 01384 233664
www.homoeopathytraining.co.uk

The Lakeland College
Postal Building
Ash Street
Bowness on Windermere
Cumbria LA23 3EB
Tel. 01539 447666
www.thelakelandcollege.co.uk

The New College of Homoeopathy
40A Royal Hill
London SE10 8PT
Tel. 0870 080 1976
www.new-college.co.uk

The North West College of
Homoeopathy
23 Wilbraham Road
Fallowfield
Manchester M14 6FG
Tel. 0161 2251028
www.nwch.co.uk

The South Downs School of
Homoeopathy
3 Chantry Cottages
Chantry Lane
Storrington
West Sussex RH20 4AB
Tel. 01903 744 774
www.homoeopathyschool.co.uk

Osteopathy

The Osteopathic Centre for Children
(London)
The School House
15a Woodbridge Street
London EC1R 0ND
Tel. 020 7490 5510

The Osteopathic Centre for Children
(Manchester)
Phoenix Mill
Piercy Street
Ancoats
Manchester M4 7HY
Tel. 0161 277 9911

The European School of Osteopathy
Boxley House
The Street
Boxley
Maidstone
Kent ME14 3DZ
Tel. 01622 671558
www.eso.ac.uk

Centres Dealing with Developmental Learning Difficulties

Body Brushing (Developmental) Therapy
Tel. 07956 678777
www.bodybrushing.co.uk

Davis Dyslexia Association UK
Dyslexia Kent
Unit 3a Slaney Place
Headcorn Road
Staplehurst
Kent TN12 0DT
Tel. 01580 892928

DDAT Centres
Tel. 0870 7370011
www.ddat.org

Acupuncture

British Acupuncture Council
63 Jeddo Road
London W12 9HQ
Tel. 020 8735 0400
www.acupuncture.org.uk

Ayurveda

(An ancient system of herbal and dietary medicine that complements homoeopathy)

Ayurvedic Medical Association UK
The Hale Clinic
7 Park Crescent
London W1B 1PF
Tel. 0845 009 4171

Counselling

British Association for Counselling and Psychotherapy (BACP)
BACP House
35-37 Albert Street
Rugby
Warwickshire CV21 2SG
Tel. 0870 443 5252
www.bacp.co.uk

Reflexology

(A system of massage on the feet and hands based on the association of body parts to zones on the extremities. The massage seeks to redress imbalances in the system.)

Association of Reflexologists
27 Old Gloucester Street
London WC1 3XX
Tel. 0870 5673320
www.aor.org.uk

Shiatsu

(An ancient Japanese system of acupressure treatment that uses the meridians or energy lines of the body to rebalance the whole; it complements homoeopathy well.)

Shiatsu Society (UK)
Eastlands Court
St Peter's Road
Rugby
Warwickshire CV21 3QP
Tel. 0845 1304560
www.shiatsusociety.org

Homoeopathic Books and Supplies

Helios Pharmacy: see page 354

Minerva Books
173 Fulham Palace Road
London W6 8QT
Tel. 020 7385 1361

Homoeopathic Supply Co.
The Street
Bodham
Holt
Norfolk NR25 6AD
Tel. 01263 588788

Useful Publications

The Informed Parent (a subscription review of vaccination and health issues)
PO Box 4481
Worthing
West Sussex BN11 2WH
Tel. 01903 212969
www.informedparent.co.uk

What Doctors Don't Tell You (a useful subscription review of medical practices and how to find your way around the alternatives)
77 Grosvenor Avenue
London N5 2NN
Tel. 0800 146054
www.wddty.co.uk

Health Insurance Agencies that cover Homoeopathy

HSA (The Hospital Saving Association)
Hambleden House
Andover
Hants SP10 1LQ
Tel. 0800 0721000
www.hsa.co.uk

HSF (The Hospital Saturday Fund)
24 Upper Ground
London SE1 9PD
Tel. 020 7928 0446
www.hsf.eu.com

BIBLIOGRAPHY

BLIGHT, Jean & COULTON, Chris: *Practical Guide to Specific Learning Difficulties*. Egon Publishers Ltd (2004)

BERKOW, Robert (editor): *The Merck Manual of Medical Information* (Home Edition). Merck & Co., Inc. (1997)

BOERICKE, William: *Materia Medica.* Boericke and Runyon (1901)

BORLAND, Dr Douglas: *Homoeopathy in Practice;* edited by Dr Kathleen Priestman. Beaconsfield (1981)

– *Pneumonias.* British Homoeopathic Association (1939)

CASTLEMAN, Michael: *New Healing Herbs.* Rodale Press (2001)

CASTRO, Miranda FSHom.: *The Complete Homoeopathy Handbook.* St. Martin's Press (1990)

– *Homoeopathy For Pregnancy, Birth and Your Baby's First Year.* St. Martin's Press (1993)

CLARKE, John H. MD: *The Prescriber.* CW Daniel Co. Ltd (1972) (First published by Keene & Ashwell in 1885, rev. 1925)

–*A Dictionary of Practical Materia Medica* (3 volumes). Homoeopathic Publishing Company (1900–1902)

D'ADAMO, Dr Peter J.: *Eat Right For Your Type.* Putnam (1996)

DETHLEFSEN, Thorwald (& Rudiger Dahlke MD): *The Healing Power of Illness.* Element (1990) (First published by C. Bertelsmann Verlag GmbH, Munich in 1983)

FOUBISTER, Dr Donald: *Tutorials on Homoeopathy.* Beaconsfield (1986)

GASCOIGNE, Stephen: *The Manual of Conventional Medicine for Alternative Practitioners.* Jigme Press (1993)

GIBSON, Dr D. M.: *First Aid Homoeopathy in Accidents and Ailments.* British Homoeopathic Association (c.1970) 17th edition 1997

HAHNEMANN, Samuel: *Organon of Medicine,* 6th edition. Victor Gollancz (1983)

HAY, Louise L.: *Heal Your Body.* Eden Grove Editions (1994)

HUME, Ethel D.: *Pasteur Exposed; The False Foundations of Modern Medicine.* CW Daniel Co. Ltd. (1988) (Previously published in 1923 as *Bechamp or Pasteur?*)

KARPASEA-JONES, Joanna: *Everything There Is To Know About Vaccination; The Essential Guide For Parents.* Vaccine Awareness Network UK, PO Box 6261, Derby, England DE1 9QN (1999 rev. 2002)

KOEHLER, Gerhard: *The Handbook of Homoeopathy – Its Principles and Practice.* Thorsons (1986) (First published as *Lehrbuch der Homöopathie* by Hipokrates Verlag GmbH, Stuttgart 1983)

LESSEL, Dr Colin B.: *The Biochemic Handbook; A Guide to Using Dr Schuessler's Biochemic Tissue Salts.* Thorsons (1984)

LILIENTHAL, Samuel, MD: *Homoeopathic Therapeutics.* Boericke & Tafel (1878)

LOCKIE, Dr Andrew: *The Family Guide to Homoeopathy: The Safe Form of Medicine for the Future.* Hamish Hamilton (1989)

MENDELSOHN, Robert S., MD: *How To Raise A Healthy Kid…In Spite Of Your Doctor.* Contemporary Books Inc. (1984) (Reprinted by Ballantine Books in 1987)

MURPHY, Robin, N.D.: *Homoeopathic Medical Repertory.* Hahnemann Academy of North America (1993)

PHATAK, Dr S.R.: *Materia Medica of Homoeopathic Remedies.* IBPS, Bombay (1977) (Reprinted by Foxlee-Vaughan Publishers in1988)

– A Concise Repertory of Homoeopathic Medicines. Homoeopathic Medical Publishers, Bombay (1963)

REHMAN, Abdur: *Encyclopedia of Remedy Relationships in Homoeopathy;* edited by Abdur Rehman. Haug (1997)

REICHENBERG-ULLMANN, Judith N.D., M.S.W., and ULLMAN, Robert, N.D.: *Ritalin Free Kids.* Prima Publishing, Roseville, CA (2000)

RODALE, J.I.: *The Complete Book of Minerals for Health*. Rodale Books Inc. (1972)

SCHEFFER, Mechthild: *Bach Flower Therapy, Theory and Practice*. Thorsons (1986) (First published as *Die Bach Blumentherapie* in 1981, revised in 1984, by Heinrich Hugendubel Verlag, Munich)

SCHEIBNER, Dr Viera: *Vaccination* Minerva Books (1997)

SCOTT, Tom and GRICE, Trevor: *The Great Brain Robbery*. The Publishing Trust, NZ (1996) (Reprinted in UK by Aurum Press Ltd. in1998)

SHEPHERD, Dr Dorothy: *Homoeopathy in Epidemic Diseases*. Health Science Press (1967)

– *Homoeopathy for the First Aider*. Homoeopathic Publishing Co. (1945)

– *Magic of the Minimum Dose*. Homoeopathic Publishing Co. (1946)

– *More Magic of the Minimum Dose*. Homoeopathic Publishing Co. (1949)

– *A Physician's Posy*. Health Science Press (1951)

SPEIGHT, Phyllis: *Homoeopathic Remedies for Ears, Nose & Throat*. CW Daniel Co. Ltd. (1990)

– *Homoeopathic Remedies for Children*. Health Science Press (1983)

WINSTON, Julian: *The Heritage of Homoeopathic Literature*. Great Auk Publishing (2001)

Index